Men and the ...

Is obesity really a public health problem and what does the construction of obesity as a health problem mean for men?

According to official statistics, the majority of men in nations such as England and the USA are overweight or obese. Public health officials, researchers, governments and various agencies are alarmed and have issued dire warnings about a global 'obesity epidemic'. This perceived threat to public health seemingly legitimates declarations of war against what one US Surgeon General called 'the terror within'. Yet, little is known about weight-related issues among everyday men in this context of symbolic or communicated violence.

Men and the War on Obesity is an original, timely and controversial study. Using observations from a mixed sex slimming club, interviews with men whom medicine might label overweight or obese and other sources, this study urges a rethink of weight or fat as a public health issue and sometimes private trouble. Recognizing the sociological wisdom that things are not as they seem, it challenges obesity warmongering and the many battles it mandates or incites. This important book could therefore help to change current thinking and practices not only in relation to men but also women and children who are defined as overweight, obese or too fat. It will be of interest to students and researchers of gender and the body within sociology, gender studies and cultural studies as well as public health researchers, policy makers and practitioners.

Lee F. Monaghan is Senior Lecturer in Sociology at the University of Limerick, Ireland.

Men and the War on Obesity

A sociological study

Lee F. Monaghan

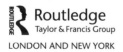

Routledge
Taylor & Francis Group

LONDON AND NEW YORK

First published 2008
by Routledge
2 Park Square, Milton Park, Abingdon, Oxon OX14 4RN

Simultaneously published in the USA and Canada
by Routledge
270 Madison Ave, New York, NY 10016

*Routledge is an imprint of the Taylor & Francis Group, an informa
business*

© 2008 Lee F. Monaghan

Typeset in Times New Roman by
Keystroke, 28 High Street, Tettenhall, Wolverhampton
Printed and bound in Great Britain by
T.J. International Ltd, Padstow, Cornwall

British Library Cataloguing in Publication Data
A catalogue record for this book is available from the British Library

Library of Congress Cataloging in Publication Data
Monaghan, Lee F., 1972–
Men and the war on obesity : a sociological study / Lee F. Monaghan.
p. ; cm.
Includes bibliographical references.
1. Obesity—Social aspects.
2. Weight loss—Social aspects.
3. Overweight men. I. Title.
[DNLM: 1. Obesity—psychology. 2. Diet, Reducing—psychology.
3. Men—psychology. 4. Social Perception. 5. Weight Loss.
WD 210 M734m 2008]
RC628.M596 2008
616.3'98—dc22
2007037745

ISBN10: 0–415–40711–7 (hbk)
ISBN10: 0–415–40712–5 (pbk)
ISBN10: 0–203–92957–8 (ebk)

ISBN13: 978–0–415–40711–3 (hbk)
ISBN13: 978–0–415–40712–0 (pbk)
ISBN13: 978–0–203–92957–5 (ebk)

To my parents, Frank and Maureen Monaghan

Contents

Tables

Acknowledgements

Many people have made this book possible. I would like to thank everybody who has either directly or indirectly enabled me to complete this project. First, my parents, Frank and Maureen Monaghan, deserve my heartfelt thanks. It was because of their love, guidance and support over many years that I was able to enter the world of academia with its relative luxuries and freedoms for imaginative work.

Second, I owe a big thanks to all of my ethnographic contacts. To preserve anonymity I will not name people. However, without their help and willingness to share their views, this book would not have the real world relevance that it has. Any book seeking to explore the world as lived and experienced cannot be written in an ivory tower, and people who kindly gave their time to this study provide a real grounding to what would otherwise be an abstract and sterile undertaking. This book presents their understandings while also connecting with more formal, published knowledge. It critiques certain organizational practices and claims that contribute to the wholesale pathologization of fat, but it is not critical of specific individuals. Throughout I remain respectful towards people who often put themselves out to help with this research even when they themselves were committed to fighting fat.

This study was funded by the UK's Economic and Social Research Council (ESRC, grant number: RES-000-22-0784). I wish to acknowledge the ESRC for their financial support and flexibility in allowing me to keep this study going after I moved from England to Ireland in 2005. While I undertook most of the research reported here, additional data were generated by Gary Pritchard. His diligent work as a researcher was facilitated by Robert Hollands. They are based at my former workplace: the School of Geography, Politics and Sociology, University of Newcastle upon Tyne. I wish to thank Newcastle University and other people who are working or have worked there for their advice and support. Names include: Liz Stanley, Janice McLaughlin, Diane Richardson, Victoria Robinson, Nicki Carter and Brad Robinson.

I am currently at the Department of Sociology, University of Limerick. This has been a good place to work with the former head of department, Brian Keary, and now Eoin Devereux, doing much to make this a supportive, productive and friendly environment. I am especially grateful to Brian for sponsoring a forum

I organized on the obesity debate and easing me into my post and Eoin for supporting the need for personal space when undertaking research. I would also like to thank other members of the Sociology department for their interest and occasional references, which were either taken directly off their bookshelves or which appeared in my pigeonhole and email inbox. Names include: Brendan Halpin, Orla McDonnell, Stiofán de Burca, Mary O'Donoghue, Patrick O'Connor, Carmen Kuhling, Pat O'Connor, Amanda Haynes and Breda Grey.

It is difficult to list everybody who has provided intellectual insight and support. However, Michael Hardey deserves a big thank you for his ongoing encouragement, insights and emails that let me know he was thinking of my research. The same applies to Lucy Aphramor, a health professional who is more directly involved in this area of study. Lucy is an incredibly compassionate, intelligent, modest and brave woman who, in her role as a cardiac rehabilitation dietician, has encountered irrational barriers when promoting an alternative paradigm to health and weight (Health at Every Size). Nonetheless, her efforts to change ill-founded institutional practices are starting to make a real difference in her clinical work, with positive effects for those she encounters. Lucy is very modest (I only learnt recently, and indirectly, that she is a highly accomplished marathon runner) but she is, without doubt, a real diamond. I am privileged to know Lucy and grateful for the insights she has shared with me, including her excellent knowledge of the primary scientific field.

Following a series of papers appearing in the November 2005 issue of *Social Theory of Health*, which Lucy contributed to, I would also like to thank Emma Rich and John Evans. It is reassuring to know people of their calibre are also critical of the war on obesity. I would also like to acknowledge several other people who have expressed an interest in my work and have read and commented on previous drafts of (some) chapters; namely: Michael Bloor, Dennis Waskul, Phillip Vannini, Debra Gimlin, David Brown, Karen Throsby, Therese Remshagen, Irmgard Tischner, Marilyn Wann and Michael Gard. Their suggestions have been valuable and encouraging, though, of course, I ultimately take responsibility for what follows.

My gratitude also goes to the staff at Routledge. In writing this book I am especially indebted to Grace McInnes for her receptiveness to the initial idea and her editorial support, plus Faith McDonald for her diligent work as production editor. The three anonymous reviewers were also very helpful. Their constructive criticism on the book proposal prompted me to clarify or refine certain arguments. They also encouraged me to believe that this book could make an important contribution to the current conceptualization of fat- and weight-related issues, not only in relation to men but also women and children.

This book elaborates and extends my thinking on a topic that has been a preoccupation for the past three years. While there is much that is original in these pages, some empirical materials and theoretical ideas overlap with or reproduce work previously published in academic journals. These journals are: *Body & Society*, published by Sage and edited by Mike Featherstone and Bryan Turner; *Social Theory & Health*, published by Palgrave Macmillan and edited by Graham

Scambler, Paul Higgs and Richard Levinson; *Sociology of Sport Journal*, published by Human Kinetics and guest edited by Margaret Carlisle Duncan (special issue on the Social Construction of Fat); and, *The Sociology of Health and Illness*, published by Blackwell and edited by Clive Seale, Pascale Allotey, Jonathan Gabe, Daniel Reidpath, Steven Wainwright and Clare Williams. The following articles, all single authored, should therefore be acknowledged:

Discussion Piece: A Critical Take on the Obesity Debate, *Social Theory & Health* 2005, 3 (4): 302–14.

Weighty Words: Expanding and Embodying the Accounts Framework, *Social Theory & Health* 2006, 4 (2): 128–67.

Body Mass Index, Masculinities and Moral Worth: Men's Critical Understandings of 'Appropriate' Weight-for-Height, *The Sociology of Health & Illness* 2007, 29 (4): 584–609.

McDonaldizing Men's Bodies? Slimming, Associated (Ir)Rationalities and Resistances, *Body & Society* 2007, 13 (2): 67–93.

Men, Physical Activity and the Obesity Discourse: Critical Understandings From a Qualitative Study. *Sociology of Sport Journal* 2008, 25 (1): 97–128.

Finally, I want to thank Faye Louise Bulcraig. Over several years Faye shared with me her emotional and sharply reflective understandings on the pains and ambivalences associated with the social and cultural degradation of fatness. This book focuses on men but I believe women and girls are generally hit hardest in a society where literally millions of people, even in the seemingly most caring of moments, are made to feel unacceptable because of the size, shape, weight and general appearance of their bodies. For some, this socially inflicted pain persists even when they embody our culture's visible yet superficial indicators of goodness, health and beauty. This is a lesson that I have learnt from Faye and it gives poignancy to my readings of feminist literature, fat activism and burgeoning critical weight studies that repudiate the war on obesity. It has also meant that I have listened carefully to men's views in a way that was critical of messages and practices that tell people their bodies are inadequate, rather than critical of so-called overweight, obese or fat people.

There was something on the news not that long ago. People were phoning in saying 'fat people shouldn't be treated on the NHS [National Health Service] because they're a burden to us'. What a load of bollocks. It makes you feel annoyed that you're being pushed into this section of people and you think to yourself, 'Well, I don't belong there. I'm happy being big. I'm relatively healthy. I've got a loving family. I've got a good job. I earn good money. I've got my own house. And I'm happy the way I am. So why does somebody want to piss on my bonfire? Why do they want to put me down?' And this is why I think people get depressed. Because they're being made to feel as if they're a burden on society. Because we're overweight. It's almost as if you're breaking the law because you're overweight.

(Big Joe, aged 33, a husband and father and working two jobs.)

1 Introduction

Beyond militarized medicine

Fat fighting, resistance and the relevance of men

Big Joe presented himself as physically and emotionally strong. However, he almost felt under siege when discussing a TV programme where members of the public telephoned in and berated those whom medicine might label overweight, obese or even morbidly obese. As a counterpoise to 'being pushed into this section of people' who were deemed undeserving of healthcare, Big Joe talked about being happy with his size, his relatively good health and his masculine credentials or social fitness. In short, this hardworking family man resisted the imposition of what Goffman (1968) calls a 'spoiled identity', though such resistance would appear fraught and contested. This is because medical authorities and proponents of public health are drawing from and amplifying the Western cultural fear and loathing of fatness, or fatphobia, with claims about a global 'obesity epidemic' (WHO 1998). This is defined as a 'disease' – attributable to 'sedentary lifestyles and high-fat, energy-dense diets' (WHO 1998: xv, xvi) – that should be tackled, or aggressively fought, by militarized medicine.

Medicine's military metaphor, as explained by Sontag when discussing the war on cancer, first became popular in the 1880s and has 'a striking literalness and authority' (1978: 70). Consider the declarations of former US Surgeon Generals, men who have been touted as the country's leading health educator. C. Everett Koop popularized the expression 'war on obesity' in 1997, citing an alleged annual death toll of 300,000 Americans (Mayer 2004: 999). Robert Carmona (2003) then called obesity '"the terror within", a threat that is every bit as real to America as weapons of mass destruction'. US medicine is known for its 'aggressive approach' (Gimlin 2007a: 45). However, the Surgeon Generals' ruggedly masculine rhetoric is also echoed in other nations with military imagery offered alongside alarmist claims about the 'ills' of 'weight' (a crude proxy for fatness). In Ireland, *The Report of the National Taskforce on Obesity* (2005: 6) calls 'body weight the most prevalent childhood disease (sic)' in Europe. This report repeatedly uses the words 'target' and 'tackle' and cites physiology literature with titles like 'Waging War on Physical Inactivity: Using Modern Molecular Ammunition against an Ancient Enemy'. The UK House of Commons Health Committee's report is equally moralizing and bellicose: as well as featuring a chapter titled 'Gluttony or Sloth?', it quotes the Chief Medical Officer, who calls obesity '"a health time bomb" that must be defused' (UK Parliament 2004: 8). Slenderness, it seems, is obligatory in wartime.

Amidst this aggressive moralizing, and its uptake and recycling in various contexts (Rich and Evans 2005), it is understandable why Big Joe felt annoyed and complained 'it's almost as if you're breaking the law for being overweight'. Some readers may feel the same, though they may not be aware of the uncertain and contested status of the scientific field from which obesity epidemic claims emanate, alongside recent literature that urges a rethink of this issue (for example, Campos 2004, Gard and Wright 2005, Monaghan 2005a, Oliver 2006). In such a context, I think Big Joe's resistance was reasonable. It could even be considered healthy. It provided an alternative to dieting, which is seldom successful and is risky (Aphramor 2005), the use of weight-loss drugs and other medical technologies that may be worse than the 'condition' they purportedly 'cure' (Kassirer and Angell 1998; also, see Ernsberger's preface to Campos 2004). Big Joe's words also provided a shield that deflected possible attacks on him as a person (Cahill 1998), which was important given the bombardment of larger people with the medically and government ratified message that their bodies are unacceptable. Sounding like a fat activist, who treats this issue in political terms, Big Joe redefined the problem: people actively make fatness into a problem for others and this is not really motivated by a genuine concern for their health and well-being. My contact obviously condemned members of the public, though, as seen later in the book, he also challenged government endorsed obesity fighting campaigns. Yet, scientists might justify the attack on medicalized fatness using dichotomous reasoning that separates the person from the body. The title of Friedman's (2003) article is illustrative: 'War on Obesity, Not the Obese'.

Such definitional practices, which manufacture fatness as a correctable problem and fuel fatphobia on an unprecedented scale, are problematic. They do not invent fat hatred afresh but they clearly reinforce and actively foster cultural disdain towards adiposity, a feminized body tissue. In this book I will maintain that institutionalized fat fighting is questionable, if not objectionable, but also more or less resistible even among people with a personal investment in it. The following is thus critical, rather than supportive, of obesity warmongering and the battles and hatred it mandates and incites. A critical approach is necessary for many reasons. Among other things, people are and have bodies (Turner 1992). Rather than objectified bodies to be aggressively targeted and tackled, people are embodied subjects living in a symbolically meaningful and divided social world. This point fits with understandings from embodied sociology, which is attentive to the ways in which bodies are the source, location and medium of society (Shilling 2003). Other social scientists recognize this. When discussing the US war on obesity, Herndon (2005) warns about 'collateral damage' from 'friendly fire'. After remarking '[a]dvocates of the war against obesity imagine themselves engaged in a battle for our nation's health', she adds: '[w]hat many doctors, public health officials and concerned journalists writing in support of the war against obesity fail to recognize, however, is that war against obesity also means a war against fat people' (129). In a related vein, Rich and Evans (2005) challenge what they call 'the obesity discourse', i.e. institutional knowledge and practices, dominated by medicine, which categorize/constitute bodies and carry a moral agenda that 'can lead to forms of size discrimination and oppression' (341).

Social scientists often conceptualize the attack on fat in gendered terms, with feminists typically challenging fat hatred because of its negative impact on many women and girls (for example, Bartky 1990, Bordo 1993, Orbach 2006, Wolf 1991). Female fat activists and fat acceptance scholars, some of whom identify as feminists, also critically extend such thinking with reference to 'really' fat women who often encounter prejudice, discrimination and oppression in everyday life and clinical settings (Brown and Rothblum 1989, Cooper 1998). Lucy Aphramor, a health professional, has also told me about her recent focus group research among large British women, some of whom were spat at in public (personal communication 2007). However, in *seemingly* contradicting the feminist argument that it is female fat that is despised, men also risk social censure if they are seen as fat in everyday life. Little is known about this within the current academic literature, though I would maintain that the relevance of researching men extends beyond the empirical and could augment feminist and fat activists' efforts to challenge 'intolerance and insensitivity: in a word, sizism' (Joanisse and Synnott 1999: 49). This is not meant to imply that men and women are equally victimized, though it does mean being open to similarities and possible shared interests within a gender order where masculinity is constructed relationally and in opposition to femininity

There are recent calls within social studies of the body to explore such issues. As maintained by Bell and McNaughton: 'So widely is the net of deviance and its attendant gaze being cast, that it is impossible to continue to deny or downplay the impact of the war on fat on both women *and* men' (2007: 126, emphasis in original). The degradation of men's bigness as unhealthy fatness is not historically peculiar (Gilman 2004, Huff 2001, Schwartz 1986, Stearns 1997) but it is currently reproduced on an unprecedented scale by biomedicine, the dominant organizing framework of modern medicine. This is amplified in 'public health' discourses with reference to men's imagined fatness; i.e., men's discursively constructed, rather than real, bodies that are assumed to be fat and risky. Inseparable from a larger gender order that seeks to rationalize bodies (for example, through calculability and efficiency), this degradation could be termed 'symbolic violence' or communicated violence (Bourdieu 2001). Given the role of experts in communicating risk (Beck 1992, Giddens 1991), this violence is often deemed acceptable, if not laudable. However, in departing from Bourdieu's (2001) concept of symbolic violence, this degradation and associated masculine domination is not always subtle and gentle. Declarations of war are a case in point, though the following 'informative' quote is also noteworthy because it ridicules men's imagined fatness when explaining the standard measure of overweight and obesity. This is from a male doctor on a British Broadcasting Corporation (BBC) health web page, with the vocabulary of health (risk) and personal responsibility providing a sugar-coated rationale for his militant irony:

More than half of the men in the UK are denting their seats because they're too fat – and that number is increasing. You can work out whether you're a healthy weight or putting your health at risk by calculating your body mass index (BMI). Use our BMI calculator or work it out using this formula: Take your weight in kilograms and divide it by your height in metres and then divide the result by your height in metres again. Underweight = BMI less than 18.5. Healthy weight = 18.5 to 24.9. Overweight = 25 to 30. Obese = 30 to 40. Severely obese = 40-plus.

(BBC Online 2007)

The BBC is not unique in using the idea of men's fatness to amplify fatphobia and sizism, which, as I will maintain, are likely to hit women and children hardest. Health organizations, researchers and other 'claimsmakers' (Best 1995) routinely define men as overweight, obese or fat and especially vulnerable to illness and early death. No punches are spared as men's apparently ubiquitous 'fat' and 'unfit' bodies are set up for a violent-sounding tackle – presumably because 'real men' can take this and it is supposedly in their best interests. Thus, during its UK Department of Health sponsored conference, *Tackling the Epidemic of 'Excess' Weight in Men*, the Men's Health Forum (MHF 2005) bemoaned men's greater tendency than women to exceed a 'healthy' weight. In their policy report they state that two-thirds of men in England and Wales are overweight or obese and claim a large 'waist' is 'hazardous'. Promotional leaflets for their conference also visually supported this message with a photograph of a man's fat stomach and taut shirt. Within this idiom, men's intra-abdominal or central obesity is especially risky – and, if it was not, then the harms of fatness would surely have to be invented to justify this not-so-subtle symbolic violence. Similarly, a recent book from a US weight-loss researcher focuses on men's stomachs and advises men to 'get rid of that potbelly' – something that renders men pregnant according to the book's cover (Schauss 2006). The National Audit Office's *Tackling Obesity in England* (NAO 2001) also immediately targets men's fatness. Featuring an image and quote from fat Falstaff, a character in Shakespeare's *Henry IV*, the report's front cover proclaims fleshy men are frail. Here fat is deemed corporeally polluting and emasculating: it spoils men's appearance, identities and, like a cancerous growth, poses a life-threatening risk for the unaware male. 'Watch out!' exclaims the front cover of Schauss's (2006) book, 'That potbelly can kill you!'

In this book I will bring in men's own voices and interpret these using a critical framework. Theoretically and politically informed, I am critical of instituted meanings and practices that define bodies as objects to be cut down in size, rather than critical of 'big' men who may have already suffered the slings and arrows of a fatphobic society. My aim is to promote healthy scepticism and productive dialogue among interested parties in ways that are open to the mutual imbrications of the biological and social. I will elaborate upon my methodology and other contextual concerns below but centrally this is a qualitative study that explores health- and weight-related issues among a small sample of men mainly living in England. It includes observations from a slimming club, in-depth interviews (N=37) and other data (for example, informal conversations with men in everyday life). Most research participants were at a reported weight-for-height that biomedicine labels 'excessive' and while many were slimming, others were not. Rather than ridiculing and advising these men within a larger context of masculine and class-related domination, I will do something different. I will offer an 'appreciative understanding' (Matza 1969) of their views and efforts to reclaim and enact socially fitting masculinities – a case of being seen as regular fellas rather than deviant and woman-like.

'Bringing in' men is important for empirical, theoretical and political reasons. Empirically, social scientists express an interest in the human consequences of the war on obesity but there are big gaps in the knowledge base. Little is known about how men live and experience their bodies, how they discuss weight-related issues and how they present themselves in the midst of a putative crisis (Bell and McNaughton 2007). Researching men could be considered especially important because men's health has attracted considerable media, if not social scientific, attention in recent years with reference to their supposed ignorance about their bodies and rising obesity (Watson 2000). Others also note the paucity of socio logical research on men's talk about body matters more generally (Gill *et al.* 2005). I therefore heed Bell and McNaughton's (2007) point that men's experiences cannot be ignored, though I do not call any of my contacts 'fat' given the potential offensiveness of this term. Another reason is that what is considered 'fat' in everyday life is a contingent social judgement rather than an objective scientific fact, with most men who are medically labelled overweight or obese on the BMI probably rejecting this measure (*cf.* Monaghan 2007).

This study is theoretically informed, as elaborated below, but I also seek to inform social theory. In line with a sociologically imaginative approach that views personal troubles and public issues as inextricably linked (Mills 1970), studying men and the war on obesity furthers efforts to rethink various oppositional dualities that have implications for discussion and practice inside and outside of sociology. Thus, mention was made above to the unsatisfactory separation of the person from the body as a rationale for warmongering. This separation is part of a larger series of dichotomies in Western thought that shape the truncated obesity debate such as: good/bad, fitness/fatness, biology/society, mind/body, reason/ emotion, object/subject and sex/gender. These ride roughshod over the richness and complexity of the real world where oppositional dualities are blurred despite considerable investments in maintaining them (Williams and Bendelow 1998). For example, consider how bodies sexed as male are positioned as feminine because of the social meanings of their real or imagined fatness, and how this subordination may evoke an emotional yet insightful response that could be considered personally healthy even if not socially transformative.

Undertaking empirically grounded and theoretically informed research also offers political gains. I am not offering what Connell (2000: 193) calls a '"compet-ing victims" rhetoric' but, as made clear by Big Joe, men also risk getting hurt in the war on obesity and this should prompt those who care about public health to reflect more on their actions. This is a message that female fat activists have long expressed (Freespirit and Aldebaran 1973) and their words have largely fallen on deaf ears. I should stress that I did not begin this research with an explicit political agenda that aimed to challenge institutional sizism. Big Joe might have sounded like a fat activist when addressing the politics of gendered identity but I never expected my small sample of men, many of whom were recruited at a slimming club, to 'do politics' and promote fat acceptance. This task is difficult enough even for feminists who are personally seduced by fat activism and experience size discrimination (S. Murray 2005)! However, by undertaking research, participating in online groups and reading and writing, this study has taken me down an unexpected road. A study on men has prompted me to critically draw from fat politics, which is mainly formulated by women in order to challenge the sexist trivialization of anti-fat prejudice and 'fat oppression', i.e. 'hatred and discrimination against fat people, primarily women, solely because of their body size' (Brown and Rothblum 1989: 1). While I would qualify social oppression views and reject some fat activists' arguments (see Chapters 2 and 3), this book is intended as a critical complement to such thinking. During this research I have learnt to see fat oppression as a real, emergent process that is not tied to female bodies though it is aimed at bodies that are positioned as feminine (disgusting, despised, dependent, passive, unhealthy) regardless of their biological sex. Within this field of masculine domination – which is potentially injurious not only for particular women but also men whose bodies supposedly symbolize 'failed' manhood – it is hardly surprising that fat oppression is often trivialized. This book aims to challenge that trivialization and sensitize more people to what has been called 'one of the last "safe" prejudices' (Smith 1990).

In terms of theory and politics, this book also connects with and helps expand a new wave of studies that challenge obesity epidemic thinking and obesity warmongering (for example, Aphramor 2005, Bacon 2006, Burns and Gavey 2004, Campos 2004, Campos *et al.* 2006a, b, Cogan 1999, Cohen *et al.* 2005, Gaesser 2002, Gard and Wright 2005, Herndon 2005, Jutel 2005, LeBesco 2004, Mayer 2004, Miller 1999, Oliver 2006, Rich and Evans 2005, Robison 1999, 2005a). This literature complements, extends and is sometimes indebted to feminisms, fat activism and the Health at Every Size paradigm – a clinically informed approach, which focuses on improving people's biomedical health and well-being without weight-loss being a necessary condition. Such writing challenges the institutional attack on medicalized fat and associated narratives of shame and blame. Contributors maintain that obesity science is overly reductionist, equivocal, largely ineffective, counterproductive, ethically suspect and depoliticizing. Largely written by people outside of sociology (for example, dieticians, nurses, exercise physiologists, physical educators), such work nonetheless recognizes the sociological wisdom that things are not as they seem (Berger 1963). This prompts me to critically explore the human significance of fat fighting and the idea that this really is the best way to promote health and well-being. Taken together, this amounts to a concerted effort to rethink current conceptualizations, promote productive dialogue and perhaps a paradigm shift that could foster more peaceful relations. This dialogue should occur throughout the social hierarchy and include health professionals and policy makers who have the potential to improve institutional practices as they affect men, women and children in their contexts of everyday life.

The remainder of this chapter has five objectives. First, the characteristics of a sociologically imaginative approach are outlined. Second, difficulties associated with exercising critical judgement are noted but the importance of this is underscored by connecting with relevant literature. Third, some words are offered on potentially offensive terms such as 'fat' and 'obesity'. Fourth, the research is described. Finally, the chapter content is outlined.

A sociologically imaginative approach: From interpretivism to critical realism

Familiarity with the social world as presently constituted means that sociology can be difficult for newcomers. 'Like a "fish in water" [that] does not feel the weight of the water" (Bourdieu and Wacquant 1992: 127), people habitually take the world for granted rather than treat practical circumstances as matters of theoretic interest. However, we are obviously not fish oblivious to surrounding water. For people who are curious about the life worlds we collectively construct, share and use to drown others with, sociology is an exciting and consciousness altering discipline. It has the potential to instil passion and interest in an often alienating world where, as Karl Marx once said, all that is solid melts into air.

Sociology comprises many approaches for systematically exploring the human condition as collectively lived and experienced. It embraces a myriad of concerns and comprises lively debate. Among other things, sociology considers how interpretations of the social *and* natural world are products of social activity. Hence, knowledge is socially constructed even when referring to something very real such as the body and the impact of social organization on life chances and health. Sociology makes clear that knowledge, meanings and actions do not arise in a social vacuum devoid of human interests and values, though some knowledge claims are more credible and socially just than others. Thus, some medical sociologists employing a realist epistemology (theory of knowledge) consider how increasing health inequalities are a product of core capitalist executive action and politics. In neo-liberal societies, which champion the individual, emphasis is placed on personal responsibility in ways that obscure the larger social dimensions of health and illness while benefiting 'Greedy Bastards', i.e. core executives and elite power groups (Scambler 2001, 2002).

When framed as a humanistic discipline, sociology is concerned with the question of what it means to be human and to be human in particular situations. Berger (1963: 189–90) explains that 'sociology's data are cut so close from the living marrow of human life that this question comes through again and again, at least for those sociologists who are sensitive to the human significance of what they are doing'. Sociology makes sense of people's sometimes joyous but also painful lives as experienced with and among others. Sociology is also debunking and provides the intellectual tools for challenging the taken-for-granted. When discussing the relevance of sociology, Berger (1963: 198) discusses how those encountering the discipline may 'become a little less stolid in their prejudices, a little more careful in their own commitments and a little more sceptical about the commitments of others'. Similarly, Stanley (2005) characterizes sociology as a discipline that rejects 'god's eye science' and refuses to acquiesce to what is authoritatively defined as real, truthful, good, virtuous, natural or inevitable. She adds that sociology offers unsettling, potentially subversive yet ethical and relevant commentary. Rather than about simple irreverence this is about the possibility of seeing the world differently and perhaps more compassionately.

This is not guaranteed when discussing weight-related issues, such is the deeply ingrained nature of anti-fat prejudice and fatphobia. Similar to psychologists who are well-intentioned but still promote the 'fight' against 'obesity' (Brownell 2005: 6), some sociologists compound dominant images of this issue without discussing the contested and potentially corrosive nature of these representations. Giddens (2006), for example, offers politically conservative ideas and broad-based claims without undertaking research or citing nascent critical literature that challenges obesity epidemic thinking. He also legitimates the war on obesity, given ethically suspect concerns about Britain's fitness on the battlefield – though, as an aside, the British army 'welcomes' men with a BMI of $32kg/m^2$ (BBC News Online 2006) and who are thus 'diseased' according to the WHO's (1998) criteria. Connell (2000), similar to Giddens (for example, Giddens 1991, 1992), generally makes valuable contributions to sociology, but he also reproduces anti-fat prejudice. This is in an otherwise carefully qualified discussion on the general *comparability* of men's and women's health. He simply defines 'overweight' as one of those 'risk factors' where 'men as a group really are worse off' (Connell 2000: 193; though, see Flegal *et al.* 2005). Crossley (2004) is also worth mentioning. Given reported increases in obesity rates, he defines fat as a sociological issue. This is an important call and his paper contains vital insights, but he also takes statistical representations more or less at face value and reiterates questionable assumptions concerning the putative causes and consequences of this 'crisis' (*cf.* Campos *et al.* 2006a, Keith *et al.* 2006). However, I want to stress that pathologizing accounts are not an inevitable outcome of sociology and non-sociologists may learn much from the discipline that challenges, rather than reconfirms, pervasive societal phobias and prejudices.

Sociology is not an afterthought or marginal add-on for other disciplines. All studies relating to the social, cultural, economic and political aspects of life benefit from what Mills (1970) calls the sociological imagination. This imagination is a quality of mind and usable set of analytic traditions. It is seen in the writings of classic social theorists who developed sociology over a century ago and exert an enduring influence. Those exercising the sociological imagination recognize that neither the life of an individual nor the history of a society can be understood without considering their mutual intersections and imbrications (Mills 1970). The sociological imagination is vital when critically engaging the war on obesity and the manufactured crisis surrounding millions of people's bodies, lives and identities. As Mills (1970) elaborates, public issues and personal, private troubles are inextricably linked. This means that the social penetrates the very core of what is intimate in people's lives, how people relate to themselves and others.

The broader relevance of sociology is evidenced in the delivery of medical school curricula, though this is often highly constrained by the pragmatic demands of the students' education. Future clinicians often receive an introduction to medical sociology, which is a large and productive subfield (Williams 2003a). This introduction is necessary because bodies are not only biological entities – they are also socially lived and experienced. Furthermore, knowledge about health is itself socially produced and, while there is more to health than formal care, health professionals are an integral part of the social contexts of health and illness. Future clinicians, if they are to be culturally competent and caring, cannot afford to be fish in water that do not feel the weight of water.

Sociology comprises many usable traditions, which vary in their relevance given the questions asked and the level of analysis (for example, the collective health and life chances of various groups or what it means to live with chronic illness). When researching everyday life, interpretivism or interactionism is valuable. Such studies often explore face-to-face interaction, for instance people's impression management on the social stage and ways of coping with institutional degradation and stigma (Goffman 1961a, 1968). Interpretivism is relevant given my empirical focus on daily life, the social actor's presentation of self or personhood (Cahill 1998) alongside the practical accomplishment of gender, which entails 'doing' difference during social interaction (West and Zimmerman 2002). Also known as 'everyday life sociology' (Adler *et al.* 1987), it includes phenomenology and symbolic interactionism: perspectives well suited to the social study of bodies/ embodiment (Waskul and Vannini 2006). Everyday life sociology explores how people collectively or intersubjectively construct, make sense of, act and talk within their life worlds (Schutz 1962, Scott and Lyman 1968). It is also attentive to emotions (for example, Hochschild 1983), which are 'at the heart of the matter: the animating principle, so to speak' (Williams 2003a: 1).

Such theorizing works well with qualitative research methods, such as participant observation or ethnography. These methods seek to obtain people's points of view and offer 'thick descriptions' of social life. Some of the feminist writings I draw from also use interpretivism and qualitative methods. These studies, which cannot be ignored in a book that challenges the larger war on obesity, explore women's bodily concerns, involvement in slimming clubs, experiences of dieting, oppression, sense of worth or inferiority, the embodiment of identity and emotionally fraught attempts to embrace fat activism (for example, Bartky 1990, Chapman 1999, Germov and Williams 1996, Gimlin 2002, 2007b, Heyes 2006, Honeycutt 1999, S. Murray 2005, Skeggs 1997, Stinson 2001). This work is empirically, theoretically and politically valuable even when confined to personal or auto-ethnographic reflections. For example, using phenomenological insights, S. Murray (2005) provides a useful embodied approach to understanding the difficulties of 'doing' fat activism and personal fat acceptance. Her contribution is important because, as elaborated in Chapter 2, I critically draw from fat activism to supplement my sociological imagination.

Interpretivism, which does not impose on researchers the choice of studying the interpersonal at the expense of the institutional, complements more structural and historically informed analyses. These include Bourdieu's (2001) study on gendered power. His ethnographic and feminist informed scholarship challenges masculine domination. Such domination works through the gender order, sexually differentiated/differentiating bodies and androcentric (i.e. male biased and institutionalized) schemes of perception, thinking and feeling. Such theorizing transcends the face-to-face minutiae of social life to engage broader instituted concerns that shape and constrain embodied lives in ways that may simply be considered part of the natural order of things. These structures comprise enduring social relations which, analytically speaking, have ontological depth, i.e. they persist beyond the local and particular and exert effects that may not always be realized by social actors themselves (Porter 1993). Subsequent chapters are grounded in qualitative data generated face-to-face but my analysis also goes beyond these data. A theoretically informed and eclectic stance is taken when critically engaging the everyday and institutional fight against fat.

Such a stance is politically important. While interpretivism and ethnography are primarily concerned with understanding people's perspectives, some ethnographers seek critically to evaluate the social. Porter (1993) offers a good example in his critical realist ethnography of racism in a hospital setting. He endorses critical realism as a way of overcoming 'the Achilles heel of phenomenological ethnography', adding: '[u]nderstanding actors' viewpoints may be a necessary condition for social knowledge, but it is not a sufficient one' (Porter 1993: 596). This fits with Mills' (1970) position where individual biographies must be understood within a larger social structural and historical scene. This is because people may not necessarily be aware of the broader sea of collectively constructed meanings and institutional practices that shape their lives and perhaps colour them with emotion and personal significance.

This does not mean people are puppets on a stage whose actions, or identity-forming 'body projects' (Shilling 2003), are determined by external social structures. People are active, they exercise agency. Yet, this is not free-floating, just as there are real biophysical processes set in motion by embodied social experiences (for example, stress and experiences of inequality) that have little to do with personal intentions, actions and choice (Freund 2006). Thus, Bourdieu (1984, 2001) uses the idea of the 'habitus' or structured dispositions to bridge the agency/structure divide. The socially acquired habitus is embodied. This means people's physicality, comportment and tastes are the interactional products and symbolic bearers of class location and distinction. It also means that social inequality is reproduced on, in and through bodies, though I should stress that this is not the same as saying people in poorer socio-economic circumstances necessarily embody and favour all that is judged pathological.

Other sociologists offer compatible views on the relationship between social structures, human agency and risk. As Scambler (2002: 95) explains with reference to health inequalities research – including Graham's (1995) study on women and smoking in the context of gender and class oppression – there is an 'indebtedness of agency to structure', i.e. cultural/behavioural factors (lifestyles) are inseparable from material conditions of existence. For critical realists, people's practices and bodies are influenced/shaped/affected by structures such as class, ethnicity and gender. These structures are at the heart of social interaction (Bourdieu 2001) and cannot be ignored in studies that challenge social injustice. Mounting such a challenge, as elaborated in the next section, is nonetheless difficult. Among other things, social structures generate tendencies, sometimes exercised unrealized (as with institutional racism or sizism), and they permit ideological rationalizations that legitimate iniquitous practices that have real effects (Porter 1993). However, because people are more or less able to exercise agency, there is always the possibility of manoeuvrability, critical reflection, humour and efforts to challenge forms of oppression.

Williams (2003b) has discussed the value of critical realism in accessible terms. He states that many medical sociologists, when drawing from research on social structures and health, either implicitly or explicitly use critical realism. There is much to commend in Williams' (2003b) paper because social structures patently have a massive impact on health and illness. This is regardless of whether or not people are 'really' fat or follow lifestyles assumed to cause what medicine calls overweight and obesity. Health inequalities literature, which shapes my critical stance towards 'blame the victim' narratives, makes clear that personal behaviour explains less than a third of the social gradient in health, i.e. the consistent inverse relationship between social standing, morbidity and mortality (Marmot 2004). This is independent of whether or not people recognize these structures and define them as real. Indeed, adults, particularly from lower socio-economic groups, often believe they are personally responsible for their (poor) health. However, if 'victims blame themselves' this does not mean they are 'really' blameworthy (Blaxter 2004; also, Williams 2003b: 47). This is noteworthy given the pervasive blame and shame attributed to so-called obesity and people's internalization of this as part of what Neckel (1996) would call 'the social production' of 'individual inferiority'.

Critical realism enables sociologists to cautiously 'bring in' and debate biology (Freund 2006, Williams 2003b, Williams *et al.* 2003) and its relation to gender and health. This is important for an embodied sociology that takes the flesh and blood body seriously, though Connell (1995: 52) explains that this does not mean adding 'social determinism' to 'biological determinism' as part of a two level analysis. Rather, it means attending to 'the body inescapable' or how the body feels, adopts 'certain postures', its physical shapes alongside people's memories of 'bodily experience' (Connell 1995: 52–3). There is, of course, more, such as the visceral or physiological (see below). Nonetheless, Connell (1995: 61) usefully explains that bodies are 'both objects and agents of social practice' or 'body-reflexive practice'. This is within an open and emotionally charged field comprising 'patterned or "structured" forms of difference which involve elements of perceived conflict and actual struggles' alongside similarities between men and women (Carpenter 2000: 48–9).

Critical realism, whether explicitly or implicitly adopted by medical sociologists, thus draws attention to the social and biological dimensions of health, illness and related practices. A critical realist analysis would, for example, recognize that life expectancy emerges from the 'interactions' of relational bodies and historically unfolding societies and the patterned accumulation of (dis)advantages through the life course for different groups. Interestingly and critically, I would mention here that while men are positioned as especially vulnerable within the obesity discourse, life expectancy has reportedly been increasing in the UK at a greater rate for men than women over the past three decades (Annandale 2003)! As this example illustrates, thinking critically and realistically (sensibly) means taking a non-reductionist approach. Thus, while social constructionist insights are important (for example who claims what in regards to health), there is no suggestion here that biology can be reduced to socially constructed meanings and discourses (Williams 2003a). By the same token, social life cannot be reduced to a 'naturalistic' or biological body (Shilling 2003). Hence, critical realism, or its recent uptake in body studies advocating a position of 'corporeal realism' (Shilling 2005), does not endorse common foundationalist accounts of the body. That is, accounts that naturalize oppressive practices and power, for example the idea that men should dominate women because of higher testosterone (Connell 1995), or people should lose weight because adiposity is a malign body tissue that causes, or is associated with, stigma and psychological problems. The latter point is worth stressing given the sociologically unimaginative call to fight obesity because of stigma. As if such calls did not publicly reproduce and amplify that which they ostensibly seek to redress, with potentially damaging effects for real biological bodies as socially lived and experienced!

Bringing in and debating biology is important, then, because the physical body is a socially consequential reality just as society is consequential for the body. In Shilling's (2005) work this translates to an analytical focus on the body as 'the multi-dimensional medium for the constitution of society'. Whether referring to Shilling (2003, 2005) or other writings on the body (for example Williams and Bendelow 1998), it is clear that embodied sociology must engage the corporeal rather than simply the discursive (as with extreme Foucauldian accounts of the body). Some of the literature I draw from is attuned to the body's fleshy materiality, including sociological writing on masculinities and health. Given space constraints I will not review this literature here, or other work that deals with male bodies, weight and fatness in a social and historical context (for example Gilman 2004, Grogan 1999, Grogan and Richards 2002, Huff 2001, Joanisse and Synnott 1999, Textor 1999). However, a study that has particular relevance and should be clearly flagged is Watson's (2000) research on male bodies. Drawing from and extending theorists such as Connell (1995), Watson (2000) discusses various modalities of male embodiment. These include: the visceral or physiological (hidden depths that can be medically visualized), the experiential (for example sense of well-being), pragmatic (the working body) and normative (size, shape, weight). Other sociologists researching men's health have used this framework (Robertson 2006). Such work is useful in ways that go beyond sociology. By exploring sexed/gendered embodiment in its various dimensions, sociologists have the opportunity to engage other disciplines that study bodies and which work at the interface between bodies, selves and society.

Promoting sociologically imaginative dialogue with other disciplines accords with Stanley's (2005) characterization of sociology as hybridic. This book is distinctively sociological but it crosses boundaries. As a single author I do not pretend to be deeply immersed and versed in various disciplines outside of sociology, but I will draw from and speak to others in a critically informed way with the hope of promoting healthy scepticism and productive dialogue. Relevant areas of study and practice include medicine, public health and health promotion, psychology, social policy, nursing, clinical therapies, physical education, exercise physiology, epidemiology, dietetics and nutrition. Other academic fields, which sociology may inform and vice versa, include: history, anthropology, cultural studies, law, political science, human geography, philosophy, women's studies and writings on men and masculinities. Readers outside of sociology should find much that is relevant, engaging and perhaps mind-changing in these pages. Like the human body, and the sociological imagination, this book is not confined to any single discourse, practice or academic discipline.

Exercising critical judgement rather than taking sides

I have previously written a paper that endorses a sociologically imaginative approach to the 'obesity debate' (Monaghan 2005a). It makes direct reference to the science legitimating the war on fat and challenges arguments offered by those playing a key role in constructing this as a massive public health problem. The paper emerged following an invitation from the UK's Men's Health Forum during their preparations for a conference on 'tackling male weight problems' (MHF 2005). The short piece I originally wrote for their magazine was titled by the editor 'Taking Sides', alongside a question concerning whether or not fat was good or bad. The contributor to the 'other side' of the debate, a general practitioner and Chair of the National Obesity Forum, then presented an opposing argument. My dissatisfaction with the limited space and dichotomous format meant that I expanded the article for the journal *Social Theory & Health*, with the aim of highlighting the subtleties, uncertainties, controversies and problems with obesity science and anti-obesity campaigns (Monaghan 2005a). This is an important issue and I did not want to be a lone voice. Hence, I was fortunate enough to obtain the agreement of three other people, also working in this area, to write two papers to accompany mine (Aphramor 2005, Rich and Evans 2005).

I will not reproduce the arguments offered in these papers, though I will briefly flag some central themes and make reference to additional literature published at about the same time or that has emerged since. This is a rapidly growing literature and it is reaching a critical mass. For readers who want a quick way into some of this, I would recommend two books: *The Obesity Epidemic* (Gard and Wright 2005) and *The Obesity Myth* (Campos 2004). Other literature is available, including earlier feminist writings that critique obesity science and the reasons why 'women are at war with their bodies' (Seid 1989), but these two books are good places to start for anyone wishing to obtain a critical and balanced understanding of the current war on obesity. In the following I will also reflect on the reception of alternative thinking and possible reasons for resistances. This provides further context to my study and promotes greater reflexivity vis-à-vis socially constructed barriers that constrain critical dialogue at societal, institutional and individual levels.

The *Social Theory & Health* papers sought to expand the truncated obesity debate, which focuses on proposed solutions to a taken-for-granted problem rather than questioning whether this should be defined as such a massive problem to begin with. My paper outlines scientific evidence that challenges the idea that so-called 'excess' weight or fat is necessarily problematic for health and longevity. The paper could be compared to Campos's (2004) book except I was more constrained in the materials I could review in a journal article and my more immediate goal was to bring some of this alternative thinking to the attention of health professionals and policy makers in a way that made sociological sense. Hence, my paper did not deny the materiality of bodies and ignore biological arguments, though I underscored the need to theorize the visceral in non-reductionist terms while citing scientific evidence that challenges the wholesale pathologization of overweight/ obesity/fatness. I also responded to some of the 'opposing' arguments offered in the MHF magazine's 'Taking Sides' article, such as '[t]he facts are indisputable. The medical profession's obsession with obesity is not a moral nor a social judgement, purely a clinical one' (Haslam 2005: 9). One only need refer to Campos (2004) and Gard and Wright (2005) to recognize that this claim is not empirically supported. Medical sociologists also make clear that medicine does not work in a hermetically sealed vacuum outside of the social; rather, medicine is a thoroughly social and moralizing activity just as health itself is not confined to anatomy and physiology.

The paper by Aphramor (2005), a registered dietician, challenges the idea that promoting weight-loss improves health. Indebted to feminist thinking and promoting social justice, she offers a sociologically imaginative piece that critiques mainstream dietetic anti-obesity guidelines. She maintains that the existing 'weight-centred health framework' naturalizes offensive stereotypes, is ineffective (there is a 95 per cent chance of regaining lost weight), depoliticizing and risky. Citing relevant literature, she lists various risks such as weight fluctuation, increased cardiovascular risk, reinforcing a sense of failure, poor body image and increased risk of smoking. She warns dieticians could face litigation if weight-loss is recommended to patients without imparting knowledge of risks and the improbability of losing weight and keeping it off. A subsequent review of the evidence has since provided further support to her point concerning the ineffectiveness of diets (Mann *et al.* 2007).

The third paper was written by Rich and Evans (2005), sociologists working in the area of physical education. Their contribution explicitly focuses on ethical issues raised by the socially constructed and publicly represented discourses about an obesity crisis. They state that while these discourses are expressed with certainty to the public there is actually considerable uncertainty. Similar to Gard and Wright

(2005), they maintain that efforts to 'erase uncertainty' around the meanings of bodies, weight, etc. may not only increase oppression but also have the unintended consequence of promoting 'disordered relationships with food, exercise and the body' (Rich and Evans 2005: 341). Evans *et al.* (forthcoming) elaborate upon these and other themes and their book is also recommended to readers.

Shortly after the *Social Theory & Health* papers were published I organized a forum, *Expanding the Obesity Debate*, mainly for health professionals and academic researchers. Aphramor (2006) and Rich and Evans (2006) also presented papers. Other presenters offered more usual accounts that pathologize fatness (Harrington and Friel 2006), and were included partly to provide the possibility of a balanced debate but also because it is difficult finding researchers who think outside the usual parameters. This was a learning exercise and I soon realized that promoting critical and productive dialogue is extremely difficult. For example, when talking at the forum and to the media I was positioned as taking an opposing stance against medical authorities, with the explicit or implicit assumption that I was arguing it is good to be fat (a difficult position to maintain when people are routinely discriminated against because of the social meanings ascribed to their bodies). While I have received positive responses I have also encountered much resistance and belligerence from those who seek to define obesity as a massive public health problem. I assume they take much of this as an attack on their professional competence and respond in a way that does not facilitate productive discussion. Although much could be said here (for example, the role of emotions in the social relations of science, which entail competition and recognition), I will simply reflect on *some* reasons for resistance within and outside of science and why obesity warmongering within public health discourses strikes me as unreasonable. From what has already been said, however, Bourdieu (2001) provides some insight in his writings on masculine domination, which is violently reproduced in ways that are often deemed acceptable – what he calls 'the *paradox of doxa*' (2001: 1, emphasis in original).

When exercising critical judgement I never initially expected to elicit some of the deeply antagonistic responses that I did. In retrospect I was perhaps naive to assume I would encounter a receptive audience who would welcome scientific evidence that so-called overweight and obesity may not be as bad as we are often told, or be relatively benign, and biomedical health may be improved without obsessing about weight or fatness. As indicated by the metaphors employed by militarized medicine, this is a hostile terrain and one that Lucy Aphramor is familiar with as a practising dietician. Treated by other health professionals in a way that 'defies dialogue' and is 'more combative than collaborative', Lucy is well aware that such responses militate against creating 'a collaborative community of learning' and 'inviting debate' (personal communication 2007). Her use of military metaphors is apposite because she has been placed on the front line of a war that she disagrees with. Fortunately, she has since been able to promote Health at Every Size in her clinical practice. This has taken considerable perseverance and mettle when encountering other clinicians who have expressed fatphobic beliefs and sizist rationalizations that are condescending rather than caring.

One might think we were offering unfounded arguments that were irrelevant for people's health and well-being, or the literature we were citing was not peer reviewed, and had been published in poor-quality journals. However, how does one respond when, for example, you cite studies such as the following and still get a belligerent response or are ignored? Thus, recent US epidemiology published in the *Journal of the American Medical Association* reports that no excess deaths were associated with 'overweight' (Flegal *et al.* 2005). Again, from the same journal, Gregg *et al.* state that while there has been an increase in the prevalence of overweight and obesity in the USA, 'mortality rates from ischemic heart disease as well as levels of key CVD [cardiovascular disease] risk factors have declined' (2005: 1869). They add, 'obese persons now have better CVD risk factor profiles than their lighter counterparts did 20 to 30 years ago' (Gregg *et al.* 2005: 1873). Writing in *Medicine and Science in Sports and Exercise*, Blair and Brodney (1999) review available evidence and state cardiorespiratory fitness is a better indicator of morbidity and mortality risk than fatness (also, Gaesser 2005, Lee *et al.* 1999). According to these studies, physically active 'obese' people (at least up to a BMI of 35 kg/m^2) generally live longer and have better biomedical health than 'normal' weight people who are sedentary. Keith *et al.* (2006) offer another interesting article in the *International Journal of Obesity*. While reported increases in people's weight are often attributed to diet and sedentary lifestyles, these researchers maintain that scientific evidence supporting this view is equivocal and circumstantial and there is equally convincing evidence for at least ten other putative contributors to 'secular increases in obesity' (for example, side-effects from medicines and sleep debt). The usual focus on what they call 'the Big Two' – or what the UK Parliament (2004), following medical researchers, call gluttony and sloth – thus says more about quasi-religious moralizing and prejudice than established scientific fact.

Powerful social forces and vested interests constrain critical thinking and people's reception of ideas that contradict existing prejudices. These forces work through the social structure, they are part of Western culture and they have a history. Masculine domination has been mentioned, with an 'androcentric uncon-scious' (Bourdieu 2001) naturalizing the evil view of fat – symbolically violent meanings that do not necessarily operate at the level of conscious intentions but which perpetuate iniquitous sexual divisions. The political economy is also extremely powerful, which means critical thinking and the possibility of changing institutional practice will never be easy. Other writers provide useful commentary when making sense of barriers to critical discussion. Hence, I will simply point readers in the direction of some interesting work from historians and political scientists before formulating additional ideas using sociological and other sociologically imaginative literature.

After explaining the twentieth century projection of fears of abundance and vulnerability onto 'fat men' and women, Schwartz (1986) provides historical leverage on the US economy where the fantasy of 'thin bodies' has generated 'fat profits' (also, see Stearns 1997). This historian convincingly shows that what is taken-for-granted in terms of weight-loss products and marketing was unimaginable in earlier centuries. Schwartz (1986) was writing over twenty years ago but his work is not only of continuing but also increased relevance. Today, an industry of organizations and entrepreneurs continue talking up the 'ills' of 'fat' while promising to 'help' people achieve a slimmer and presumably healthier, longer and happier life. Fatness is often deemed costly but fat fighting also pays, providing employment and status for considerable numbers of people.

Oliver (2006) elaborates in a manner similar to the former editors of *The New England Journal of Medicine* when challenging medicine's ethically suspect complicity with big business (Angell 2004, Kassirer 2005; also, see Kassirer and Angell 1998). He explains that powerful organizations share a close and inter-locking relationship when claiming millions of people are too heavy/fat and this is a serious problem. This relationship comprises the vested interests of the pharma-ceutical industry, governments, researchers and clinicians. This 'health-industrial complex' (Oliver 2006: 31) engages in various definitional practices such as conflation and downward revision, which have resulted in massive inflation. Restated, while there may well be real changes in population weight (though, see Campos *et al.* 2006a), the idea of a crisis is discursively amplified by health officials who typically conflate overweight with obesity while using a downwardly revised BMI classification for overweight. In 1998 the US National Institute of Health reduced this threshold (from BMI 27.8 kg/m^2 for men, and 27.3 kg/m^2 for women, to 25 kg/m^2) with over 30 million Americans immediately becoming overweight (Oliver 2006: 22). An expanded problem obviously equals an expanded market for many interested parties who have a vested economic interest in fat hatred.

Other constraints on critical discussion are more firmly grounded in everyday life, with the health-industrial complex perhaps more accurately being seen as reinforcing the embodied dispositions of the habitus (similarly, see Bourdieu 2001: 68). Many people accept and reproduce the obesity discourse if not fully then at least in part. This is not to view people as 'judgmental dopes' (Garfinkel 1967). As indicated, there are historically transmitted and situationally rational reasons for degrees of acquiescence (Schwartz 1986, Stearns 1997). In Western nations, from about the end of the nineteenth century onwards, fat has been a problem for many people or, rather, what is contingently judged as 'fat' has actively been made into a problem by and for many people. However, contemporary social con-ditions make the 'claimsmaking' (Best 1995) of weight control especially salient. As well as neo-liberalism, where individual consumers are charged with taking responsibility for their health (Scambler 2002), the body is an index of moral worth in a rationalized 'risk society' (Beck 1992, Giddens 1991). Here collective fears and anxieties are embodied and conceptualized using a mechanical metaphor. What has been written about cancer in the twentieth century extends to fatness today: 'In our own era of destructive overproduction by the economy and increas-ing bureaucratic restraints on the individual' writes Sontag (1978: 66), 'there is both a fear of having too much energy and an anxiety about energy not being allowed to be expressed'. Regardless of whether or not fatness really is caused by gluttony and sloth and actually causes disease, it is often defined as such.

Correspondingly, millions of people seek to lose weight in order to 'fit in' with a sizist society where fatphobia is embodied.

Clearly, then, constraints are multi-faceted and directional. They are also gendered in ways that go beyond the masculinist metaphors of militarized medicine to include the (attempted) subordination of fe/male bodies on embodied hierarchies. In the remainder of this section I will formulate some sociological ideas on the difficulties associated with promoting critically informed discussion. Reference is made to six interrelated yet contestable constraints that work around, on and through bodies: medicalization, healthism, epidemic psychology, rationalization, class disdain and religiosity. This, it should be stressed, is a partial discussion.

Medicalization refers to the biomedical colonization of everyday life (Zola 1972). That is, where ever more aspects of mundane existence are defined as issues to be dealt with by biomedicine. While there are medical arguments concerning the risks of men's intra-abdominal obesity, or visceral fat (the so-called potbelly), and men's greater tendency than women to be at a supposedly 'unhealthy' weight, the medicalization of men's weight goes further. Today the ordinary and even iconic are transformed into clinically maligned categories: as explained by Campos (2004), Hollywood heartthrobs Brad Pitt and George Clooney would be defined respectively as overweight and obese according to current BMI definitions. While this highlights the possibility of meaningful resistances in everyday life (even among men seeking to lose weight), medicalization is powerful. It implies serious-ness, the need for social control and the moral obligation among those deemed 'sick' or 'at risk' to do all that they can to get better. Medicalization is amplified in the new public health where everybody is urged to play their part in the manage-ment of risk through lifestyle (Petersen and Lupton 1996). If people are not already overweight or obese then they are deemed at risk of becoming so and heir to the problems that implies. Even people at a 'healthy' weight are only two steps behind, that is, they are defined as at risk of becoming at risk of a 'disease' called 'obesity' (WHO 1998). And, as argued by Moynihan (2006a, b), it only takes 'an expert committee' with links to government, medical associations and the profitable pharmaceutical industry to shift the boundaries of abnormality and expand the problem further.

Healthism is 'a form of medicalization' (Crawford 1980: 365). The ideology of healthism elevates health to an ultimate value, a metaphor for the good life, with 'solutions' to disease ultimately seen to be an individual matter. Bearing a middle-class stamp, healthism is related to moral worth but also, following Bauman (2005), the avoidance of death, which becomes life's fundamental meaning. In that respect healthism is internalized as part of the ethical self, the 'good' citizen who owes it to themselves *and* others to engage in self-care (Edgley and Brissett 1990). Exercising critical judgement is difficult because fatness is often claimed to cause illness and constitute a life-threatening disease in its own right (WHO 1998). Accepting fatness, within this framing, is similar to accepting cancer and risky behaviour such as smoking (Saguy and Riley 2005). Just as Crawford (1980: 365) states there was 'a vocal and often aggressive anti-smoking ethic' almost three decades ago, today there is a pervasive and hostile anti-fat ethic. The more pernicious difference, of course, is that attention moves from behaviour to the physical body, with fatness becoming a medically sanctioned 'badge of stigma' (Herndon 2005: 128). Deviance is inscribed on the surface of the body, at least for those seen to be fat in everyday life. Healthism, as might be anticipated, becomes 'self-perpetuating' as people with the necessary resources try to quell 'the insecurity of the deviant, the anxiety of not fitting in' (Crawford 1980: 382). This is at a historical juncture when millions of people are medically disparaged as overweight or obese and extolled to fit in.

Medicalization has its own infectious psychology. Strong (1990), a medical sociologist, first proposed the idea of 'epidemic psychology' when discussing reactions to HIV/AIDS in the 1980s, with such reactions deemed potentially more corrosive than actual biological risks. What I term 'obesity epidemic psychology' is comparable. This psychology is mediated through channels of mass communication, language and interaction. Obesity epidemic psychology may not manifest itself in pure form in everyday life, but it comprises panic, fear, moralizing action and intense social stigmatization. It is spread by incorrect yet endlessly recycled news reports that overweight and obesity kill 300,000 Americans annually (Campos 2004) – a figure increasing to 400,000 before being dramatically revised downwards in the *Journal of the American Medical Association* to less than 26,000 (Oliver 2006: 3-4). Similar to reactions to AIDS, people endeavour to make sense of the fragile social world in response to a putative crisis. This entails the quotidian search for meaning by fallible human beings. This is an interpretive act and exercise in social labelling that (re)creates societal scapegoats.

Epidemic psychology implies a socially disorganized knee-jerk response, at least in the early stages of a perceived crisis (Strong 1990). However, it is now more than twenty years since 'the obesity crisis' reportedly began (Gard and Wright 2005), and organizational efforts to diagnose and tackle this are highly rationalized. This relates to bureaucratic concerns for efficiency, calculability, predictability and technological control. Ritzer (2004), using Weber's (1930) theory of rationalization, calls this McDonaldization. This is because the fast-food restaurant, somewhat ironically in the context of this discussion, exemplifies rationalization just as the bureaucracy did in the nineteenth century. Rationalization is more or less seductive but it also has unintended consequences or irrationalities. Some of these were mentioned above, such as reproducing stigma and possibly fuelling anxieties and disordered relationships with the body and food (Rich and Evans 2005). Obesity epidemic claims are also streamlined claims that frame and constrain academic and policy discussion. They eclipse matters pertaining to social structures and status, which are measurably more consequential for biomedical health than individual 'lifestyle choices' (Marmot 2004).

Class disdain is also extremely salient, with disparaging attention in popular renditions of the obesity discourse often focusing on 'fat people' living in poverty (for example, Critser 2003). Besides highlighting how such disdain is a conduit for covert racism among White commentators in the USA, Campos (2004) underscores the middle-class search for distinction. Restated, if fatness is increasingly common among poor people then it is incumbent for those of higher socio-economic status and aspirations not to look fat and, indeed, to condemn their subordinates' fatness, which is attributed to individual failure or pathological culture. His point meshes with recent sociological writing on how the British middle classes, or, more specifically, 'the public bourgeoisie' (those involved in mass communication such as broadsheet journalists, academics and social commentators) construct their identities (Lawler 2005). Although not focusing on obesity and its common representation as a 'lower class' problem, Lawler (2005) offers relevant commentary on how middle-class identity is constructed in contra-distinction to working-class people, who are considered disgusting. This is not simple snobbery. Such distinctions and degradations, maintained by those with the power to make their definitions count, are embodied in socially acquired and distributed taste (Bourdieu 1984). Such evaluations often relate to bodily appearance and are naturalized with a focus on individual corporeality. It is perhaps unsurprising that pathologized bodies are often working-class female bodies (Skeggs 1997). Unconsciously incorporated, this relation to the gendered/classed body feeds a male coded war on obesity. This war renders visibly 'fat' (feminized) bodies, regardless of their actual sex, 'threatening' to respectable society and calls forth oppositional thinking that creates barriers for distinguishing difference. Disdain and class distinction thus work alongside gender distinction in a visual culture. Here, distributions of fat that blur the culturally idealized male form – central obesity, which may be inversely related to socio-economic status even when BMI is not (Marmot 2004) – endangers middle-class manhood and is saturated with the fear that 'they' could look like the feminized, disgusting 'them'. Tackle, rather than rationally debate, is the mantra in 'epidemic' times.

Finally, religiosity constrains critical discussion. Writing in a medical journal on 'the obesity time bomb', Fitzpatrick (2004) compares clinicians and scientists to pious evangelists. Religious fundamentalists are compelled not to tolerate the tolerant (Williams 2003b) and intolerance is the hallmark of militarized medicine. Again, there are historically transmitted reasons for this. These include, but also extend beyond, the search for profits. Western biomedicine is historically intertwined with religion (Turner 1995), with medicine and the quest for health progressively filling the moral void left by secularization. 'Medicine', writes Fitzpatrick (2001: 6), 'has become a quasi-religious crusade against the old sins of the flesh'. Writing about the ideologies of the contemporary US health and fitness movement, Edgley and Brissett (1999: 105) locate its religious under-pinnings in 'a Puritanism that has always seen the problem of controlling others as central to its mission'. Other academics flag religion vis-à-vis efforts to self-regulate the female body, food and fat. Germov and Williams (1996: 642) state that the 'thin ideal' 'reflects a desire for secular purity of the soul through salvation from stigma. The "aesthetic body" has become the new religion, with dieting providing a form of aesthetic spirituality'. As a secular religion, medicine and the cult of slenderness exert a potent influence. A critical study could be considered blasphemous. The war on obesity is a holy war and conscientious objectors risk excommunication.

Despite such constraints I aim to encourage a critically reflexive approach that is circumspect about oppositional dualities and open to the mutual imbrications of the social and biological. A sociologically imaginative approach is mindful of socially constructed and embodied barriers but also open to productive possibilities among a range of interested parties. In all of this it is encouraging to know that if people are interested in promoting biomedical health, more so than a culturally defined image of health, there are alternatives. There is evidence that key dimensions of biomedical health and well-being can be improved by adopting the Health at Every Size paradigm, and adopting this from the outset in order to avoid possible impairment which could occur with repeated dieting and weight fluctuation (Aphramor 2007). To draw from Watson's (2000) body schema, what this means is an emphasis on visceral, experiential and pragmatic embodiment over the normative; i.e. an expanded rather than 'thin' conception of health that eschews numbers on the weighing scales, tape measure or BMI. Some clinicians use this paradigm and there is much supportive evidence. For example, a peer-reviewed journal, *Health at Every Size* (formerly, *Healthy Weight Journal*), has been in print for two decades. People *may* lose weight with this approach but weight-loss is not the expressed goal and marker of success. Rather, practitioners encourage size acceptance, bodily movement in ways that are practical, making peace with food and improving metabolic fitness (for example, cholesterol, insulin sensitivity and blood pressure) through nutrition and moderate physical activity (Bacon 2006, Gaesser 2002, Robison 2005b). They also flag social factors affecting health and challenge anti fat prejudice, discrimination and the vested interests of the weight loss industry. This converges with fat activism. I will refer to Health at Every Size throughout this book when going beyond militarized medicine, fat fighting and men's own meanings and discourses, though, at the same time, I remain attuned to men's own definitions of a life worth living (for example, sedentary pleasures, eating fatty food and drinking alcohol).

Some words about words: Being labelled 'fat' or worse?

Because words like 'fat' and 'obese' often carry a sting it is worth clarifying and qualifying how I use them. I will also explain why I use alternative words such as 'big' and refer to large men as 'big fellas' rather than 'fat boys' as evidenced in recent work (Gilman 2004).

There are obvious difficulties when talking about fat. Kulick and Meneley (2005: 2, emphasis in original) write: 'the tone with which the word *fat* is uttered is often concerned, ashamed, alarmist, or condemnatory. Fat, we are told relentlessly, is bad'. Of course, the F-word is not completely taboo. Calorific food is often considered pleasurable if not entirely healthful because it contains fat. The Bible equates fat with prosperity, as in 'the fat of the land' (Stearns 1997: 6), and religious faith: 'he that putteth his trust in the Lord shall be made fat' (Proverbs 28: 25; cited by Wann 1998: 110). Within Black American hip-hop, fat or 'phat' has positive meanings when applied to music and men's bodily appearance (Gross 2005). There are also positive appropriations in fat acceptance groups like the

National Association to Advance Fat Acceptance (NAAFA), which mainly consist of women identifying as fat. For them, '"fat" is an adjective like "tall" or "thin" and should not be offensive' (Solovay 2000: 29). And, men sometimes call each other fat in an observably good-natured and well-received manner. This is noted in Duneier's (1992: 38) ethnography of Black working-class men in Chicago where the playful insult – being called a 'little fat-faced fucker' – reaffirmed group belonging and was apparently well-received among friends. However, Kulick and Meneley (2005) also point to the fear and loathing often evoked by the word 'fat' and thus how being called fat could cause offence in contemporary Western culture.

Being reflexive about words is important because words are tools and are affective. Crossley (2001: 81) states, 'the language of a society or social group is an expression of the various emotional attitudes that its members have collectively adopted towards the world'. Emotions matter not least because they are inseparable from embodied identities, that is, how people relationally view themselves, feel about themselves and present themselves as lived bodies. For example, Lynne Murray (2005), in *The State of the F-Word: Three Letters that Still Shock*, is cautious when discussing 'fat' given its common association with negative traits and stigma. Within contemporary Western culture the discrediting attributes often associated with fatness are well known, such as laziness, gluttony, ugliness, sickness and immorality.

Even so, social scientists, similar to fat activists who challenge dominant understandings, use the words 'fat' and 'fatness' when distancing themselves from biomedicine (for example, LeBesco 2004, Sobal and Maurer 1999a, b). That is understandable, but in writing this book I do not want to betray research contacts, men who may have eschewed a 'fat identity' (Degher and Hughes 1999) or employed different terms of reference (see below). Ethical concerns should run through the research process, including the point of writing up and publishing one's study. Calling individuals 'fat' is unnecessary to my analysis, potentially stigmatizing and incompatible with a study that includes people who did not necessarily view themselves as fat even though medicine might have labelled them overweight or obese.

Given my substantive and political concerns, the F-word is nonetheless unavoidable. Rather than calling men fat, I will use the words 'fat' and 'fatness' when referring to context-dependent meanings, communicated violence and resistances. For example, bodies that are seen as fat by others, people who self-identify as fat, the institutional attack on medicalized fat, and fat acceptance groups that promote the rights of 'fat people'. Of course, proponents of the obesity discourse use biomedical terms (overweight, obesity and even morbid obesity). I will say more about these labels below. However, it should be recognized that these are fundamentally about body fat, or adipose tissue, which is deemed 'excessive' by medical authorities (WHO 1998). Also, while health workers and promoters use words like 'weight' and 'body mass', similar to so-called 'laity' they employ these often *inoffensive* terms as an efficient yet crude proxy for fat (though they may also simply define weight as a public health issue and even a disease). Within this discursive context, 'weight' usually refers to imagined fat which, interestingly, provides space for men's resistance and manoeuvrability when faced with the idea that they and/or the majority of men in developed nations really are fat.

When talking about weight, men often identified themselves, or referred to others, as big. I will use this word when directly referring to men whom medicine might label overweight, obese or morbidly obese. To be clear, what constitutes 'big' is socially constructed and is therefore relative. A man who is 30 stone (420 pounds or 191 kilograms) is unlikely to view another who is 16 stone (224 pounds or 102 kilograms) as big, while a man who is just over 12½ stone (175 pounds or 79 kilograms) at 5'10" would probably not view himself as big but medicine would consider him too big and label him overweight using the BMI. I thus use 'big' flexibly, albeit with some mind as to how particular men viewed themselves.

Bigness, unlike fatness, is a functionally ambiguous term. Hence, it is similar to the word 'weight', which might be treated as a proxy for fat but which, in reality, includes lean body mass or muscle. The word 'big' fits with the social construction of acceptable and admirable masculinities. Big male bodies vary in their organic composition, physical appearance and standing on masculine hierarchies. Not all would be considered or labelled fat by self or others. This is not only about body composition and build (for example, relative proportions of adiposity and muscle) and contingent perceptions of the physical body (*cf.* Monaghan 2001). It is also about deference, dignity and respect. Being a big man, rather than a fat man, or big fat man, is more appropriate in a fatphobic society. This is a society where masculinity is thought to proceed from men's bodies (Connell 1995) and *a certain degree of size is associated* with adult presence more so for men than women (Morgan 1993), i.e. the embodiment of gendered power (Shilling 2003). In that respect, sizism is a gendered form of bigotry that is inseparable from sexism (Smith 1990), though sizism also has the potential to hurt men who are seen as fat and are subordinated on masculine hierarchies.

While research participants are given pseudonyms, a generic referent is sometimes useful. Using everyday gendered terms, men who might exceed a medically defined 'healthy' weight are respectfully called big fellas or big men. Gilman's (2004) use of 'fat boys' is rejected. Aside from problems with the F-word and the discrepancy between medical and everyday definitions of 'appropriate' adult male weight-for-height (Monaghan 2007), to call them 'boys' is to infantilize them and subordinate them further on embodied hierarchies. Crucially, if sizism is also comparable to racism (Cooper 1998) then it is telling that race has been understood historically as a hierarchy of bodies and the hierarchical ordering of masculinities. As discussed by Connell (2000: 61) in relation to imperialism, this positioning has in some circumstances resulted in the 'feminization' of colonized men and 'in many parts of the colonized world indigenous men were called "boys"'. If big fellas are being colonized by the obesity discourse then to call them boys is, I would argue, analogous to the subordination of colonized men's bodies under imperialism. The embodiment of masculinity comprises a gender politics that is intimately connected to selfhood (Connell 2000). Substituting fella for boy is not only more respectful but also anthropologically accurate.

Given the greater licence people have towards their own preserves (Goffman 1961b), men nonetheless sometimes called themselves fat. There are various reasons for this. On one level this parallels the interactional moves of people with visible impairments who seek to put others at ease by explicitly acknowledging their visible difference (Shakespeare 1999). This identification may also be compared, albeit in a less politicized and organized way, to fat activism where 'fat people' are urged to call themselves 'fatso' in order to 'turn fat hatred back on itself' (Wann 1998: 28). British working-class men even sometimes proudly call themselves 'fat bastards' and, in so doing, unintentionally perform political work that defiantly challenges moral censure. And, while offensive to middle-class sensibilities, the word 'bastard' is compatible with typically White, British working-class masculinities as in 'he's a good-looking bastard' or 'hard bastard'. Of course, depending on context, this may also be self-deprecating as when a big fella 'confesses' his 'deviancy' and his intention to lose weight. And, when imposed by anonymous others, this can be intensely stigmatizing in line with a history of anti-fat lexicon that ridicules big men as fat slobs (Stearns 1997). Some men participating in this research, besides calling themselves fat or fat bastards, also called others fat or talked about being called fat or fat bastards. This is an empirical study, which means men's talk and forms of identification are presented verbatim.

The words 'overweight' and 'obesity' are also unavoidable. These are considered technical terms within biomedicine that can be rationally and efficiently calculated using the BMI. Yet for members of the public, the term 'obese' is often offensive. Aphramor (2006) makes this point, referring to a study of 300 patients enrolled in 'obesity treatment' (Wadden and Didie 2003). She adds that while the word 'overweight' might be less stigmatizing outside of medicine, it 'again diagnoses people, constructing a disease state which leaves no room for large people to be healthy and/or "fatness" to be viewed as a non-pathological diversity in body size' (Aphramor 2006: 19). Fat activists agree. Wann (1998: 19, emphasis in original) contends, 'over *whose* weight?' 'Obesity' is also rejected. Again this is about challenging medical degradation and associated harms. As explained by Wann (personal communication, 2007) when urging me to rethink my use of the expression 'critical obesity literature': 'please understand that the term "obesity" medicalizes weight diversity and is also a direct threat to the health of fat people. Fat people are denied medical care and targeted with, and coerced into undergoing, dangerous "cures" because of that label'.

Men contacted during this research who were not fat activists addressed the politics of gendered identity, rather than fat rights, when talking about the 'obesity' label. Some said they found the term highly insulting. One interviewee thought it referred to somebody so fat that they could not get out of their chair. Another man, a school headmaster, thought the word referred to *The Guinness Book of World Records* extreme until a nurse told him he was almost obese. I mention these examples not to support the biomedical view that 'laymen' are poor at judging if they are overweight or obese. Rather, this highlights the problematic status of these words, the empirical inaccuracy of the 'implicit value premises' of 'technical risk experts' (Beck 1992: 58) and how men contacted during this study resisted being discredited by biomedical labels that connote pathology, disease, illness, physical impairment and risk.

Other biomedical terms are also identifiable. For clinicians, somebody with a BMI ≥ 40 kg/m^2 is 'severely' or 'morbidly obese'. Oliver (2006: 55) states the term 'morbid obesity' was coined in the 1950s by a bariatric surgeon when seeking more business. Wann (1998), who reports good metabolic health and a healthy lifestyle, states she was defined as morbidly obese when refused health insurance. She complains the 'label of "morbid obesity" wasn't a diagnosis; it was discrimination' (Wann 1998: 10). Some men contacted for this research said they were labelled morbidly obese, much to their dissatisfaction. Such words were beyond the pale. Instead, and in line with Aphramor's (2006) point about the variable stigma attached to medical labels, some really big fellas self-identified as overweight. Again, this was not about their failure to perceive themselves correctly, in line with negative stereotypes about fatness and stupidity. Their alternative understandings were not about ignorance but about resisting moral opprobrium and constructing identities.

In short, labels cannot be used innocently. This parallels an approach to language within the social model of disability: a politicized response to biomedicine and those who locate faults within the physical body rather than the larger disabling society. Given the role of language in shaping meanings and even creating realities, proponents of the social model reject terms like 'spastic' or 'cripple' as well as 'handicap' as used by the WHO (Oliver 2004: 280–1). Certainly, as noted above, men participating in this study sometimes used biomedical words, such as over-weight. This is understandable given the power of biomedicine and the fact that a politicized understanding of fatness is marginalized. However, similarly to the F-word, I refer to men's use of these terms and discuss overweight and obesity when engaging medical meanings, rather than label specific individuals as such. I would follow Campos (2006) here who also uses the words 'overweight' and 'obesity' when directly engaging the primary scientific field. I endorse his point that these 'question-begging' terms 'should always be read with an implicit "so-called" modifying them' (Campos 2006: 3).

The research: Treading lightly on a potential 'minefield'

I wanted to 'bring in' men's missing voices to critical weight studies and to do so without being offensive. Researchers have an ethical obligation to their research participants. The British Sociological Association's statement of ethical practice states: 'Sociologists have a responsibility to ensure that the physical, social and psychological well-being of research participants is not adversely affected by the research. They should strive to protect the rights of those they study, their interests, sensitivities and privacy' (BSA 2002: 2). Unlike invasive biomedical research, sociological research does not tend to pose a literal threat to the life or limb of research participants. However, given the moralizing and stigmatization sur-rounding 'weight' or fatness, this topic constituted a potential minefield. As a researcher, treading lightly not only entailed using participants' vocabularies. It also meant stepping back and changing the subject if the discussion got too near to the bone.

During this research qualitative data were generated on issues that could be related to, even if not always directly about, weight or fatness. For example, there was no intention of making the topic of 'man breasts' explicit, which, as discussed by Longhurst (2005a), typically assaults men's identities and is surrounded by taboo. Between 2004 and 2006, data were generated on the meanings of health, physical activity through the life course, food and diet, the body, slimming and other sociologically relevant concerns (for example, relationships with family, friends and colleagues). These are issues that all men could talk about regardless of whether or not they were 'objectively' fat and/or had adopted a 'fat identity' (Degher and Hughes 1999). Additionally, even if men defined themselves as having a weight problem and were or had been slimming club members, there was no intention to impose a fat identity on them and breach situational proprieties. No direct questions were therefore asked about the Surgeon Generals' declarations of war on obesity and 'the terror within', though discussion did engage government claims that most men in England are supposedly 'too heavy'. This was couched in terms of a research interest in the broader topic of health as understood by men themselves, and, if relevant, an interest in their expressed views about weight/fat.

Various methods were employed and contexts explored. Research included a 'virtual ethnography' (Hine 2000) of, in and through online fat acceptance and admiration groups. These were mainly based in the USA. I was previously unaware of these groups and their meanings, practices and values. However, after typing the words 'men' and 'fat' into Internet search engines, new worlds presented themselves which ranged from the politically astute to the pornographic (Monaghan 2005b). I have engaged intermittently with online politicized groups and activists, though understandings from more playful groups, such as the gay male Bears, are also included in this book.

Qualitative data were obtained offline in various settings, at times not always dedicated to research. For example, informal conversations on men's weight sometimes occurred during everyday life. Weight-related talk is common and part of the mundane in much the same way that talk about the weather is in Western Europe (including Ireland, which is my current place of residence). If relevant data emerged when talking with men, I recorded these in a field diary and obtained informed consent whenever practicable. Television programmes, which were recorded and sometimes transcribed, also served as a supplementary data source alongside newspapers, magazines and online documents (for example, government and policy reports).

While I have various slices of data, most of the ethnography was generated in a commercial mixed-sex slimming club in north-east England. The slimming club was selected for ethical, pragmatic and theoretical reasons. Ethically, I did not want to impose 'weight problems' on people's identities and relevances. The slimming club was advantageous in that respect because overweight is already an issue for fee-paying members who publicly identify as such. Pragmatically, slimming clubs are ubiquitous, access was relatively easy to negotiate, weight-related issues are part of the front stage setting, members join for various reasons (including but not confined to medical reasons), and clubs are open to men and women. Theoretically, I wanted to include dis-confirming cases that challenged rather than proved emerging ideas and concepts. Restated, as this study progressed (formulating a research proposal to obtain funding, doing online research, talking with various people) I became increasingly sceptical about the obesity discourse. And, while it may be relatively easy to find men who disagree with weight-loss injunctions, I wanted to include men who were publicly committed to weight-loss or 'fat fighting' in order to generate a credible and robust analysis. My theoretically informed sample is unusual because men often avoid slimming clubs, but, I would maintain, this adds to the study's strength. Including male slimmers constitutes a critical case when exploring the acceptability or otherwise of 'therapeutic' interventions intended to promote slenderness, health and happiness. One might assume these men wholeheartedly embraced fat fighting. Whether they did or not was an empirical question.

Nine months' ethnography was undertaken at Sunshine slimming club (the names of research participants, places and organizations are pseudonyms). I undertook four months of fieldwork at three classes and my research associate, Gary Pritchard, undertook five months of fieldwork at two classes. Unlike Stinson (2001), who, in her ethnography of a US slimming club, followed the organization's weight-loss programme, we openly undertook fieldwork as observers rather than active participants. This is because neither of us wanted to lose weight. Ethnographic contacts were publicly informed by the club consultant that we were there as university researchers. Observations, conversations and analytic memos were written *in situ* in a field diary and then elaborated as soon as possible afterwards. These ethnographic materials are presented in subsequent empirical chapters. Unless otherwise indicated, ethnographic field notes are taken directly from my field diary.

Sunshine reported a national membership of 250,000. A rival company, Fat Fighters, was also approached as part of an overt study but they refused access. While observations were not made there, former or current members were interviewed: some dissatisfied members switched their allegiance to Sunshine, just as some Sunshine slimmers subsequently joined Fat Fighters. Weekly classes were, with the exception of one, held in a church hall. This was not formally a religious or evangelical weight-loss programme – types of programme that have been popular in the USA (Schwartz 1986) but, as will be seen in Chapter 2, religious themes were recurrent. Three classes were run by the same consultant, Sandy, who, like other consultants, also watched her weight. A male consultant, Danny, held another class in a school. Classes varied in size, with one of Sandy's groups sometimes attracting over 80 people, while Danny's seldom exceeded 20. Classes met for about one hour each week.

Women usually attend slimming clubs but one of Sandy's classes regularly attracted up to 20 men each week out of approximately 30 attendees. The typical male slimmer was from a working-class background, White, in his 40s or 50s and presenting as heterosexual. Members, the consultant and other workers (who were often unpaid members volunteering their services) 'supported' each other as they sought to lose weight through a modified diet. There were commonly shared rituals in classes. These included congratulating members if they lost weight and group 'therapy' sessions. During therapy, members shared ideas and confessed their dietary misdemeanours with the goal of obtaining practical knowledge, assuaging guilt and reaffirming individual and collective commitment. Even so, there was a high rate of attrition in line with clinical observations that dietary approaches to weight-loss usually fail (Aphramor 2005, Mann *et al.* 2007).

Data were also generated during in-depth interviews (N=37). These lasted between one and two hours and were audio-recorded and transcribed. Interviewing was an efficient method for obtaining a range of men's views and provided a wealth of data. These data are used extensively in this book. Data extracts are presented verbatim and are only edited slightly to preserve anonymity and clarity. Unless otherwise indicated, men's talk was obtained during interviews rather than, say, informal conversations in the slimming club or in everyday life. It is sometimes relevant to the analysis to know who generated these data, for example when men were talking about sport, muscularity and physical activity (see below on the embodied aspects of the research). For the most part, men were talking with me, though I will make clear in subsequent chapters which data were obtained by Gary.

I conducted 25 interviews and Gary did 12. A total of 18 interviewees were current or former slimming club members. Most of these men were recruited at the slimming club with the help of the consultant. The remaining 19 interviewees included men contacted through friendship networks, a fitness centre and asking men for an interview after striking up an informal conversation in contexts of everyday life. Men recruited outside of slimming clubs were not necessarily concerned about losing weight and did not always define themselves as having a weight problem. The ethics of interviewing these men were negotiated by stressing our interest in men's health more generally rather than weight or fatness in particular, though prior contact with some of these men, or their friends, meant that we knew whether or not their weight was of 'intrinsic relevance' (Schutz 1970) to them. And, with regard to men recruited from the fitness centre, respondents self-completed a questionnaire asking them to list their reasons for joining and to confirm their willingness to be interviewed.

Respondents' ages ranged from 16 to 79 and the mean age was 43. All were White, with the exception of two men of Afro-Caribbean origin. All presented as heterosexual except one man who was affiliated to the gay Bear subculture. Six interviewees were educated to university level (including postgraduate), though only one of these was from the slimming club. All men were either employed, in full-time education or retired. Various occupations, including a few professions, are represented such as: university researcher, nurse, teacher, mechanic, lorry driver, shop assistant, porter and doorman.

Men were not recruited for interviewing simply because their BMI was likely to equal or exceed 25 kg/m^2, though, as stated above, most were reportedly at a weight-for-height that medicine labels overweight or obese. Men's self-reported measures sometimes give additional context to their talk and quantifiable concerns (for example, discussing their dieting careers and weight-loss goals). As might be expected with men from England, all used Imperial measurements, i.e. stones and pounds. I will present their preferred measures though I appreciate readers outside the UK often prefer other measures. Hence, Table 1.1 might be useful as a quick guide. Additionally, in qualifying my use of men's self-reported measurements, two points should be made. First, the validity of these does not really matter to my analysis. The aim was not to measure objectified bodies in accord with the requirements of medicalized height–weight studies, which have been subjected to methodological critique (Knapp 1983). Rather, the aim was to understand people in accord with the humanistic requirements of interpretive sociology. Second, and following Throsby's (2007) decision in her study on bariatric surgery not to report respondents' weights – due to what she calls the 'enfreakement' of larger people – I will stress that while I share her ethical concerns, I am reporting the views of men who often sought to rationalize their bodies as part of their presentations of self as ordinary and responsible fellas rather than freaks.

These men often worked hard at presenting themselves as ordinary, but this small sample is obviously not statistically representative of British men. I am not in a position to explore the range of experiences of different men throughout the social structure (for example, different gay men or men from a wide range of ethnic backgrounds). Nonetheless, this research does offer depth and richness of data and provides some much-needed empirical insights into an under-researched topic. Qualitative data, comprising field notes, interview transcripts and other materials (for example, from websites and the media), were imported into and analysed with the aid of coding software, Atlas.ti (Muhr 1997). As recommended by grounded theorists (Glaser and Strauss 1967), data generation and analysis were concurrent processes. Data were indexed according to various thematic codes (for example, diets, physical activity, BMI). This allowed me efficiently to compare across and

Table 1.1 Weight conversion table

Stones	Pounds	Kilograms
10 to 12	140 to 168	64 to 76
12 to 14	168 to 196	76 to 89
14 to 16	196 to 224	89 to 102
16 to 18	224 to 252	102 to 114
18 to 20	252 to 280	114 to 127
20 to 22	280 to 308	127 to 140
22 to 24	308 to 336	140 to 152
24 to 26	336 to 364	152 to 165
26 to 28	364 to 392	165 to 178
28 to 30	392 to 420	178 to 191
30 to 32	420 to 448	191 to 203
32 to 34	448 to 476	203 to 216

Note: 1 stone is equivalent to 14 pounds or 6.35 kilograms

within cases and account for any that contradicted emergent analytic propositions. This approach is also called analytic induction (Bloor 1978), though, as explained by Charmaz and Mitchell (2001), using grounded theory does not bar researchers from using existing theories. Indeed, these may sensitize researchers to processes occurring in their data and perhaps prompt them to look beyond their materials.

Analytically, men's accounts were treated as '*displays* of perspectives and moral forms' (Silverman 2001: 112) and a potentially (un)reliable source of information about the world. For example, when generating and analysing data on physical activity I was more interested in how men's talk was related to their displays of social fitness or moral worth rather than determining their actual physical activity levels and physical fitness. At other times I was interested in how men talked about their decisions to go on a diet and what this said about the real world as lived and experienced by them. This meant going beyond 'misleading' polarities such as true/false or form/content and recognizing that 'when gaining access to a cultural universe [. . .] accounts are part of the world they describe' (Silverman 2001: 113).

Given the nature of this topic and demands for researcher reflexivity, I will finish this section with some biographical information. I will say something about my research career and embodied insertion into the research. As well as potentially shaping research participants' responses and presentations of self (for example, their displays of moral worth, their talk about messages that discredit weight), I aim to be reflexive about how aspects of my biography could have shaped my interpretation of findings and the larger war on obesity. However, in keeping with a critical realist approach, I would not conflate being with knowing or ontology with epistemology (Skeggs 1997) (for example, the idea that only women can acquire a feminist consciousness or only fat people really know about fat hatred).

Besides teaching medical sociology to social science students, medical students, nurses and others in the clinical therapies, I have previously undertaken ethnography among other big fellas (for example, Monaghan 2001, 2002, 2006). That research explored the social worlds of bodybuilders and nightclub security staff with an emphasis on embodied risks as understood by them – risks that had absolutely nothing to do with whether or not their bigness rendered them diseased. Indeed, their physicality was a form of capital that generated income and masculine validating recognition! Among other things, my previous embroilment in these domains means that I am not inclined to simply view bodies with a BMI >25 kg/m^2 as somehow in need of remedy. Another issue concerns my own embodied responses to forms of violence. Researching nightclub security plus a biography of boxing means that I have experience with physical violence. As part of my own masculine identity and habitus I do not think I am overly sensitive. Nonetheless, I have been shocked by the symbolic violence committed by caring institutions, which is simply rationalized away as medically justified. Anti-fat prejudice and institutional sizism may be exercised unrealized, but, from my standpoint, the occasional bloody nose inflicted by an errant bouncer pales in comparison to the not-so-subtle violence communicated by organizations and their representatives when seeking to promote a 'thin' conception of health. I empathize with fat activists and some of my contacts who are or were angered by this. At the same time I appreciate why many people acquiesce with it when presenting themselves as 'good' people on the social stage.

There are other reasons for 'bringing in' my own body. Notably, the obesity debate is characterized by 'credibility struggles' (Saguy and Riley 2005) and authors risk being discredited because of their physicality. However, I have reservations about playing a credibility game where only certain 'privileged' bodies are permitted to contribute, especially in medical circles, regardless of their professional credentials. Consider, for example, correspondence on 'the obesity problem' in *The New England Journal of Medicine* where the editors were asked about their BMI after urging a more cautious approach. The enquirer believed this was important if the editors were 'to avoid any accusations of a hidden agenda' (Imperato 1998: 1158). Implicit in this request is the sizist assumption that the editors' suspected fatness would prevent them from offering a reasoned contribution. However, in turning the tables, Campos (2004) suggests the best people to contribute are the extremely fat women who are taking a leading role in fat activism. If fat is the issue, I can also appreciate that a social researcher who is seen as fat may be better placed to generate rapport with people who identify as fat and obtain rich qualitative data as a result.

Using such criteria I lack relevant qualifications, though, unlike Gary who describes himself as 'thin' verging on an 'average build', I am a reasonably big fella. Skinny until the age of 19, I have lifted weights in gyms for most of my adult life in order to get bigger. Like many men exercising in bodybuilding gyms, I have sought to 'bulk up' by gaining and retaining muscle. At the time of writing I am relatively lean and muscular with a body mass *intentionally* exceeding BMI 25 kg/m^2. I am thus technically 'overweight', though, similar to fat activists, I reject that value-laden term as I suspect most strength athletes would. My physique has varied in size, composition and appearance though I do not imagine myself to be fat and I am generally intolerant towards fat on my own body. This is not only about embodying the dispositions of a fatphobic culture but also my emergent dispositions, i.e. an acquired subcultural appreciation of lean bodybuilding physiques which, contrary to some masculinity studies, cannot simply be theorized in terms of gender inadequacy (Monaghan 2001). Although intolerant towards fat on my own body, I would not extend that intolerance towards other people. And, in case research participants inferred that from my appearance, I wore baggy clothes to try to render my size ambiguous. I also told men that I was not part of the food police and I wanted to learn from them, though, at the same time, I was critical of official claims that most men are unhealthy, diseased or at risk because of their weight. Gary presented a similar non-judgemental self when talking with men who often identified him as thin. Of course, I recognize these identifications mean that men may have been staking out a particular identity during interviews. Masculinity is produced relationally in front of other men (Bourdieu 2001). However, regardless of whether or not they viewed us as 'privileged' bodies, men still displayed rich and diverse views. Hopefully, the full richness and complexity of these data are captured in subsequent chapters.

Chapter outline

This chapter has provided a broad introduction. After discussing the value of researching men, I outlined the characteristics of a sociologically imaginative approach, offered some words about potentially offensive terms and presented a reflexive description of the research. Chapter 2 offers a typology for interpreting weight-related accounts. It includes understandings from published studies, the media, online research, fat activism, interviews with men and ethnographic fieldwork. This presages themes pursued in subsequent chapters and clarifies the value of fat activism for informing sociology. Chapter 3 explores men's dieting careers. Reference is made to men's definitions of dieting, gendered conditions and triggers for going on a diet, efforts to sustain a (modified) diet and reasons for aborting weight-loss diets. Chapter 4 goes beyond efficient accounts of obesity causation and critically explores the manufacturing of men's fatness as a correctable problem with particular reference to the slimming club. Ritzer's (2004) McDonaldization of society thesis is used as a reference point to empirically explore the rationalization of men's bodies plus irrationalities and meaningful resistances. Chapter 5 reports and analyses men's talk about physical activity, slimming, health and fitness. Referring to, but also moving beyond, government endorsed obesity fighting campaigns, men's displays of social fitness are considered with particular reference to one mode of accountability: justifiable resistance and defiance. The conclusion, Chapter 6, draws from preceding chapters to underscore the value of healthy scepticism and 'bringing in' men to weight-related studies. It also offers several policy recommendations and finishes with some words on resisting and possibly ending the biomedical war on obesity.

Finally, to avoid potential misunderstanding, I will briefly reiterate my intentions and the overall tenor of this book. My primary aim is to promote critically informed and ultimately productive discussion among academics, health professionals, policy makers and other interested parties. I aim to do this by offering a sociologically imaginative study that is empirically grounded, theoretically informed and politically attuned. I do not dismiss the value of nutrition and physical activity for biomedical health (in a society where these are differentially distributed and more or less beneficial depending upon social structural location and other embodied concerns), but these are not viewed here as medicines for the putative disease known as obesity. Nor are they viewed as substitutes for tackling social inequalities, which have the biggest impact on population health. This study repudiates rather than promotes obesity warmongering while exploring the socially fitting identities men presented in a society where most men are reportedly overweight or obese. In contrast to those declaring and marshalling the war on obesity, biomedical bodies are viewed as embodied subjects rather than objectified bodies, i.e. people who not only have bodies but are lived bodies embedded within and co-constituting a broader social world. I will therefore 'bring in' men's previously unheard voices while offering critically informed commentary. The following has policy and clinical relevance and it is my hope, but not necessarily my expectation, that it will encourage a more tolerant and informed approach among individuals and organizations committed to the attack on medicalized fat. This study has obvious relevance for understanding men's health. However, insights are not always specific to men given that the war on obesity is directed at practically everyone. The tenor of this book is serious but there is a lighter side too. Hopefully there is much that will make readers smile without trivializing a public and private issue that is actively made into a problem by and for millions of people.

2 Bodily alignment and accounts

From excuses to repudiation

Typifying and evaluating weight-related accounts

Words about weight-related issues, like bodies, take many shapes and forms. Big Joe, quoted immediately before Chapter 1, challenged those who condemned 'fat people', though there are obviously other types of account. Consider some other men's talk:

> I suppose I'm slightly overweight with what some people call a beer belly. I call it my lorry driver's belly. Because at the end of the day I'm sat down an awful lot of the time and if you look at lorry drivers they do tend to have a [pats his stomach] paunch. (Howard)

> [Laughing] I always like the food that makes you fat. (Arthur)

> People nowadays are trying to blame McDonald's, KFC and all that for obesity. And people are now starting to sue them in America for fast-food being available, that's made them fat, as far as they're concerned. Hang on a second. Who twisted their arm and shoved the food down their throat? They did. So why blame somebody for providing you with something if you get fat? It's not their fault. It's your fault. (Jim)

> It's all in your genes. You're meant to be the way you are. It wouldn't do for us all to be the same. It wouldn't. (Freddy)

Sociologists underscore the importance of words or accounts in question situations (Hunter 1984, Scott and Lyman 1968). Accounts are 'aligning actions' (Stokes and Hewitt 1976), or socially derived vocabularies, that are intended to bridge gaps between (in)actions and expectations. Accounts include written words (Orbuch 1997) and they need not always be vocalized, instead taking the form of 'linguistic explanations that arise in an actor's "mind" when he questions his own behavior' (Scott and Lyman 1968: 46–7). Independent of their truth-value, accounts have pragmatic, therapeutic, explanatory and other functions (Burnett 1991). They may bolster social identities while drawing from, reproducing and possibly subverting dominant understandings. In this chapter I will typify and evaluate different weight-related accounts. Drawing from published studies, the media, online research, fat activism and men's talk, I will consider ways of accounting for and orienting to bodies that medicine might label overweight or worse.

Theoretically, I will use and expand Scott and Lyman's (1968) original typology. As shown in Table 2.1, this framework is structured around issues of responsibility and ascribed negativity. Scott and Lyman (1968) discuss excuses and justifications as general types of account. With excuses the pejorative status of something, such as weight and/or behaviour assumed to cause this, is accepted but personal responsibility is mitigated; with justifications responsibility is accepted but its negative status is challenged. Citing the sedentary nature of one's job might constitute an excuse-account for overweight, while somebody who loves fattening food might voice a justification. Table 2.1 includes two additional concepts: contrition and repudiation. These are grounded respectively in a discussion on slimming and fat activism. When discussing the former I will mainly use data from men who were seeking to lose weight; i.e. they accepted responsibility for their incorrect yet correctable bodies. When discussing repudiation I will outline politicized ways of knowing fatness, using fat acceptance material. This will clarify my evaluative approach to the obesity discourse and why I honour Big Joe's and other men's repudiating talk that challenged social censure with or without mitigating personal responsibility (what I will go on to describe as softer and harder repudiation). The typology structures data reporting and analysis, with more politically astute strands of fat activism used throughout this book to inform my interpretation of men's talk and the war on obesity. However, I will first critically reflect on accounts-based sociology.

Table 2.1 An expanded accounts framework

	Accept pejorative status	*Deny or challenge pejorative status*
Accept responsibility	Contrition	Justifications
Deny (relevance of) responsibility	Excuses	Repudiation

Accounts-based sociology: A critically informed reading

The theoretical development of the accounts concept in sociology can be traced to such people as Garfinkel, Goffman, and Scott and Lyman (Orbuch 1997). Orbuch (1997) notes that while Garfinkel saw accounts as a regular aspect of everyday life, this concept has largely been used in the sociology of deviance. Certainly, that was the explicit rationale in Scott and Lyman's (1968) work and there is a long tradition of accounts-based research on crime (for example, Cavanagh *et al.* 2001, Sykes and Matza 1957). Given the original intentions and common uses of this approach, I will stress that I am not comparing my contacts to deviants or criminals (also see Gimlin 2007b).

There are limitations and blind spots associated with any analytic approach. In his critical realist discussion on interpretivism and research designed to elicit people's accounts, Williams (2003b: 55–6) underscores 'the "primacy" of practice, habituated knowledge/unthinking dispositions' and thus how research on accounts may reproduce a misleading picture. For example, note the discrepancy between people's words and deeds or the tacit and experiential aspects of everyday life that are ineffable. While words are important, in remaining mindful of these concerns I would not elevate accounts and language over concrete practices and material embodiment, 'discursive consciousness' over 'practical consciousness' and so on (Giddens 1984, cited by Williams 2003b: 56). Certainly, while there are many accounts for unwanted weight, and there are multiple engines that drive fatphobia in the larger society, accounts may never arise. Indeed, if overweight, medically defined by BMI, is statistically normal in many nations (WHO 1998), and such bodies are defined as normal by self and others, then there is no gap between bodies and expectations – though that is gendered and racialized, since feminists observe that body dissatisfaction is practically normalized among White Western women regardless of actual weight (Bordo 1993, Grogan 1999). Also, accounts may be uncalled for from much larger people if their weight is treated with 'tactful blindness' (Goffman 1967). And, if somebody does adopt a stigmatized 'fat identity' (Degher and Hughes 1999) (i.e. an identity that is spoiled rather than a source of pride, as proclaimed by some fat activists), potentially problematic situations may be avoided.

It should also be noted that when people talk there are many matters that are understood but left unspoken (Garfinkel 1967). Understanding is never confined to specific utterances but a whole range of retrospective and prospective possibilities. For example, what is said after an utterance may clarify the sense of what came before, with conversation typically organized around such expectations and actions. A corollary is that subject positions are complex: people may oscillate between essentially indeterminable accounts and identities that are presented to self and others in a way that befuddles Scott and Lyman's (1968) schema, and my expanded typology. This is, then, an ideal typical model or analytical abstraction. It helps make sense of rather than fully captures messy empirical reality in all its dynamism and layered complexity.

Accounts are multifarious but whether they are honoured in everyday life depends upon cultural 'background expectancies' (Scott and Lyman 1968): the seen but unnoticed backgrounds of everyday activities that are part of the natural attitude of life, the world taken for granted (Garfinkel 1967, Schutz 1970). Thus, Garfinkel (1967: 118) underscores the 'omnirelevance' of 'sexual status' as an aspect of the 'unnoticed background' that shapes the acceptability or otherwise of accounts. West and Zimmerman (2002: 13) pick up on this with regard to the 'womanly' or 'manly nature' of accounts and thus whether or not people 'live up' to normative gendered expectations. However, while people may be more or less inclined to accept particular gendered accounts within particular interpretive communities that are themselves gendered (for example, masculinized, militarized medicine), accounts-based sociology typically displays relativistic indifference toward any particular discourse. This is problematic given the ethical implications of the obesity discourse (Rich and Evans 2005) and other issues discussed in Chapter 1.

Extreme social constructionist positions, and the predominantly social psychological focus in later work on accounts (Orbuch 1997), are problematic insofar as they deny real material considerations that work on, in and through real biological bodies. After all, embodied social structures are real in their effects independent of whether or not particular groups of people define them as real through discourse or accounting practices. The ideology of healthism and personal responsibility is pervasive and consequential in social life, shaping everyday 'body projects' and individual self-identity (Shilling 2003: 4). Yet, as indicated in Shilling's (2003) non reductionist discussion on 'the naturalistic body', biology cannot be divorced from society – a point he extends when advocating 'corporeal realism' in his more recent writings on embodied sociology (Shilling 2005). Aphramor (2005) offers compatible theorizing when stating the physiological is political. More generally, this underscores the value of a critical realist approach that engages interpretive, social structural and biological debates (Williams 2003b). I will critique obesity warmongering, and the personal battles it mandates or incites in the name of health, but I also recognize that accounts supporting the public and private fight against fat often have situational efficacy, suit various institutional ends and have currency in late modernity. Embodied sociology makes sense of this, but it should also be critical of larger structures and processes that strip people of dignity and respect all in their supposed best interests (Monaghan 2006).

Types of excuse and justification: From inactive thyroids to 'overactive' microwaves

There are many excuses and justifications for weight or fat and weight-gain. Table 2.2 offers an advanced cognitive map, with this section grounding these accounts in empirical data.

Excuses

The word 'excuse' usually implies blatant fabrication. Al, a slimmer who cited various mitigating factors for his past 31 stone, stated: 'I'm not making excuses. I'm just stating facts.' However, this concept is used here to refer to accounts where people accept the pejorative status of bodyweight or fat, and perhaps ways of living assumed to cause unwanted weight, but mitigate individual responsibility. Excuse-accounts are common in a fatphobic society where, despite the popularity of diets, people are reportedly heavier than ever. Usually offered in a retrospective sense, excuses provide discursive space for individuals to be absolved from past 'sins', while leaving the path open for personal salvation through contrition. However, not all of these excuses had currency among men negotiating masculine identities or carried sociological weight.

Table 2.2 Types of excuse and justification for weight or fat and weight-gain

Types of excuse	• Biomedical accounts: Appeal to disease, i.e. 'obesity' as a chronic disease. Appeal to disease processes, medicalized conditions, medication and biographical disruption. Examples: cardiovascular disease, untreated depression and imposed physical inactivity; medications such as anti-depressants; Prader-Willi syndrome and insatiable appetite; hypothyroidism; endocrine conditions; hypothalamic tumours; a cold-like adenovirus. • Other naturalistic accounts (for example, genetics, ageing, reduced metabolism). • Appeal to environmental and socio-cultural influences. Diet, activity patterns and weight reportedly affected by: modernization and its impact on production and consumption; socio-economic factors (notably food poverty); informal appeals to social pressures, such as gendered role obligations, boredom, family problems and associated comfort eating; other considerations: local drinking cultures and the weather, smoking cessation, crash diets. • Appeal to defeasibility, i.e. reduced knowledge, will and other contingencies. • Appeal to psychological drives and intra-psychic conflict. • Appeal to food addiction. • Appeal to physical injury, especially in relation to male-coded activity such as sport, work and other high-risk endeavours.
Types of justification	• Reject medical definitions of overweight and obesity, i.e. the BMI. • Appeal to embodied masculinity; i.e. 'you're more of a man'. • Denial of injury, for example results from medical tests and talk about Fat Uncle Norman or the Winston Churchill effect. • Condemnation of condemners, for example 'I'm fat but you're ugly'. • Appeal to sexual desirability (especially in the gay Bear subculture). • Appeal to loyalties, for example eating as an expression of an unbreakable affection. • Self-fulfilment, for example the love of food or food porn.

Similar to Scott and Lyman's (1968: 49) invocation of biology, are *appeals to disease or disease processes* – the hallmark of *biomedical accounts*. Conrad and Schneider (1992) call this the medicalization of deviance. While various medical models of obesity offer different causal accounts and invoke different disease processes (for example, hypothyroidism or underactive thyroid), health professionals secured an official disease designation *for* obesity in 1990 (Sobal 1995). In biomedical accounts obesity is 'a chronic disease' (WHO 1998: 4) affecting bodies conceptualized using a mechanical metaphor (for a critique, see Gard and Wright 2005). Biomedical reports offer what Taylor (1979: 155) calls '"non-motivated" vocabularies of motive', i.e. accounts seeking to avoid 'censorial weightings' for individuals. Discussing the shifting status of obesity in the widely-consulted *Cecil Textbook of Medicine*, Chang and Christakis (2002) state obesity is currently conceptualized there as something individuals *experience* rather than something they *do*, transforming the obese from 'societal parasites' into 'societal victims'. However, although ostensibly neutral and compassionate, biomedicine continues with its moralizing religiosity. Ritenbaugh (1982: 352), after noting how bio-medicine obfuscates responsibility for illness, writes: '[t]he etiology of obesity is described neutrally in biomedicine as a positive imbalance between energy ingested and energy expended [representing] the biomedical gloss for the moral failings of gluttony and sloth'. As noted in Chapter 1, medical and government reports explicitly focus on gluttony and sloth (UK Parliament 2004). Thus, while the 'disease metaphors of obesity' may go some way in disguising 'the more direct accusations of weak will-power and defective character, they have not refuted the nagging culture-wide suspicion [that] fat people are still their own worst enemies' (Edgley and Brissett 1990: 262).

No respondents, even if they would be medically labelled obese, said they suffered from this 'disease' and were thus explicitly or implicitly deserving of sympathy. This is understandable in a culture where public health discourses are amplifying the putative 'ills' of medicalized fat and associated moral opprobrium. As noted in Chapter 1, obesity might be a technically 'neutral' term in biomedicine but it is a stigmatizing concept in everyday life. It is typically associated with physical extremes and the 'Other', such as the person who is seriously impaired because of their size. Situational proprieties constrained discussion specifically on this issue during interviewing. Nonetheless, the idea that an otherwise acceptable and functional body is diseased because it has reached an arbitrarily defined mass (i.e. a body that is imagined to be excessively fat within biomedical discourses), clashed with men's embodied and perhaps clinically supported understandings: men talked about feeling, looking and, according to various biomedical markers, being healthy even if they were technically overweight or obese (see justifications below).

Whether validated by medical tests or not, such talk was related to the underlying negotiation of masculine identities. It was protective given possible assaults upon selfhood. As stated by Shriver and Waskul (2006: 475): '[m]asculinity – widely associated with strength, toughness, and vigor – is significantly damaged by the weakness and dependence of disease and illness'. Hence, men's tendency to eschew the idea that they were intrinsically diseased, because of their 'bigness', followed a common gendered script. This also follows the historical definition of 'endo-genous obesity' as a woman's problem caused by 'inherently weak' biology rather than 'sensuous' overconsumption (Schwartz 1986: 137). As reported below, some men still appealed to diseases when excusing their unwanted weight-gain, though they did not see their 'excess' weight or fatness as a disease in and of itself.

Again, this made sense in terms of men's negotiation of masculine identities. 'Hegemonic' or dominant masculinity (Connell 1995) is not only associated with strength and vigour but also responsibility, action and control. Men's reported ability to 'live up to' and embody these manly qualities was sometimes compromised by what they considered to be genuine medical conditions, the onset of which was totally beyond their control and which mitigated personal responsibility for their unwanted weight. *Disease processes* alongside *biographical disruption and imposed physical inactivity* were thus invoked by some men when negating the cultural suspicion that people with 'weight problems' are their own worst enemies. That included Ernie, a slimming club member in his 50s, who had an arthritic hip and limp (so did his brother who was much lighter than Ernie, who was about 17 stone). Phonetically playing on words, Ernie said he became 'a beast' due to hereditary arthritis that restricted his mobility. Three interviewees also reported gaining unwanted weight, or regaining previously lost weight, *after* suffering heart attacks and becoming sedentary. In effect, they had no choice about expending fewer calories. Jim, my lightest interviewee, who was close to his target weight at about 12½ stone, joined Sunshine after suffering a heart attack and gaining 2 stone. When accounting for his past weight-gain, Jim also blamed his depression and ineffective medication (other men said prescribed drugs directly caused them to gain unwanted weight). Depression had 'objective' salience for Jim, a psychiatric nurse, though he ultimately sought to control this along with his weight. Similar to other men, Jim also talked about a biography of physical activity. That was a gendered presentation of responsible selfhood that mitigated responsibility for his heart attack and subsequent weight-gain:

> When I had the heart attack I was frightened to do anything. So you stop exercising, you become very, very careful of how much you're gonna do cos you think to yourself 'if I put too much effort into it I'm gonna cause myself to have another heart attack'. And I went through a period of depression for about six to nine months where my doctor was convinced that the depression I'd slipped into was never gonna let me get back to work. It wasn't the fact that I didn't want to go back to work. The medication that he put me on just didn't help me initially. And then you start to give yourself a kick up the backside and start thinking 'hey, hang on a second. Stop letting it control you, you control it'. That's what I did. But unfortunately by then I'd become a couch potato and I'd gone from 12½ stone to 14½ stone.

Ironically, given the mantra of anti-fat rhetoric, cardiovascular disease may be a cause, rather than a consequence, of overweight and obesity. Other diseases, which may account for more expansive bodies, also have aetiological significance, such as endocrine conditions, various genetic disorders and hypothalamic tumours. However, the WHO (1998: 146) states: 'these are extremely rare causes of obesity, accounting for only a small proportion of obesity in the population'. Another rare condition is Prader-Willi syndrome. As part of its clinical sequela, this chromosomal disorder causes hyperphagia (increased appetite) and rapid weight-gain (Allen 2004). At the time of this study a BBC television programme called *Not My Fault I'm Fat* followed young people diagnosed with Prader-Willi. The programme included a young man who weighed 31 stone and entered residential care to control his diet. While interviewing one of my largest respondents, Roy, we discussed this programme after he said he was always hungry and unable to maintain a previous 11 stone weight-loss. However, Roy doubted whether a local general practitioner in his small town could diagnose rare medical conditions. That may have been preferable for Roy; he referred to those in this TV programme as 'poor buggers'.

There are more common biological or 'naturalistic' (Shilling 2003) accounts that side-step the idea of disease and, as seen later, sometimes inform repudiation. One strategy is to appeal to natural genetic variation, with such talk having currency in the popular imagination and media (Crossley 2004). Obesity scientists reject genetic explanations when explaining population trends in bodyweight (WHO 1998), though there is evidence that 'greater BMI is associated with greater reproductive fitness yielding selection for obesity-predisposing genotypes' (Keith *et al.* 2006: 4). In terms of negotiating identities and social fitness, 'genetics talk' had salience at an individual level for some men who identified with 'weight problems' (and who sought to excuse their unwanted weight or fatness). Regardless of its validity, such talk mitigated responsibility for body types that 'ran in the family', as with Ralph, who was about 17 stone and focused on mothers even though he said his son took after him: 'I would say nine times out of ten, it's genetics. If your mother was big, nine times out of ten you're going to be big. I mean, I've got a son who's not thin, a big lad. He's the double of me. He's heavier than me now.' Andy, of similar size, said: 'my dad was thin as a rake but my mam was on the fat side. I must take after my mam' (laughs).

Others invoked 'natural' ageing processes with reference to reduced metabolism and 'middle-age spread'. As with Ralph and Andy's talk, 'invoking the principle of basic biological nature' (Scott and Lyman 1968: 50) was relatively normalizing talk. It avoided some of the pathologizing tendencies of certain organic accounts, where responsibility is denied at the expense of rendering the 'sufferer' biologically flawed or diseased. In that respect, these men were similar to older women in Gimlin's study who saw weight-gain as 'inevitable' rather than 'a marker of personal failure' (2007b: 411). Freddy, aged 59, at about 22 stone and not dieting, mentioned 'natural' ageing after I had shown him health promotion material urging middle-aged men to lose weight: a concrete example of how public health discourses ultimately attribute responsibility for obesity to individuals (or groups of individuals as social categories) and expect contrition through lifestyle change (*cf.* Gard and Wright 2005: 182). Freddy mainly voiced excuse-accounts. Elsewhere, Freddy called himself a 'slob' because of his weight and attributed his weight 'problem' to his genetics plus enforced inactivity due to health problems and work constraints. However, taken in isolation, the following cannot be neatly typified as an excuse. Responsibility for the 'undesirable' was denied but negativity was tempered. He explained bodies naturally 'deteriorate' with age and health promoters should not expect otherwise. Albeit in embryonic form, Freddy leant towards softer repudiation. Yet, this was not fully realized because his weight was ultimately deemed problematic in a society that valorizes slimness and youthfulness:

> They [health promoters] come out with these things. And they just say 'well look at him at 40, his belly is bulging out'. But everybody has mid-drifts bulging at 40. It's part and parcel of getting old. He's had his body for 40 years. He can't be the slim dashing young fellow he used to be. Your hair recedes. You lose your teeth. Your skin goes saggy. You know? You can't be that person. You just can't. It's just part and parcel of living.

Scott and Lyman (1968: 49) state that biology is 'part of a larger category of "fatalistic" forces which, in various cultures, are deemed in greater or lesser degree to be controlling of some or all events'. Moving from the endogenous (glands, genetics, metabolism), obesity scientists currently emphasize external factors, echoing and expanding the early twentieth century definition of men's fatness as exogenous and a more correctable problem than women's endogenous obesity (Schwartz 1986). Here obesity scientists *appeal to environmental and socio-cultural influences*, i.e. the 'obesogenic environment' that reportedly leads to sedentary living and overconsumption. This account feeds off Western cultural anxieties about the 'excesses' of modernity (Gard and Wright 2005). It also feeds the obesity, health and fitness industry that profits from 'lifestyle solutions'. Understandably, then, this type of account has greater currency than the virologists' view where much obesity could be caused by a cold-like adenovirus (Dhurandhar *et al*. 2000).

Stressing 'energy-in/energy-out' (Gard and Wright 2005) or 'the Big Two' (Keith *et al*. 2006), many social-structural and cultural conditions reportedly affect diet, physical activity and weight. Some respondents used these words to account for population trends (depersonalized accounts) at a time when such words were often expressed in the media. For example, men talked about convenience food and/or decreased physical activity associated with modernization. Reference was also made to changing social structures affecting the gendered division of labour in and outside the home. Under such conditions, Doug said, 'people can't say no to convenience', with particular reference to the inconvenience of food preparation for working parents, and walking instead of driving. After saying 'you live in a society that is quicker, everything is done at speed, you're working to a deadline', Mike complained with a more personal, but also depersonalized, reference: 'you get something to eat at home, and then you get out quick because you've got to do this, you've got to do that, and everybody's doing that. Everybody.' Some men's talk compared to formal epidemiological accounts that invoke 'the wider determinants of obesity' (Harrington and Friel 2006). These 'environmental discourses' assign responsibility to larger 'social forces' while imparting notions of right/wrong, good/bad and normal/abnormal in a way that accepts and reproduces the pejorative status of fatness (Rich and Evans 2005: 350).

Such accounts, especially liberal versions that underscore the constraining effects of poverty, have been critiqued by fat activists for associating fatness with an 'inappropriate relationship with food' (Cooper 1998: 81). This criticism could also be extended to relatively sophisticated social scientific writing that challenges 'unidimensional' causal accounts (biological, structural, political) but which still perpetuates the idea that people become 'obese' by (over)eating 'debilitated' food (Guthman and DuPuis 2006: 445). Although carefully framed, these excuse-accounts also ignore other putative contributors that go beyond the big two (Keith *et al.* 2006). An additional point, which connects with some of the discussion in Chapter 3, is that discrimination may lead to poverty for 'fat persons' rather than poverty restricting people's access to 'nutritious food' and making them fat (Fikkan and Rothblum 2005: 22–3). Even so, environmental discourses emerge in everyday life. Interestingly, this does not mean such accounts elide more critical talk as directed towards people seen to profit from socially determined fatness, intolerance and collectively sustained ignorance. The following recounts a conversation with Shamus before appearing on a TV show about food and fat. Shamus, a single parent struggling on a low income, ran an Internet support group for other single parents:

Field diary, TV station in Ireland: Shamus, who told me he had lost a lot of weight despite still being 'obese' on the BMI, excused his past weight by saying he was living on a very low income and had to buy the cheapest food available, which was also the most calorific. He extended his excuse-account to explain childhood obesity: 'I mean, we teach our kids to be careful with money but in the shop a low-fat bag of crisps costs four times the amount of a normal bag. So what do you think they'll buy?' There was a woman sat opposite us who was a busy working mum. She developed a branded ready meal because she said she was working 60 hours a week and unable to cook 'healthy food' for her family from scratch each night. She had some of the packaged meals with her. Shamus asked her how much they cost. After she told us (about €3.50) he said: 'Nobody can afford that'. She assured him that sales were healthy, to which he replied: 'Well, somebody like me couldn't afford that and thousands of single parents I know couldn't either'. Once the woman had left he said, with an air of indignation, most people at the TV station had no idea what it was like for ordinary people.

In the UK, the diets of those on low incomes may not be that different from the rest of the population (Food Standards Agency 2007), though concern about food poverty, and especially its impact on single mothers, has been a policy issue there for some time (Acheson 1998). I would add that if food poverty is considered relevant (Harrington and Friel 2006), then this issue may be addressed without being diverted by fatness (not all people on a low income are clinically obese) and eclipsing social structural factors that have a more significant impact upon health. Restated, social organization, not obesity, could be described as the real problem albeit without writing out biology. This has policy implications (Chapter 6).

Following Doug and Mike, there are also *informal appeals to social pressures.* As discussed by Watson (2000) and Robertson (2006) in relation to men's health, these 'pressures' include gendered role obligations associated with marriage, fatherhood and work – pragmatic concerns that may constrain men's physical bodies. Hunter (1984) states gender-specific 'type scripts' and masculine role requirements bolster such accounts. Certainly, such words had resonance for Howard, the lorry driver quoted at the start of this chapter, who compared himself to other truckers who spend long working hours seated and who are said to have a 'belly' as a result. (Leaning towards softer repudiation, the negativity of his overweight was also partially resisted; rather than talking about looking pregnant he appealed to dimensions of working-class masculinity, i.e. beer and trucks, while also patting his stomach as if it was a faithful companion.) Lorry drivers aside, these gendered type scripts are part of a larger cultural stock-of-knowledge where the male body is 'a tool or instrument used to fulfil gendered social roles' (Robertson 2006: 438). Reiterating energy-in/energy-out, the following account is from a slimming magazine and was attributed to a 37-year-old businessman who had peaked at over 30 stone but who had since lost 14½ stone. Presented alongside 'before and after photos' (including images of a much slimmer man in rugby attire), this account was published in a media where excuses are routinely offered for becoming but not remaining fat. Analytically, it can be seen that organizational interests and the search for profits bear upon the framing and honouring *of* accounts and provide gendered material *for* accounts:

> I've been running my own company since I was 17 and the nature of the business made it easy for me to gain weight. Before that, I was a county athlete [rugby player] but from the age of 21 onwards, the business began to take over and my weight rocketed. Working it out I gained a stone a year for 20 years. I live on the road and I was doing a lot of entertaining and spending a lot of time in hotels.
>
> (Walters, quoted by Weight Watchers 2003: 76–7)

Other social pressures may also shape men's diets and reportedly excuse their unwanted weight. Stan, peaking at 24 stone and registered disabled, blamed his past 'comfort eating' on boredom: 'cos you got nowt else to do'. Others ate as a way of coping with boring jobs. Mike talked about his past monotonous work as a security guard, comprising 16 hour shifts with limited physical exertion. He complained: 'There was nothing to do. I was working on building sites. And there was nowt to do during the night. So we were just sitting and picking [at food]'.

When voicing 'social pressure' accounts, some men mentioned bereavement and relationship difficulties. As with Stan's reference to 'comfort eating', food sometimes provided solace under distressing social circumstances. Depressed after splitting with his girlfriend, Ryan said it is 'nice to eat away your depression. It's stupid but that's one way of doing it.' Stepping beyond these men's words, contributors to the sociology of food offer politically salient commentary. Probyn (2000: 2) states that talk about 'comfort food' is a 'sugar coated' reference that 'camouflage[s] widespread loneliness or disappointment in life'. As with food poverty, then, it would appear that the reductionist war on obesity is way off target. Of course, under present social conditions, it is unsurprising that there are no equivalent campaigns to tackle loneliness or the health-damaging effects of social inequality and stressful or tedious work.

Stan also mentioned comfort drinking as part of a depersonalized excuse-account for weight-gain. Although a discrediting overgeneralization, alcohol was considered a calorific sedative for others assumed to be dissatisfied with their lives. Yet, it is clear that drinking alcohol, similar to eating, is not only or necessarily about disappointment and loneliness (see next section on justifications). Some men also appealed to regional drinking culture and other contingencies that were external to, and even controlling of, their personal decisions. Reflecting on his past weight-gain and work in a brewery where he drank plenty of free Guinness, Al, in his 50s, said: 'there's a lot of talk about binge drinking now but at my age I grew up in a culture where, as opposed to binge drinking, it was a macho culture where you had to drink'. Al was from north-east England. I have heard similar talk, comprising a meteorological dimension, in Ireland. There the socio-cultural and natural environments mitigated men's unwanted weight with pub culture and drinking attributed to the wet weather.

Other considerations could also be subsumed under the rubric of socio-cultural factors. In a healthist, neo-liberal culture people are often extolled to 'do the right thing' for their health, albeit with possible contradictory results. Thus, some men mentioned smoking cessation that reportedly resulted in increased appetite or unwanted weight-gain even without necessarily eating more. Quitting smoking was an indicator of moral responsibility given the harms associated with tobacco but also a way of mitigating personal responsibility for becoming heavier (also, Keith *et al.* 2006). Other men talked about going on unsustainable 'crash diets' that lead them to regain lost weight plus some more. Gard and Wright (2005: 46–7) also cite studies where people reported 'dieting to lose weight, either frequently or infrequently, [but] put on significantly more weight by the end of the research period' even when doing more physical activity.

An appeal to defeasibility is another excuse-account. This is 'the capacity of being voided' which fits with 'the widespread agreement that all actions contain some "mental element"' (Scott and Lyman 1968: 48). Here 'knowledge' and 'will' are constrained by a lack of information. Bernard, a slimming club member who later became a consultant, emphasized how lack of information prohibits people from successfully losing weight. Indeed, while Bernard talked about having a slow metabolism, being brought up on 'bread and dripping after the war' and becoming 'desk bound' when working as an engineer, he excused his previous inability to lose weight, given his lack of technical know-how. Bernard extended this account to 'overweight' people in general, 'because the information on how to control your weight is not easily available', adding, 'the little diet sheet' offered by doctors 'is not even a half-hearted attempt at giving you the information'. Such talk reflected the organizational interests of a commercial slimming club. It defined 'overweight' people as 'poorly informed' and poorly serviced by clinicians, while suggesting they would benefit from the services of slimming consultants. Of course, this is derogatory – it suggests people are 'dietary dupes' in need of rescue by the more wisely informed entrepreneurs of the commercial obesity industry (Dennis Waskul, personal communication 2007).

An *appeal to psychological drives* is a reductionist type of 'fatalistic' account. Rather than blaming society or social pressures, personality characteristics reportedly cause obesity. Reviewing relevant literature, Cash and Roy (1999: 216) write: '[a] traditional, psychoanalytic perspective often regards obesity as a symptom of some unconscious intrapsychic conflict or a self-protective, defense mechanism [. . .] Thus obesity is viewed as a consequence and not a cause of psychological disturbance'. While some men talked about depression as a consequence of social circumstances, poor physical health or relationship difficulties, none presented their unwanted weight as a direct consequence of psychological disturbance. This extends the previous point about illness, masculinity and vulnerability in a society where 'mental illness' is highly stigmatized. Cash and Roy (1999) also reject psychoanalytic accounts. For them, such accounts merely reflect the cultural bias against fatness; a cultural bias that, I would add, means that if there is any 'psychological disturbance' associated with fatness then one should not ignore the power of stigmatizing fat oppression (discussed further below and in Chapter 3). When interpreting 'psy' perspectives from within the accounts framework I would also question Cash and Roy's (1999) point that these blame fat people. As with psychological explanations for illicit drug use (Weinstein 1980: 581), such accounts suggest individuals cannot avoid their behaviour because they do not have 'free will', are unable to exert self-control and are largely powerless to implement effective change. What Cash and Roy (1999) do indicate, though, is how common background expectancies shape the honouring of accounts. This is in a society where self-control is a dominant theme (Ritenbaugh 1982) as well as an index of masculinity and moral worth.

An *appeal to food addiction* is another type of excuse-account. While addiction is perhaps 'the ultimate excuse' for illicit drug taking because 'everybody knows' various psychoactive substances cause unwanted dependency (Weinstein 1980), this excuse does not necessarily translate well to food. After all, everybody is dependent on food. Yet, this supported Paul's addiction account, with him claiming food is a drug:

> I feel that food's a drug. The only problem is you have to have food to live. You don't have to have smoking. I think it'll probably be easier to give up smoking [he's a non-smoker] because you can say 'right I'm not having them' but you have to have food to live.

After I immediately asked whether people could get addicted to food, Paul replied: 'Oh I think so, definitely. I think I was. I think I was. But it's a habit. Maybe not an addiction, more of a habit, yeah. But yeah, I think you can be addicted.' It is worth adding that Paul was a slimming club employee. His outlook contrasted with other men, employed in more masculine occupations, when offering other types of excuse-account (see below on injury). Of course, Paul's account was not peculiar: Overeaters Anonymous, which offers a therapeutic environment for eating disorders, subscribes to the idea of food addiction (Lester 1999). The film *Super Size Me* (Spurlock 2004) and many online reviews also claim McDonald's products are addictive. Yet, reported profits from McDonald's British restaurants fell by 71 per cent in 2003 (Laville 2004), placing a question mark not only over McDonald's but also the idea that their products are addictive. Fast-food accounts for obesity are taken as my point of departure in Chapter 4.

While addiction accounts were uncommon among men contacted during this research, their unwanted weight was often excused through an *appeal to physical injury*. This was clearly related to the social construction of masculinities when injuries, resultant physical inactivity and their overweight (or what clinicians would call obesity, Chapter 1) were caused by male-coded action, i.e. passivity and adiposity resulting from institutionally endorsed activity, rather than fatalism and apathy. Andy, aged 52, and weighing around 18 stone when I first met him at the slimming club, told me he was lean when younger but he broke his leg when in his 20s while parachuting in the Territorial Army. He said he 'piled' the weight on after the accident to the extent that he could not fit into his uniform when returning to work as a prison officer. Dom, aged 42, a mechanic and another slimming club member, told me he had been 'big' all of his life. Offering an appeal to 'natural' body build, he said he was 21 stone when in his early 20s despite exercising most days, i.e. he was not personally responsible for his weight because he remained heavy even when physically active. However, he peaked at 33 stone 10 months before our interview, gaining this additional weight over several years following a serious occupational injury. He told me that while working under a bus the axle fell off and nearly crushed him. Ralph, aged 68 and describing himself as 'a big fat lad', told me he had an artificial knee following an active boy-hood and rugby injuries in his youth. This retired electrical engineer said he tried to lose weight by exercising in a gym. However, he joked about his unsuccessful efforts: 'I go on the weights to try and lose a bit of weight off my chest and some of those [lifting exercises]. Just to lose weight off here and here [upper body and legs]. But you've only got so many bends in that false knee'.

Talk about the risks of army life and manual labour, or the vicissitudes of ageing and sports-related orthopaedic injuries, obviously differs from the vocabulary of addiction and psychological drives. One explanation for these men's preference for these types of account is that working in masculine domains (for example, the army, prison service, mechanics and engineering) rendered physical injury talk more honourable. In short, these accounts fitted with their gendered concep-tions and presentations of themselves as previously very physically fit, hardworking and active men who were often willing, if not always able, to control their weight. This also fits with sociological research on the negative effects of patriarchy for men in paid work and sport (Annandale and Hunt 2000, Connell 1995).

Justifications

With justifications, responsibility for the questioned is accepted but the pejorative status is denied partially or totally (Scott and Lyman 1968). Some justifications for weight-gain, or having a body that medicine would label overweight or worse, are discussed below.

One strategy is to *reject medical definitions of overweight and obesity* by critiquing the BMI. The BMI, which is about imagined fat rather than real fat, is the lynchpin of the obesity industry. As explained in Chapter 1, the BMI is based on a measure of weight and height, not adiposity, and it is used by health authorities when claiming the majority of men in developed nations are overweight or obese (WHO 1998). I have discussed men's critical talk about this index elsewhere (Monaghan 2007) and will only briefly mention their views here. In line with the analysis presented in Chapter 4, the BMI could be described as an irrational aspect of rationalization, i.e. the efficient use of calculations that do not necessarily make sense. Few men actually endorsed this measure and intended complying with it even though such talk could enable men to present a moral self-image. 'Ridiculous' was a recurrent word, both inside and outside of the slimming club. Whether talking to Gary or myself, men expressed incredulity with some laughing when stating the BMI defines World Cup winning English rugby players as obese. Others mentioned Arnold Schwarzenegger, given his former status as an elite bodybuilder and muscular Hollywood action hero. Mitch, who told me at the slimming club that his BMI was between 28 and 30 after losing 6 stone, added: 'I mean, when you consider Arnold Schwarzenegger's BMI is over 30 it makes a complete mockery of it all really'. These men were not bodybuilders, or strength athletes, and they were not suggesting they were extremely muscular (also see Chapter 5). Rather, they were saying the BMI clashed with their understandings of appropriate adult male weight-for-height. Here men accepted responsibility for their weight (which is not simply fat), and perhaps sought to lose (some) weight, while rejecting medical measures that classify most men as overweight or obese, i.e. implicitly, or explicitly, 'too fat' (BBC Online 2007).

Gender and sex-specific corporeality are mediating factors when rejecting medical definitions, or at least accommodating a larger body. While justifiable resistance occurred in the slimming club, this extended beyond slimming clubs and was evidenced in everyday accounts that placed masculinity in the foreground. *An appeal to embodied masculinity* emerged among men who used bigness as a referent, instead of fatness, and whose size was institutionally validated. For Big Joe, a doorman who was not slimming, his size quite literally meant being more of a man:

> If you're a big guy, if you're a guy on the biggish side, it's seen as a masculine thing, a manly thing. You're more of a man. Whereas it is not the same with women. I mean, you're not more of a woman. Because you perceive being feminine as being petite and small.

This resonates with Connell (1983), who states, '[t]o be an adult male is distinctly to occupy space, to have a physical presence in the world' (cited by Morgan 1993: 72). Big Joe's point also fits with feminist work on the 'thin ideal' which is understood as a 'body backlash' to women's demands for more space in the public realm (Williams and Germov 2004: 345–6). Germov and Williams (1996: 636) explain that there is, in effect, a 'double standard' with women facing 'a far narrower "acceptable" weight range', though that does not exempt men completely from fat fighting and body dissatisfaction. This is one reason why I maintain that while men risk getting hurt during the war on obesity, women and children risk being hit hardest. Bell and McNaughton (2007) hint at this when acknowledging the differential impact of the 'tyranny of slenderness' (Chernin 1981) on the sexes, while adding that men are not completely immune from body concerns as indicated by the valorization of larger but also lean muscular male bodies.

The social construction of masculinities, especially among younger working-class men, figures in the accommodation, cultivation and validation of 'big' bodies that comprise various proportions of muscle and fat. According to BMI, all the men below would be classed as overweight or obese, some even injected anabolic steroids and lifted weights at a bodybuilding gym to build extra mass (also see Monaghan 2001). Only one man, John, who had a different type of social body, was defined as having a fat body. John initially denied this negative typification, which subordinated him on a gendered hierarchy that values 'hard', muscular (masculine) bodies over 'soft', fat (feminized) bodies. However, his denial was immediately followed by his admission ('OK, yeah it is') before a mitigation of personal responsibility, as with excuses. Interestingly, John then changed tack. He *justified* his weight by referring to a past photograph where, weighing several stone lighter, he said he looked ill (also see Chapter 3 on aborting diets). Again, it is such mixing and matching of elements common to excuses and justifications that leads me to expand upon Scott and Lyman's (1968) typology shortly:

> *Field diary*: I stood at a pub entrance with three doormen, Mick, Jack and Luke. A ticket collector, John, was also present. Mick, singing the praises of Luke, said he was 'really good' on the punch bag at the gym, especially when weighing 18½ stone. Jack asked Luke whether he still went to the gym because he was obviously much lighter. Luke said he still went but lost weight (implicitly, muscle) because he was stressed (an excuse-account for unwanted weight-loss). John, the ticket collector, then said: 'I'm about 17 stone' to which Jack jokingly replied: 'Yeah, but it's fat!' John laughed and then said defensively: 'No it isn't.' He then admitted: 'OK, yeah it is. I've put 4 stone on since working here. It's all those late night takeouts from over the road [a fast-food shop was directly opposite]. I'll bring in my driving license and show you the photo. It doesn't look like me. I look ill on it.'

Talk about looking ill when lighter and, by implication, looking healthier or more acceptable when heavier, constitutes a *denial of injury* (Scott and Lyman 1968).

This is not just about physical appearance or 'normative embodiment' (Watson 2000). So-called 'excess' weight may also be accepted because it need not impact negatively on biomedical health, activities of daily living and longevity. Paul, who, at about 13½ stone and 5' 9" tall, would still be medically defined as overweight after losing a third of his original weight, said he would 'have every test going . . . because I believe I am healthy. And I believe I am very healthy.' Similar to some steroid-using bodybuilders interviewed in South Wales, Paul expressed faith in medicine and biomedical health screening even when challenging medicine (Monaghan 1999).

Much larger men similarly denied injury with reference to biomedical health, including Big Joe. It would be misleading to say that 'overweight' women do not also deny injury (*cf.* Gimlin 2007b) but Big Joe differed from women interviewed by Carryer (2001). For these women, 'being large precluded good health' with 'socially imposed restrictions' constraining their sense of 'deservedness' in healthcare settings (Carryer 2001: 91). My respondent buttressed his account, rendering it more honourable, with reference to a recent medical examination for life insurance. Although he said 'I'm never, ever ill', the media focus on obesity meant that he was initially worried about his weight being a massive health risk. This prompted him to question his medical tests, but he added that his doctor assured him that he was not at 'death's door' in an account that invoked 'visceral embodiment' (Watson 2000):

> So we did the medical, and the doctor said to me, 'for a guy who is so big, you are healthy'. I didn't have high blood pressure; my chest was all right considering I had asthma as a kid. But I mean, that surprised me, it really did. Because I am massively overweight. There wasn't anything wrong with me. I mean, I've had blood tests done. They test for things like diabetes and cholesterol, [surprised tone of voice] nothing wrong with them at all! And you say, 'Well, hang on a minute. This isn't right this. According to the TV and what the doctors on TV are saying, I should be at death's door.' But my doctor says, 'Yeah, OK, you're overweight, you're massively overweight, but as a rule you're generally healthy.'

Even illnesses commonly attributed to, but not necessarily caused by, obesity need not constrain such talk. As stated by Al, who peaked at 31 stone before deciding to lose weight because, among other things, he was excluded from various everyday activities and stigmatized:

> I've never had a real physical health problem. As I said, I've got diabetes but it's always been managed very well. There have never been any issues around that. And a thin person may say 'Oh he should lose weight because it's a strain on your heart' and a fat person will say, 'Well how many joggers drop dead?'

Other big fellas, who embraced physical activity and currently accepted their size, similarly denied injury. Edward, aged 73, who would be medically labelled obese based on reported weight and height, joined a fitness centre six months before I interviewed him. He intended losing 2 stone but his weight remained unchanged. This was not defined as a personal or medical problem. Similar to Big Joe, Edward referred to a medical exam and good metabolic health:

> The only reason I wanted to lose weight; well it's supposed to help you. But I'm pretty fit. I go to the gym when I want to. Go to the doctors, the first thing he does, he tests me blood pressure. 'Oh that's all right.' Test it. Move on. Everything's he's tested is all right. So I said, 'Well, carrying a bit of weight didn't seem, you know, to cause me a problem.'

Similar to Davison *et al.*'s (1992) research on 'lay' understandings of coronary heart disease candidacy, some men invoked the 'The Fat "Uncle Norman" figure' who lives a long life even when smoking and drinking. Edward talked about his uncle who was 'a big lad, a big fella' who drank three pints of beer every night and 'lived until he was 90 odd'. Oliver, my oldest contact at 79 and technically obese, also talked at the slimming club about his mother who ate cream and butter but lived to 106. He also talked about much larger people who 'are all right', which prompted him to pause and ask, tongue-in-cheek, 'What am I doing here?' Echoing the reference to Fat Uncle Norman, Marmot (2004: 10) calls this 'the Winston Churchill effect' – the British wartime prime minister who would have been classed as obese, who drank and smoked heavily yet lived a long life. Marmot's (2004) point is that while an epidemiological link exists between lifestyle and disease at a population level, this may be contradicted at an individual level. And high social status and control over one's life may confer health benefits that mean the usual suspects for an early grave will be far less injurious than commonly assumed.

Condemnation of condemners is another justification. Like denial of injury, this account is part of Sykes and Matza's (1957) 'techniques of neutralization'. Here people shift the focus of attention away from their putative deviance to the motives and behaviour of disapproving others. 'Using this device', write Scott and Lyman (1968: 51), 'the actor admits performing an untoward act but asserts its irrelevancy because others commit these and worse acts, and these others are either not caught, not punished, not condemned, unnoticed, or even praised'. I would revise this statement, adding that people do not *necessarily* need to admit that their bodies or (in)actions are untoward. Certainly, Big Joe's size was an economic resource in the night-time security industry: the degraded status of being, in his words, a 'fat bloke' was also overshadowed by a cultivated reputation for hardness. He told me he not only condemned but also justifiably assaulted men who identified him as fat and used this label, along with various expletives, to insult him. Such action, and talk about this action (presented as highly controlled and a calculated means of saving face, honour and respect), was about embodying masculinity in an occupation where physical violence is a commercial resource for regulating unruly bodies (Monaghan 2002).

Other men also condemned condemners. Richie, a slimming club member of three years who weighed about 20 stone and reported good metabolic health, was critical of clinicians who told him to lose weight. For him, violence was an imagined rather than an actual response to health professionals who assume 'overweight' people are ignorant. After stating 'the overweight person knows more about trying to lose weight than most doctors and most dieticians', he complained, 'when you get a doctor or a dietician telling you what you should be eating and what you should do, it is so patronizing and belittling that you want to chin them'. The unhelpful delivery of such advice also impacts men's dieting careers, as discussed in Chapter 3.

Condemnation of condemners was common among much larger men. Roy, who, like Big Joe, was one of my largest contacts, referred to imagined condemners as 'skinny gets'. He also mentioned the possibility of weight-loss, which he did in the past, but the impossibility of those with a problem with his weight to correct their lifetime of ugliness. Roy added that he was happy and described his general health as good, with particular recourse to his physical work as a mechanic. However, accounts are temporally 'phased' in response to subsequent questions, answers and the ongoing negotiation of identities (Scott and Lyman 1968). Thus while Roy justified his bigness, he later told me he was worried about his future health and was awaiting bariatric surgery (also see Chapter 4). Aged 36 and recently becoming a father, Roy said he wanted to be mobile, active and healthy in middle-age, thus enabling him to continue being a good father. Subject positions, and associated accounts, are complex and shifting. For those constructing normative masculinities, mouthing justifications for becoming, being and remaining 'big' does not preclude contrition through whatever means. However, when referring to anti-obesity campaigns and government officials who 'pick on overweight', Roy was condemnatory: 'I think somebody's sitting there in the government getting a hell of a big pay cheque with a big department below them, just thinking "How can we tell people what they already know?"'

Condemnation of condemners is particularly common in online fat acceptance groups, where, more in line with repudiation and the rejection of slimming, responsibility for one's weight is either denied or the relevance of responsibility is denied. Nonetheless, some condemnatory themes worth mentioning here include: the societal double standard that typically allows 'slim' but not 'fat' people to escape judgement when eating calorific food and remaining sedentary; harms associated with medical interventions and the slimming industry more generally (for example, metabolic problems caused by restrictive dieting, malnutrition and deaths associated with bariatric surgery); named scientists who perpetuate 'fat myths' but who undermine their credibility because they are remunerated by the diet industry; and more personal jibes where condemners are condemned for their own perceived physical shortcomings. Saguy and Riley (2005) discuss some of these themes. They characterize this as a credibility struggle, with those contributing to the polarized obesity debate seeking to discredit others during 'framing contests' over the nature and consequences of 'excess' weight/fat.

Another justification is an *appeal to sexual desirability*. This overlaps with the commodification of men's heterosexual fantasies, as exemplified in the porn industry with a rotund Ron Jeremy perhaps the most famous of male porn actors.

While this US actor's long-standing success and popularity among male viewers could partly be attributed to the hope that men's fatness does not impede promiscuous sexual conquest (with emphasis given to hopes rather than expectations), this contrasts with Gilman's (2004: 23) statement: 'It is hard to imagine a sexual fat man in modernity'. Going beyond the celluloid, Big Joe's justification was embedded in his work experiences providing security in the night-time economy. Rejecting the beautification of men's bodies in men's magazines, he stressed, 'it's not what you are but who you are' when discussing the different pressures on men and women in the heterosexual mate market. After saying men do not have to worry about having a suntan, six pack and trendy hairstyle to attract women, he claimed if he was not married he could have 'umpteen women' given the macho image of being a 'big' doorman. Yet, Big Joe still expressed internal doubts about the sincerity of some women who complimented him at work (also see Chapter 3 on dieting triggers and sexualities):

> You get women coming onto doormen. Because it's an image thing. They like to be seen with somebody who's a bit of a big guy. I have women coming up to me sometimes and saying 'Oooh, you're nice and big!' And you think to yourself, 'Are you taking the piss love?' And a lot of them aren't. Some of them are. But the majority of them aren't. I think they see it as, they feel more protected if they're with a big guy.

An appeal to sexual desirability extends beyond male heterosexuality. Big gay men are also eroticized in certain contexts and this sexual economy is highly organized. Barry belonged to the gay Bear subculture, which 'includes many big men deemed fat and denigrated by the mainstream of gay male social and community networks' (Textor 1999: 223). Barry won an international Mr Bear competition, which he described as 'like Miss World', and told me he was subsequently asked to star in a gay porn film and magazine (he declined the offer, but was flattered). Critical of what he called 'body fascism' in gay male culture, Barry expressed no desire to be thin and said about gay bars: 'In the mainstream clubs I would never bloody take my shirt off, ever, because I would just get looked at and people would bitch really. But in the Bears' bars, well, you get asked to take it off.' Territoriality, explored by Lyman and Scott (1970), helps sustain contexts where bodies, that may otherwise be discredited, are discursively and physically credited. Barry described how 'skinny twinks' (slim gay men with sexual currency in the gay mainstream) sometimes enter Bear bars and openly laugh at Bears but in so doing they risk being told to 'bugger off out of our bar' (condemnation of condemners).

Online size acceptance and admiration groups also justify men's bigness or fatness with an appeal to sexual desirability. As discussed elsewhere (Monaghan 2005b), heterosexual men are typified as Big Handsome Men and receive (at least some) social validation from Big Beautiful Women and Female Fat-Admirers. Re-signification is well articulated in cyberspace among gay men and weight-gain is celebrated. Gay male 'gainers' and 'encouragers' (Textor 1999) collaborate in constructing these positive meanings, partly in response to HIV/AIDS and associated emaciation. 'Feedees' and 'feeders' are the heterosexual equivalent. Scott and Lyman's (1968) *appeal to loyalties* captures this. Fatness and efforts to become fatter are permissible or even right because these serve the interests of another to whom one owes an unbreakable affection.

Self-fulfilment, or pleasing oneself, is the final justification described here. This could relate to sedentary living and was expressed by some men when discussing physical activity (Chapter 5). This is also evidenced in an online study of male computer programmers. Here men resisted discrediting talk about physically inactive lifestyles, fleshy bodies and masculinity using justifications that celebrated 'large and sedentary bodies' (White 2006: 404). Of course, self-fulfilment takes other forms. Following the references to pub culture, self-fulfilment is an apt justification for drinking alcohol and developing what is often called a 'beer belly'. All of this is socially embedded. For Sean, drinking and weight attributed to pub life were justifiably related to conviviality and good mental health in a nation that has a high male suicide rate:

> *Field diary, friend's home in Ireland*: Sean told me that he felt he was about a stone overweight (based on his own comfort zone, rather than the BMI) and gains weight when he goes to the pub. This emerged in the context of a discussion about the weather. After he joked 'It rains twice a year in Ireland: once for six months and then again for another six months' I mentioned the 'rain excuse' for going to the pub, drinking and gaining weight. Laughing, he re-framed this excuse as a justification: 'Any fucking excuse! Good living. You can't beat it'. After attributing his 'overweight' to the pub, he added: 'But I enjoy the pub. It's good seeing your mates. What's the alternative? Stay in, or maybe jump off a bridge?' Sean's justification about 'good living' was visually supported. He was wearing a favourite and much admired T-shirt featuring Homer Simpson. It celebrated beer drinking and lying on the couch.

Food also provides calorific and discursive material for self-fulfilment. In his autobiography, which deals with issues such as social injustice and the war on fat in the USA, Oscar Zeta Acosta expresses self-fulfilment when responding to doctors who urged him to diet: 'What value is life without booze and Mexican food . . . Shit, I couldn't be *bland* if my life depended on it' (quoted by Chamberlain 2001: 101, emphasis in original). Arthur, quoted at the start of this chapter when saying he liked fattening food, added: 'I put weight on because I just eat. I don't comfort eat. I don't eat because I'm hungry. I eat because I enjoy it. Put it that way.' Arthur and Oscar's talk is unlikely to be accepted within 'civilized' (Elias 2000) society given the middle-class demand for rational risk avoidance, the regulation of appetite and bodily boundaries. Even so, sociologists of food, besides discussing the stigma of obesity and the ambivalence surrounding consumption in a risk society, underscore the 'passion, delight, and pure hedonism with which food is intimately associated' (Germov and Williams 2004: 21). As also observed during virtual ethnography, self-typifying male gluttons, who do not find anything 'wrong' with being fat or becoming fatter, celebrate the pleasures of eating in cyber communities (Monaghan 2005b). There an 'overactive' microwave, rather than inactive thyroid, is the most likely account for fatness. Moving offline, the love of food, of which George Bernard Shaw said '[t]here is no sincerer love' (cited by Germov and Williams 2004: 20), emerged when interviewing others contacted outside of slimming clubs. Discussing his love of take-away food, Victor talked about regularly taking a doner kebab home at night while sober and extending it to the morning after (he did not use alcohol as an excuse-account for his actions). Victor said he would reheat leftover kebab meat in the microwave for breakfast because he enjoyed it so much. If Campos (2004) talks about 'food porn' then doner could be described as a cheap, casual lover who is so good partly because she has a reputation for being so bad.

Contrition and repudiation: Slimming and fat activism

Categories implied by, but not incorporated into, Scott and Lyman's (1968) typology include two other modes of accountability or aligning action: contrition and repudiation. *Contrition* occurs when people accept responsibility and blame while typically tempering this with an offer of reparation. *Repudiation* occurs when full responsibility for the 'questionable' is denied, or the relevance of responsibility is denied, and imputations of deviance are challenged. These are discussed further in relation to slimming (contrition) and fat activism (repudiation).

Contrition: 'Forgive me, for I have sinned'

Much 'body talk' in Anglophone culture asserts the pejorative status of fatness and individual responsibility. The taken-for-granted view is that adults typified as fat are ultimately responsible due to gluttony and sloth and they should take corrective action by making the body a 'project' (Shilling 2003). This is an individualizing, moralizing and methodical attitude to the body. Rich and Evans (2005: 351) refer to this as the 'rational ascetic' when discussing the obesity discourse, personal responsibility and blame. They add that this perspective is aimed at making bodies disciplined and predictable, in line with other rationalizing principles (see Chapter 4).

Defining fatness in these terms pathologizes literally millions of people in order to engender and often gender compliance to healthism and the cult of slenderness. Providing the necessary conditions for weight-related accounts and other forms of 'remedial work' (Goffman 1971), this blame-giving reproduces the wrongs of fatness and discredits people deemed fat (irresponsible). Some men contacted during this research, who were doing contrition, similarly endorsed this at a personal and generic level. Jim, from Sunshine, told me this informed his general philosophy on life. Analytically, people doing contrition enact an expected yet depoliticized version of social fitness. Here men were effectively saying 'I know I have erred but I am a good person who seeks to redress this through lifestyle changes.' As elaborated below, this empirically supports Schwartz's (1986: 12) point that '[b]etween the mirror and the scale lie acts of confession and repentance' though, as an account, contrition need not be verbally expressed (Scott and Lyman 1968), just as public confessions do not depend on really being contrite (Karen Throsby, personal communication 2007). Finally, Jim's reference to the media, which was recurrent in other men's talk, is worth highlighting and will re-emerge in Chapter 3. The dissemination of obesity epidemic psychology via the media contributed to existential anxiety and panic among some men:

> Some people don't take responsibility for what they do and look after themselves. But nobody else can do it for them. My main outlook on life has always been that. If there's anything wrong in my life I can't blame anybody else but me. Because I haven't taken notice of what's happening. I haven't listened to what is going on in the media. I haven't read what's going on in the media. But more importantly I haven't taken a damn good look at myself and thought, 'Hang on a second, I didn't used to be like this. I used to be like something else. What's changed?' and then address the problem. And that's what I do constantly.

Here Jim endorsed what Germov and Williams (1999), in their study of dieting women, call 'the body panopticon' – a Foucauldian informed concept where the person subjects their own body and other people's bodies to constant surveillance. Following the slimming club's emphasis on dietary intake, men's attention typically focused on food. Eating throws into sharp relief the relations between lived bodies, embodied identities and society. And, somewhat harshly, some men invoked animalistic stereotypes. Such words immediately discredited larger people, and, by implication, themselves, even if there was a biomedical excuse-account or they were slimming. I was sometimes struck by the highly moralized opprobrium in such talk. During contrition, the stylized slimmer basically accepts sizist discourses. These render 'fat people' inferior, though, unlike racially marked bodies, male-coded 'exogenous obesity' (Schwartz 1986) is attributed to volitional and changeable personal action: a case of inferiority as 'deficient individuality', rather than 'collective status', which reproduces social inequality through an 'emotional nexus' (Neckel 1996: 17). Jerry, who lost 3 stone over the past five months at Sunshine but still weighed over 19 stone, and had evidently internalized fat oppression, said the following to Gary:

> If it's genetics, it's the glands, that can't be helped. But if it's purely and simply about just being a pig then you can lose the weight. You can change. I've proved it myself. You can change the way you eat. So if anybody has got something wrong with them, well, that's fair enough. But if it's just purely gluttony and greed and just overindulgence then you can change. There's just no need for it. You can change.

Contrition shares with justifications an acceptance of responsibility for (gaining and/or maintaining) weight/fat but differs with regard to its pejorative status. The point at which contrition and justifications diverge is the point at which excuses and contrition converge: negativity is accepted and reproduced. Honeycutt (1999: 173, emphasis in original) provides an example from a woman who was not a slimmer: 'I *could* lose weight if I wanted to. I've done it enough in the past. I mean, I can't blame people for being disgusted [at my weight]. I'm disgusted with myself sometimes.' Following Honeycutt (1999), and Neckel (1996) on the production of gender and class inequalities, emotions take centre stage and are intimately related to bodily regulation. Guilt, shame and misery are socially constructed and personally experienced emotions among people who, sometimes from childhood onwards, are made to feel inferior. This is not an intrinsic property of fat. It is about social degradation/regulation and, similar to fat activists, some interviewees were acutely aware of this. Jason, who was not part of the slimming club sample but was told to lose weight by his doctor, complained to Gary: 'There is something about weight-gain and the whole weight issue which is about making people feel guilty.' Internalized oppression – what Bartky (1990: 22) calls 'psychological oppression' or 'the internalization of intimations of inferiority' – has negative implications for psychosocial health and well-being. Oppression, inequality and reduced social status undermine experiential embodiment and could have adverse consequences for the visceral (Freund 2006, Robertson 2006). Jerry, who said others called him a fat bastard and, as evidenced above, disparaged other inexcusable big people, reasoned: 'some people will put themselves down for being overweight and obese which makes them unhealthy'.

Contrition may be emotionally abrasive but men also expressed less self admonishing responses (for example, resignation, indifference, half-hearted compliance). Furthermore, there was space for comedic laughter, with laughter having redeeming qualities for those living in oppressive social circumstances (Berger 1997). Resonating with some of the slimming club sketches on the BBC's comedy *Little Britain*, two male slimmers informally talked about resistance and concealment. These men drank in the same pub as their consultant, Sandy. Referring to surveillance, they joked during fieldwork with Gary about ensuring 'all crisps and nuts are out of sight and dusting off any crumbs from our jumpers' when Sandy entered the pub. One could imagine Sandy, like Marjorie Dawes from *Little Britain's* slimming club, telling them to eat dust. However, that was not part of Sandy's repertoire. And such injunctions were unnecessary since, as evidenced above, and argued by fat activists, many 'fat people' have already been made to feel like dirt.

Other men refused to be crushed by fat oppression when publicly doing contrition. At a slimming class mainly comprising women, Jim sought to lose weight (admittedly not a large amount) but displayed 'coolness' (Lyman and Scott 1970) when his weight remained constant or if he gained. Here, constructing unperturbed masculinities entailed 'role distance' (Goffman 1961b) among a larger group of women, some of whom were not particularly big but publicly announced feeling 'devastated' when they did not lose weight. This is understandable from a feminist perspective, given the blame and shame associated with fatness, with shame defined as 'the distressed apprehension of the self as inadequate or diminished' and 'one of the most insidious means by which women come to recognize, regulate and control themselves through their bodies' (Skeggs 1997: 123). Other male slimmers publicly constructed unperturbed masculinities when joking and laughing about their common deviations, for example: 'My plan has gone pear shaped, like my body!' This was in a predominantly male group where Sandy advised: 'You can lose weight and you can make excuses, but you can't do both at the same time.' Stan attended this class. After I mentioned the 'pear shaped' joke during our interview he explained: 'You've got the responsibility to put your-self down. It's you that's got yourself in that state to start off with, being fat, and then you start losing it and you can start joking about it.'

Masculine role distance aside, contrition is comparable to the public apology (Goffman 1971). The person accepts the idea that they have done wrong and should make amends. During this recurrent process, dissociation from, and vili-fication of, one's objectively separable fatness may occur alongside claims of really being a 'good' person inside (Honeycutt 1999). At the experiential level, Cartesian dualism may be replicated while being totally dependent on the inter-twining of relational bodies, minds and society. In Goffman's (1971: 113) words, there is 'a splitting of the self into a blameworthy part and a part that stands back and sympathizes with the blame giving, and, by implication, is worthy of being brought back into the fold'. Paul told me this splitting of the self was spatially organized at Fat Fighters: 'they have an overweight corner, where if you've gained, you go in a separate part'. After I joked, 'Do they give you a dunce's cap as well?' he replied, 'They might as well [laughs], it is classed as total humiliation.' Paul added that Fat Fighter consultants also risked public humiliation if they gained weight and, unlike Sunshine employees, risked unemployment. Interestingly, total humiliation, first self-humiliation then humiliation from others, is a recurrent theme in Orthodox Christianity where holy fools (who were canonized) imitated the humiliation of Christ before his crucifixion (Berger 1997).

Contrition is not confined to 'relations in public' (Goffman 1971). It includes private self–body relations (the befuddling of self–other and public–private dichotomies) and compares to holy folly in other ways. That includes 'religiously motivated nakedness', which is associated with the holy fool's invitation of 'disgust and vilification' (Berger 1997: 192). This religious inheritance, which, for those with faith, is a source of insight, is embodied. Because the attitudes of 'the generalized other' are incorporated within individuals, influencing their thinking and conduct (Mead 1934), social deprecation and attempts to ameliorate negative 'role-taking emotions' (such as embarrassment and shame) do not depend on the presence of others (Shott 1979). Indeed, the sorry act of accepting respon-sibility for being/remaining undesirably fat is perhaps best suited to situations of private self-reflection (naked self-criticism). Even so, talk about this during public confessionals could serve as evidence of genuine contrition, with self-deprecation deemed highly motivating for those seeking 'positive' (righteous) change. An Australian big fella said the following while successfully slimming and, in so doing, used language similar to Jim quoted at the start of this chapter when condemning people who blame the fast-food industry for their fatness. This man rejected excuses for being 'overweight' as expressed by others – and, by implication, his past self – and explicitly vilified his current self though this was tempered by his displayed commitment to slimming. Here, Cooley's (1983) 'looking glass self' was no mere metaphor and 'provided a distorted glimpse of *another* world' (Berger 1997: 193, emphasis in original) where he would be triumphant:

> A lot of overweight people play the victim card, and they play the victim card because it disassociates them from taking responsibility for their actions, and they look for the sympathy vote. But the problem is the sympathy vote is never there because throughout the years they shovelled the food in their faces that got them in that position. When I feel that I've got it [weight-loss regime] sorted, and I get slightly cocky, I take off all my clothes, I go and find a full length mirror at home, and I jump up and down in front of it stark bollock naked. That keeps you absolutely on the straight and bloody narrow, let me tell you. That's motivating.
>
> (Discovery Health 2004)

Contrition includes other remedial tactics. 'Proclaimers' (Hunter 1984: 161) are prospective aligning actions that are oriented toward the positive, emphasizing personal responsibility (entitling proclaimers) and/or the putatively positive character of the yet to occur act (enhancing proclaimers). Slimming, according to this rhetoric, becomes an avenue to a better life. As noted by Martin (2002), there are good (economic) reasons why some slimming organizations co opt accounts that emphasize improved health and appearance rather than guilt and shame. Yet, immediately after telling me about Fat Fighters' 'overweight corner', Paul said Sunshine's positive approach was unusual: 'We will bend over backwards not to humiliate, and that is unique to Sunshine.' While Paul extolled his club's merits (in practice consultants also enacted stigma: see Chapter 3), enhancing proclaimers have wider currency. This is in a moral economy where those assumed to be gluttonous and slothful attempt to project middle-class ideals of moral worth. The ideal typical slimmer becomes a 'disciplined body' (Frank 1991) who projects a positive identity to self and others. This entails proclaiming the value of being or becoming slim and resolving to 'take control' through lifestyle changes.

By publicly and/or privately aligning oneself with slimming culture, positive future perfect states are intimated with 'contradictory results: social approval and self-derogation' (Hunter 1984: 165). Here actors are typecast in a valued, 'self-authored' role that simultaneously denigrates fat while placing the means for salvation within their hands. Sunshine did not have an overweight corner but those losing a large amount of weight were called 'big losers' (also note the US TV show called *The Biggest Loser* where participants attempt to lose weight). Bernard, co-opted as an advisor into several classes by Sandy because he was her biggest loser, told me not long after I first met him that he still had 3 stone to lose and disparagingly called himself a fat bastard. However, Bernard was happy to act as a source of advice and 'support' for others after going from 26 to 16 stone, and took no offence when Sandy publicly called him a 'big loser'. As an aside, fat activists state many people are 'losers' because of fat oppression. Here self-deprecation is attributed to social expectations that are inseparable from the free market economy and medical science that has 'a vested interest in furthering fat hatred' (Cooper 1998: 33).

Slimming clubs capitalize on fat hatred and reward those conforming to its logic. Big losers, like Bernard, gained social approval when successfully losing weight. He had seen the light and exerted a halo effect at the slimming club. Given the recurrent religious theme, and following Chapter 1 on constraints on critical discussion, it is clear that fat fighting is not a simple matter of economic exploitation: it is a quasi-religious stance that proffers, however ephemerally, a feeling of salvation in response to suffering. It is what Bourdieu (2001: 74) calls the *illusio* – a game, imposed from without, that personally matters because it is in the mind and body. For those embroiled in this *illusio*, contrition entails 'worshipping at the shrine of slenderness' (Brumberg 1988: 257). It makes a virtue out of conscientiousness and, at least ideal typically, prohibits behaviour construed as sinful. While Sunshine's staff rejected religious connotations, in north-east England weekly meetings were often held in churches. Sunshine's slimming book was also informally called a bible, members counted the 'syn' value of calorific foods and there were other quasi-religious themes, for example, emotional stories about the disabled walking, talk about resisting temptation, asking whether new members had a last supper before joining and the consultant urging members to bask in the glory of weight-loss.

I mentioned the religious theme to Paul, who joined Sandy's class with his wife. He said the following though added they were merely joking: 'I'll be honest. We have a little joke, me and Liz, cos if we do go off the rails we'll go oh sort of like "Forgive me Sandy for I have sinned."' This might have been a joke and thus not considered real, but religion was inescapable. For example, Sandy lent me a folder with newspaper articles featuring 'big losers'. The folder's cover was titled: *Slimming Editorials: Sandy's Slimming Angels at St. Peter's*. It also featured a cartoon image of a slim man, with matchstick legs, standing in front of a mirror looking at a fat body. This religiously framed picture struck me of anorexia; the person with imagined fat who sees a mirror image that others cannot see. 'Religious asceticism' plays a role in women's experiences of anorexia (*cf.* Gremillion 2005: 20) and it clearly played a role in some men's and women's experiences of slimming in north-east England. This also parallels observations among women in Stinson's (2001) ethnography of a commercial weight-loss group in the USA.

More generally, contrition comprises multiple atoning technologies for people seeking to wash away their sins, as manifest in real or imagined fat. These 'technologies of life' (Rose 2004) are intertwined with a political economy of hope, vitality and a promissory culture. They are intended to neutralize fat bodies or the unwanted fat on 'self-caring' bodies, leading to the Promised Land where slimness supposedly guarantees happiness and healthiness (rather than a perpetual state of fear about easily regaining weight and being stigmatized as fat). These somatic techniques of constriction and contraction – rationalized diet, physical activity and perhaps pharmaceuticals and surgery – are the very stuff of intentional weight-loss. In accord with the logic of expansive consumer capitalism, these are also marketed to people who do not necessarily accept responsibility for gaining unwanted weight in the first place. Indeed, many of the previously noted excuse-accounts were voiced by slimmers when referring to their past selves, though they could also be used to excuse recurrent or future deviations during an often long and meandering weight-loss journey. Such accounts provide a safety net for those walking the slimming tightrope while supporting the often ineffective yet profitable weight-loss industry.

Techniques that cut 'sizeable' bodies down in size are Foucauldian 'truth games', ostensibly allowing the thin person inside the fat body to escape (Frank 1991). Here the guilty discursively if not practically seek to realign socially disjointed bodies and identities by endorsing these constraining yet enabling techniques. Similar to accounts described by Scott and Lyman (1968), such words are ritually significant, helping shore up the timbers of fractured sociation if well timed and placed. They may even help re-animate previously eclipsed social bodies, leading to a metaphorical re-birth of the social self and a renewed love of life. However, it should be stressed that the promise of salvation may never materialize; if enacted, techniques of contrition may actually become a dissatisfying source of attrition not only for women but also men (Innanen 1999). Additionally, a discrepancy may exist between proclaimed intentions and physical actions, between word and deed. Sociologically, such proclamations, especially for those going to slimming clubs, may help deflect the moralizing 'concerns' of others even if the speaker has no real intention of losing weight (or the ability to do so) (Karen Throsby, personal communication 2007). In situations of bodily co-presence, contrition could thus include emotionally expressive 'face compliance' which may never manifest itself in the embodied actions and materiality of fat bodies (Degher and Hughes 1999). The success of this ritualistic rather than restitutive strategy (a displayed orientation to rules rather than actual compensatory action) is thus likely to depend on various factors, including: social distance between interactants and attendant biographical knowledge, the use of rationalized technologies (for example, the weighing scales) and the actors' displays of sincerity as read through 'shared vocabularies of body idiom' (Goffman 1963). Even then, there is ample evidence that dietary approaches to weight-loss do not have their intended effect and are counterproductive, and this says more about the interventions themselves than the individuals seeking to lose weight (Aphramor 2005, Mann *et al.* 2007). Contrition contains elements that inform a politicized and corporeally grounded repudiation of fat fighting.

Repudiation: 'FAT!SO?'

Wann (1998), a fat activist, expresses repudiation in her book *FAT!SO? Because You Don't Have to Apologize for Your Size!* I will outline fat activist accounts and politicized ways of knowing as interpreted through my typology. This will then critically inform a more empirically grounded, politically attuned and theoretically informed analysis of men's accounts in subsequent chapters.

Most readers will probably be unfamiliar with fat activists' accounts, which are not part of the cultural mainstream in the same way that excuse-accounts and contrition are. Activists' accounts are marginalized because they reject the tenets of a fatphobic culture and the ideology of personal responsibility vis-à-vis the possibility and desirability of becoming thin. Nonetheless, repudiating accounts are obtaining greater visibility and, as will emerge in subsequent chapters, men expressed variants of these, albeit with an emphasis on the gendered politics of identity. Rather than seeking to educate the public, change laws and achieve social change, big fellas engaged in gendered identity work when presenting 'appropriate' masculinities to self and others. And, in traversing ideal types, some expressed repudiation even when slimming.

Fat activists take various stances when expressing repudiation, though, like many feminists, theirs is a 'vocabulary of anger and injustice' (Skeggs 1997: 23). Some assert they are 'pissed off', even in academic books (Mitchell 2005), and challenge narratives of blame by denying the *relevance* of personal responsibility. Alternatively, if the issue of responsibility is accepted as relevant, then repudiation shares with excuses the view that people labelled fat are not fully responsible for their weight. However, repudiation differs from excuses regarding the pejorative status of bodies medically categorized as overweight or worse. The point at which repudiation and excuse-making diverge is the point at which justifications and repudiation converge: social censure is challenged.

This is not a simple case of 'fat people' having their cake and eating it. The acceptability of accounts or aligning actions depends on power, status and stereotypes (Hunter 1984). If, according to common cultural background expectancies, fat people are deservedly discredited, then it is difficult to convincingly challenge this without contradicting taken-for-granted tenets that homogenize, essentialize and pathologize, i.e. fat is bad and ugly, fat people are responsible for their weight, therefore fat people are uncivilized and unworthy of ritual courtesy. Aphramor (2006), in her report on size discrimination, observes that such stereotypes are so pervasive that they are simply taken for granted and permit public insults, even towards people of high social status. It is thus unsurprising that many people, more usually women who are denigrated as inappropriately fat, feel crushed by the weight of societal disapproval (Honeycutt 1999). Yet, fat activism offers collective resistance through repudiating talk. This seeks to transform shame into acceptance and possibly even 'pride' (Cooper 1998) through intervening emotions such as anger.

Following the discussion on contrition, fat activism could be considered blasphemous. As noted in Berger's (1997: 192) discussion on holy fools who invite humiliation for Christ's sake, '[t]he worst sin is pride; everything must be done to avoid this'. However, fat activists have no interest in holy folly. Size or fat acceptance groups provide alternative vocabularies, interpretive schemes and background expectancies that render forms of repudiation normal, reasonable and sensible. In line with Foucault's (1978) point that where there is power there is resistance, fat activists offer 'reverse discourses' that 'lead to the "production of alternative forms of knowledge"' (Weedon 1987: 11, cited by Germov and Williams 1996: 644). Largely comprising 'the own and the wise' (Goffman 1968), such groups offer social support for fat people in physical and cyberspace. Unlike the commodified support at slimming clubs, this is not dependent on slimming. Size acceptance or 'fat politics' is about 'generating better self-esteem without weight-loss being a condition' (Cooper 1998: 192).

Repudiation comprises elements contained in Goffman's (1971) discussion on remedial work. These elements include denial, demands and blame. For example, activists may deny the relevance of individual culpability when demanding civil rights and blame social prejudice or fatphobia for the negativity ascribed to fatness (as well as possible health problems given, for example, discrimination in healthcare and risky weight-loss practices). In the remainder of this section I will elaborate on how the issue of personal responsibility is negotiated by fat activists and fat acceptance scholars plus the perceived inappropriateness of fatness. To borrow from Skeggs (1997), a feminist sociologist, these politicized formulations entail rejecting 'shameful recognitions' which shape how 'fat people' relate to themselves and others as embodied subjects. Analytically, I will also draw from sociological or sociologically imaginative literature when typifying and evaluating politicized arguments, which, in turn, may inform sociological analysis.

Regarding personal responsibility, fat activists sometimes claim there are 'good' fat people who are physically active and care about their dietary intake. For all practical purposes, they may be compliant with everyday healthist injunctions. They may have also repeatedly tried to lose weight and attempted to keep it off. However, they do not embody the 'thin ideal' (Germov and Williams 2004), or a weight that medicine deems healthy. According to this discourse, people remain fat for 'good' reasons beyond their control. Concordant with recurrent observations in weight-loss research, fat activists assert that exercise and calorie restriction are largely ineffective in making fat bodies thin (Campos 2004, Miller 1999). A person could be a 'model' citizen wedded to healthism but the fleshy body becomes an unreliable marker of possible or actual compliance and even measurably good metabolic health (Gaesser 2002).

Appealing to 'the naturalistic body' (Shilling 2003), as with biological excuse-accounts, fatness is attributed to physiological or genetic factors (though, on the interactions of biology and global inequalities, see Aphramor (2005)). Cooper, for example, dedicates her fat activist book to her inherited 'fat genes' while also remaining ambivalent for various reasons, such as the future possibility of eugenics to eliminate bodies that should be considered 'part of a wide spectrum of body types' rather than an aberration (Cooper 1998: 77–8). In their ideal typical description of fat acceptance, Saguy and Riley (2005: 870) call this 'a body diversity frame' that 'present[s] fatness as a natural and largely inevitable form of diversity'. Such words, in speaking directly to the issue of personal responsibility, make 'identity claims' that contest the audience's actual or possible disapproval (*cf.* Hunter 1984). Of course, as noted under excuse-accounts, scientists often discount genetic explanations for an obesity epidemic. Yet, such words have salience for some people when mitigating responsibility for their weight/fat and negotiating identities. Here, to draw from Campos's (2004) legalistic metaphor, individuals are innocent rather than guilty and should not be unfairly prosecuted in the court of public opinion.

Before outlining other aspects and permutations of repudiation, three additional points are worth making about the 'body diversity' discourse. First, it would be hypocritical for obesity scientists to dismiss such talk since, as noted by Gard and Wright (2005), obesity scientists simultaneously assert the irrelevance of genetics at a population level but the importance of genetics at an individual level. Second, and without reifying the idea of genetic inferiority and implied Health Nazism (Edgley and Brissett 1990), appeals to body diversity serve as a useful counterpoise to the new public health. That is, the idea that people have a duty to exercise self-care (read: embody a supposedly 'healthy' weight) if they are to be accorded full rights of citizenship (Petersen and Lupton 1996). If bodies 'naturally' vary then it is unreasonable to propose that everybody at a given height should fall within a narrow weight range. Third, when fat activists discuss genetics, those subscribing to 'set point theory' stress how the naturalistic body interacts with social pressures to diet, which, as already noted, often results in additional weight-gain. Cooper (1998: 12–13) describes set point theory in terms of the biological body's 'weight-regulating mechanism' (also Tenzer 1989, Orbach 2006). This is, in part, genetically inherited but may be altered by dieting which increases the body's propensity to store fat. This discourse has important identity effects. Cooper (1998: 12–13) states this theory 'moves beyond' individual blame narratives that vilify 'fat people' as 'villainous gluttons' and instead draws critical attention to 'diet industries for creating a population of fat people whilst exploiting and denigrating their own market'. This overlaps with Campos (2004) on the US cultural obsession with weight and the industries that help to manufacture and sustain this by blaming its consumers rather than its products.

However, there is a different tack. While responsibility for fatness may be shifted elsewhere, as part of what LeBesco (2004) calls the 'will to innocence', repudiation may entail challenging the wider relevance of responsibility – a less palatable position when seeking alignment with a potentially sympathetic audience. There is complexity because human agency is structured and embodied: 'innocence' accounts, or *softer repudiation*, may be politically potent and sensitive to the social situation of larger people if critical attention is directed at political economic forces, constraints and irrationalities associated with fat fighting. However, what could be called *harder repudiation* makes a somewhat different but important point; namely, whether people are wholly 'culpable' for their corporeality is irrelevant when demanding equality and rights. This moves beyond Cooper's appeal to genetics or blaming the 'unscrupulous' diet industries for making people fat, though she also expresses harder repudiation when stating 'fat people have as much right to be greedy, lazy, unfit or smelly as thinner people' (1998: 43).

Abandoning the will to innocence may be defined as harder repudiation for two reasons. First, it implies emotional indifference to and even rejection of audience sympathy. Second, in a context of obesity epidemic psychology (healthism, neo-liberalism, masculine domination, etc.), it is less likely to be honoured. Nonetheless, harder repudiation aims to be socially transformative and fits with the messiness of human embodiment. As discussed by LeBesco (2004), the lived experience of fatness, similar to human embodiment in general, is contradictory. It incorporates health and illness plus moments of self-control and abandonment. And, while individual bodyweight *may* be more or less controllable, this 'shouldn't preclude one's protection from discrimination, from the opportunity to live a happy and full life' (LeBesco 2004: 115). This position, obfuscating arbitrary distinctions between 'good' (responsible) and 'bad' (irresponsible) fat people, is a non-essentialist alternative to excuse-accounts that trace fatness 'along a bio-logical path to bad genes or horrible hormones, or along a social path to traumatic childhood experience' (14).

Various arguments also challenge the inappropriateness of fatness and social meanings that discredit people who are seen as fat. Fat activists vary in their views but, in exercising their sociological imaginations, they maintain that forms and levels of fatness have often been, and continue to be, valued and desired in a historical and cross-cultural context. Certainly, this is evidenced online where people identifying as fat create supportive and eroticized domains, which cater to men and women of various sexual orientations (Monaghan 2005b). Fat activists also assert that fatness is stigmatized because of prejudice, ignorance and 'junk science' and powerful commercial interests are inseparable from such processes. Weight-based discrimination, or sizism, rather than actual bodily size, is the real problem for fat activists 'doing' repudiation.

Within this politicized discourse, sizism is considered nonsensical. Although rhetorically glossing over other forms of discrimination (for example, wheelchair users experience discrimination), Smith (1990) defines sizism as one of the last 'safe' prejudices in societies where other forms of oppression are unacceptable (also, see Chapter 3). Formally, some of this reasoning compares to the social model of disability where oppression is considered the problem, not the body per se. This model has been critiqued within disability studies for, among other things, equating disability with oppression rather than the socio-cultural experience of impairment (Shakespeare 2006, Williams 1999). Nonetheless, the social model is explicitly used by some fat activists and scholars (Cooper 1997), and recommended to others (LeBesco 2004). This makes sense not least because *the negative experiences of fat embodiment in Western culture may have very little to do with physical impairment.* Yet, I would highlight complexity lest some medical sociologists critique this as a form of social reductionism that denies human corporeality. To borrow from Thomas (2001) who discusses the social model of disability in general, rather than fat activism in particular, 'impairment effects' typically associated with *much larger bodies* are not ignored. However, fat activists emphasize the social relational aspects of disabling environments and attitudes (Solovay 2000). Illness and impairment may certainly restrict bodies but these are contextualized so that it is broader discriminatory meanings and practices that are deemed particularly problematic. These may also have real material effects; for example, and to connect back to softer repudiation, repeated dieting could result in impairment because people usually end up gaining more weight. This fits with Aphramor's (2007) pragmatic endorsement of the Health at Every Size paradigm, and adopting this from the outset in clinical practice (Chapter 1).

At the risk of oversimplification, challenging the pathologization of fatness, and, by association, people deemed fat, thus comprises two main threads: positive and negative. Positively, activists underscore the acceptability and perhaps desirability of forms and levels of fatness. Mitchell (2005: 222), in anticipating and seeking to counter media misrepresentations of fat activism, stresses the importance of slogans such as: 'Fat Doesn't Necessarily Mean Unhealthy', 'Fat Doesn't Mean Lazy' and, innocently, 'Everybody is a Good Body', which is juxtaposed with 'the most outrageous: Fat is Sexy'. Here fat acceptance merges with admiration, though, contrary to some misrepresentations of fat politics within sociology (Crossley 2004), this is done knowing that fatness is often disparaged rather than a body ideal in late modernity.

Negatively, but still serving valued ends, activists blame institutional meanings and practices for the 'wrongfulness' of becoming, being and remaining fat. This is not just about the irrationalities of dieting or a disabling built environment. The social environment is also considered a hotbed of fallacious or medically ques-tionable reasoning, damaging stereotypes, discrimination and anti-fat prejudice. Some activists, as discussed in relation to disability studies, might overstate their case in an attempt to challenge existing ideas (Shakespeare 2006) but strands of fat activist thinking are supported by research literature (Aphramor 2006, Cooper 1998, Solovay 2000). While some activists again claim they are being victimized, condemnatory accounts emerge that forcefully grapple with sizism. For example, LeBesco (2004: 59) describes 'the reinvigorated effort to wipe out obesity as a sort of modern day eugenics campaign', citing a survey of married couples in which 11 per cent reported they would abort a child if it were known to be genetically predisposed to obesity. Outside academia, a contributor to an online size accept-ance group offered similar condemnatory words: 'I think we all get enough hassle from all those skinny people and thin-minded people and those neo-puritans – I don't believe in hassling people for no good reason!' Martin (2002), in his ethnography of NAAFA, terms these 'oppression tales', where members challenge a size-biased society. This explains why fat activists like Mitchell (2005) are 'pissed off', though she also expresses softer repudiation when talking to issues of responsibility. In short, she seeks to mitigate personal responsibility with appeals to 'addictive' 'junk food' and the contradictions of capitalism shortly after extolling the sexiness of fat (Mitchell 2005: 216).

To reiterate, repudiation is not easy. Sociological research undertaken among women at NAAFA shows they had real difficulties accepting the organization's redefinition of fat (Gimlin 2002). An academic feminist, who reports being seduced on the level of personal size acceptance by Wann's (1998) 'political arsenal' (but found this unrealizable in a society where she was fair game for public insults and various injustices) explains this by stressing identity is embodied rather than in the mind (S. Murray 2005). That is, subjectivity is constituted through bodily immersion in a larger social world where tacit 'ideas are ingrained in our very being' (S. Murray 2005: 275). Unsurprisingly, then, even fat activist leaders sometimes publicly doubt themselves, vocalizing internal contradictions and 'I'd-rather-be-thin sentiments' (LeBesco 2004: 95).

Mixing and matching elements common to excuses and justifications may thus be experienced as a fraught and contested process for those personally doing repudiation: something related to everyday background expectancies, social reactions and the embodied habitus (Bourdieu 2001) rather than the coherence or otherwise of fat activism. As stated by Lyons (1989: 72), who promotes size acceptance among women and endorses physical activity, without weight-loss, as part of a broader activist agenda: 'it takes courage to challenge a world that tells us to get thin or get lost'. Difficulties persist even when talking with significant others who (unsuccessfully) try to minimize the salience of being 'inappropriately' fat. Somebody on a fat acceptance weblog wrote the following (emphasis in original). In so doing, the author provides reflexive and affective commentary on the vicissitudes of accounting for fatness, and thus oneself, in a fatphobic culture. This argument is not gender specific. However, it is to be anticipated that gender and other axes of power shape the perceived need for such words, and their reception, in 'a nation of meddlers' (Edgley and Brissett 1999):

> When I talk to those close to me about being part of the fat acceptance movement & trying to educate people about the truth about fat/health/ genetics/metabolism, etc., they want to know why I care about this stuff, what's the big deal, 'because YOU'RE not fat'. Of course, some of them go on to put both feet in their mouths by saying things such as, 'YOU aren't like those lazy slobs who eat at McDonald's all the time, shovel stuff into their faces around the clock, & never exercise'. Yes, that's [the] point, isn't it? That our culture promotes the belief that ALL fat people eat huge amounts, ALL fat people eat junk, ALL fat people never exercise, ALL fat people run up the cost of medical insurance, ALL fat people die young, &, for that matter, the belief that it is anyone else's BUSINESS if a particular individual never exercises & spends his or her days eating lard & Twinkies. I am torn between justifying myself by pointing out that I have a pretty healthy lifestyle [. . .] & knowing that doing so is somewhat beside the point, but we shouldn't HAVE to justify our existence or prove that we are GOOD fat people who are always trying to be thin, we shouldn't have to have perfect habits in order to be treated well & given full rights in our society.

Participants in these communities often find themselves in an arena of detailed argument and discussion. Expressions are offered that could be typified as justifications, others as excuses, and sometimes unwelcome interjections proclaim the benefits of intentional weight-loss. As discussed above, such words imply different things about responsibility and the moral status of fatness. It is unsurprising, therefore, that fat acceptance communities are emotion whirlpools. However, repudiation, in its various forms, is wholly meaningful and has political value. Repudiation entails disavowing opprobrium, promoting association with the fat body (Honeycutt 1999) and other people adopting a fat identity. And there is an unapologetic demand for respect and ritual courtesy as well as a rejection of the so-called self-deprecating 'fat shuffle' (Gimlin 2002: 129). Activists respond to the 'problem' of fatness by demanding social change (for example, greater public understanding) rather than often ineffective and potentially dangerous efforts to change the fleshy body, i.e. a personal solution to a socially constructed problem. In short, the potentially problematic is externalized rather than internalized, challenged rather than accepted.

Finally, it is worth recognizing that in a visually oriented culture, where female bodies are routinely objectified, physical appearance bears upon the honouring of talk (Scott and Lyman 1968). Cooper (1998) calls this looksism, or appearance-based prejudice. In this context, anti-obesity researchers and others usually discredit fat activists (who are often very large women) because they are fat (Saguy and Riley 2005). Yet, researchers do not acknowledge that they themselves may be biased due to organizational affiliations, research funding from the weight-loss industry, efforts to promote their careers, their own internalization of fatphobia and psychosocial investments in being thin. Small wonder then that fat activists welcome, sometimes in a critical and experientially informed way, research from lean people who have symbolic and cultural capital and are willing to empathize with the fat activists' worldview.

Concluding remarks: Toward a sociological repudiation of obesity warmongering

Accounts are socially situated. Different accounts suit different purposes in different situations. Without denying the situational efficacy of all of the accounts presented above for specific individuals in specific circumstances, from a critical realist position some accounts are more sociologically credible than others. This not only relates to everyday and fat activists' accounts. It also relates to academic and scientific accounts that engage with and perhaps reproduce the idea of an obesity epidemic and authorize/challenge aggressive intervention. Whether referring to excuses that reiterate the wrongfulness of 'excess' weight/fat while ostensibly mitigating individual responsibility (such as biomedical accounts), justifications that challenge its pejorative status while accepting responsibility (such as rejecting the BMI) or some other permutation, some accounts or aligning actions carry more sociological weight than others.

Weight-related accounts are multifarious and this book reports qualitative data in their richness and complexity. Gender is a key substantive concern, or, more specifically, men's talk about weight-related issues and how they constructed masculine identities in a society where fatness is routinely discredited as female or feminizing filth. Accounts are a central resource for 'doing' gender, or being seen as a regular fella who is ordinary rather than deviant and woman-like. However, this book does not simply report on the empirical world. Ethnographic description and other qualitative data are important given the paucity of empirical research on this topic but data reporting is insufficient. Analytically, I want to offer a well-informed and sociologically imaginative interpretation of various weight-related accounts, (in)actions assumed to contribute to fatness and everyday remedial work. To reiterate, some accounts are more sociologically sensible than others, regardless of the situational efficacy of specific accounts in specific situations. Based on my reading of the literature and undertaking this research I would maintain that aspects of fat activism could inform (but not do the work of) sociology. In repudiating obesity warmongering, and the battles and hatred it mandates or incites, fat activism provides a reverse discourse that offers subjugated but often insightful and more or less reflective knowledge. Fat activism is a fitting response to not-so-subtle symbolic violence as communicated by powerful institutions seeking to combat medicalized fatness. This war is aimed at practically everybody while hitting hardest people who are seen as fat in everyday life.

I am not a fat activist campaigning for civil rights. Nor am I personally seeking to make fatness more liveable. I am a sociologist primarily seeking to contribute to knowledge and stimulate debate in a field of masculine and class-related domination, politics and social injustice (Bourdieu 2001, Connell 1995). However, there is much about fat activism, and what I call repudiation, that is sociologically and politically sensible. While some arguments advanced by some activists are questionable, such as addiction accounts or the idea that 'fat people' are passively exploited by the weight-loss industry, fat activism has the potential to change how weight/fatness is commonly understood. Such thinking is vitally important in a divided society where the science, morality, ideology and economics of the obesity discourse are under scrutiny (Gard and Wright 2005, Rich and Evans 2005) and where powerful organizations draw from and authoritatively reinforce intolerance on an unprecedented scale. From the perspective of medical sociology, repudiating accounts are also fitting because the war on obesity perpetuates a misleading, or at best oversimplified, understanding of what determines health. This is a pernicious manifestation of depoliticizing and individualizing healthism in neo-liberal societies where victim blaming is often the name of the game. It is therefore something that sociology, using various understandings gleaned from fat activism, is well positioned to critically engage.

Grounded in data and connecting with relevant literature, subsequent chapters repudiate the larger war on obesity, the hatred and intolerance it draws from and amplifies and institutional efforts to fight fat. This fits with my broader concern to offer a sociologically imaginative study of this public issue and sometimes-private trouble. This is not about simply taking sides in an ethically and scientifically suspect battle, that is, of arguing 'fatness' is intrinsically good or bad. Nor is it about swallowing things whole as espoused by various interested parties. It is about exercising critical judgement in an informed and ethically responsible way. There are several strands to my repudiating stance. These relate to the pejorative status of what medicine calls overweight and obesity, the issue of personal responsibility and the wider relevance of responsibility.

Subsequent chapters question *the pejorative status* ascribed to overweight/obesity/fatness. This is important given the repeated invocation of health as a justification for the war on obesity and, by unavoidable association, people labelled obese. As with critical weight studies, this entails questioning reductionist reasoning and malevolent assumptions where real or imagined fatness is the enemy rather than, say, discrimination, stress, broader environmental concerns and risky weight-loss practices. Obviously, then, this is not the same as saying 'fat people' are always healthy. Indeed, given the social subordination of many people labelled obese or worse, it is to be expected that their health may not be as good as it could be. However, if attention is directed at biomedical health, the visceral over the normative (size, shape, weight), then the point to recognize is that 'the physiological is the political' (Aphramor 2005: 322): the social impacts upon and works through the physical body in ways that disproportionately advantage and disadvantage different groups of people as reflected by morbidity and mortality rates. Certainly, this means I would challenge the idea that most men in Western nations are ill, diseased or at risk *because of their weight or fatness*. The real world is far more complex, just as so-called 'obesity-related problems' disproportionately affecting super size people are never simply the result of the physical body or adiposity abstracted from society. And, if attention focuses on health as lived and experienced, rather than measured, then ways of living that are assumed to cause fatness may also be a justifiable source of self-fulfilment and pleasure rather than suffering and misery.

Of course, many people are willing if not able to lose weight by foregoing certain gustatory pleasures and employing other means like exercise. Such alignment is understandable under current social conditions where obesity is defined as a massive problem and 'good' citizens are obliged to take *personal responsibility for their weight* (an efficient yet unreliable marker for adiposity and health). Grounded in data, and theorizing from bodies while also going beyond bodies, my analytic framework contains elements of softer repudiation. This means I do not necessarily dismiss accounts that mitigate personal responsibility for weight or fatness. No doubt, there are good reasons why people cannot achieve slenderness. If one is to assume bodyweight is reliably determined by lifestyle (itself a questionable assumption), it is clear that people differently located in the social structure are not always able to engage in 'corrective' bodywork. 'Failure' to do the 'right' thing, as conventionally defined, is less about ignorance and more about socially distributed means, abilities and priorities. Also, without denying the ways in which social location and practices materially affect bodies (for example, childhood nutrition and its relation to health and physicality), there is a rich diversity of 'naturalistic' (Shilling 2003) bodies with some betraying what may otherwise be considered a healthy lifestyle. Whether explained in terms of genetics or other naturalistic accounts (or the interplay of society and biology), bodies are not pure social constructs and weight or body composition is not fully open to individual control.

However, I would also question *the relevance of responsibility for weight or fatness*. I do this given the complexity and contradictions of human embodiment, the suspect nature of militarized intervention and the degree to which key dimensions of health are affected by social structural factors rather than personal choice and behaviour. Of what relevance is it, and to whom, if somebody is not at a so-called 'healthy' weight or does not try to achieve this? As with fat activists, I would ask: so what if somebody is fat? So what if that person does not always have 'perfect' habits? Does anybody? Because the majority of adults in developed nations are supposedly overweight or obese, are most people expected to change their ways and become a 'model' citizen who is model-like and thin? Does that mean the so-called overweight, obese or fat should be denied healthcare and be discriminated against by health professionals? Hence I also express harder repudiation, which is not dependent on the 'will to innocence' (LeBesco 2004). This stance is not about bowing to medicalized dictates and searching for audience sympathy and approval. It is about exercising healthy scepticism, justifiable resistance and empathizing with everyday people who may not always acquiesce with fat fighting in particular and healthism more generally. This stance fits well with interpretive, embodied sociology and its attempts to understand people while critiquing the larger inequitable social structure (Monaghan 2006).

Harder repudiation may seem indifferent to audience approval and may seem confrontational, contradicting the idea of promoting productive dialogue. However, like fat activism, it aims to promote size acceptance and social justice without the need to prove worthiness as arbitrarily defined by privileged groups who exercise power/knowledge and often make fat profits in the process. Harder repudiation, at the minimum, promotes tolerance of bodily diversity, though I am also aware that activists such as Wann (1998) demand fat rights and liberation. Sociologically, harder repudiation does not mandate scientifically contentious, largely ineffective and culturally insensitive 'meddling' (Edgley and Brissett 1999). Promoting tolerance and justice is important in a risk- and body-oriented society where the physical body is intimately tied to people's relationships, identities and sense of moral worth. It may also be a matter of life and death in contexts like the hospital: large or 'fat' people suffer the same health problems as everybody else and are equally deserving of compassion, support and care (Cooper 1998).

In sum, in aiming to promote productive discussion, and hopefully change institutional practices, I think it is vitally important to repudiate the war on obesity. This metaphorical war glosses over the complexities, uncertainties and controversies within obesity science (Gard and Wright 2005). It also glosses over the ways in which health is socially constructed and experienced, comprising pleasure and emotional well-being. And, it pays scant attention to the potential risks and irrationalities of trying to lose weight and keep it off. Most disturbingly, and with no grasp of sociology whatsoever, obesity warmongers and other proponents of the obesity discourse totally miss the point that stigma is not an intrinsic property of fatness. It is an emergent property of social relations, organization and structures. Theoretically, empirically and politically informed, subsequent chapters challenge the supposed intrinsic wrongs of overweight/ obesity/fatness, the symbolic violence exercised in the name of health and the putative direct benefits and effectiveness of commonly proposed remedial work – specifically, dietary approaches to weight-loss and physical activity. The substantive focus is on men, given the gender bias within the existing academic literature (Bell and McNaughton 2007), but it should also be clear that my critical thinking extends beyond men, with this book challenging the larger war on obesity as directed at 'everyone everywhere' (Gard and Wright 2005: 17).

3 Smoking guns, wartime injury and survival

Men and dieting

Dieting and contemporary masculinity

Dieting is common in manly sports like boxing, where competitors reduce their calorie intake in order to reach their fighting weight. In contrast, everyday dieting to become 'fashionably thin' is typically equated with women. Germov and Williams (1996) refer to this as 'the sexual division of dieting', while other feminists describe dieting as 'the essence of contemporary femininity' and the antithesis of masculinity (Wolf 1991: 200). While intentional weight-loss through whatever means is not exclusively female territory, and gender differences should not be exaggerated, there is evidence of a sexual division. Crossley (2004: 225) confirms feminist literature with reference to a UK survey: women were almost twice as likely to be 'trying to be slim' as men (41.1 per cent compared to 22.6 per cent).

Feminists explain this sexual division in terms of increasing female autonomy and the diminution of traditional sources of social control, such as the church and family. In short, dieting and other forms of bodywork help to ensure women's obedience in male dominated societies (Bartky 1990, Wolf 1991). Bell and McNaughton (2007), in asserting gendered similarities over differences, maintain that such theorizing is constrained by its emphasis on patriarchy, with feminists largely denying men's weight concerns. While I would question aspects of Bell and McNaughton's (2007) work (for example, it is misleading to state women have never been more than 15 per cent concerned with their weight than men when some surveys suggest women may be up to twice as likely as men to be trying to be slim), they usefully highlight men's historically recurrent concerns about their fatness. For example, William Banting, in mid-nineteenth century England, was a famous follower and advocate of dieting (Huff 2001). So too was George Cheyne, in the eighteenth century (Schwartz 1986). More contemporaneously, many men are conscious about being too 'heavy' with dieting also considered acceptably masculine. Mike, who was not from the slimming club, reasoned: 'I think if you spoke five years ago about men going on diets they would have probably laughed at you. Nowadays I think it's more acceptable'. Mike attributed this increasing acceptability to invitations from major slimming clubs. However, as recognized by Mike and others, this is also about the everyday, and medically ratified, unacceptability of fatness.

Superficially and clinically, much dieting could be attributed to the desire to 'improve' physical appearance plus health concerns (Sobal *et al*. 2003). If fashion and looks strike some men as too feminine or vain, biomedical health (risk) has everyday relevance in a context of mass medicalization and healthism. Thus, health takes centre stage in de Souza and Ciclitira's (2005) qualitative study on men and dieting. This relates to 'the care of the self ethic', which renders dieting meaningful and satisfying for those involved in its 'enabling moment' (Heyes 2006). While politicized writing on dieting, bodily repression and fat oppression must be complemented with an understanding of this, much dieting could also be attributed to manufactured intolerance and stigma. Writing before the intensification of obesity epidemic psychology, Brown and Rothblum (1989: 1) asserted 'the stigmatization of being fat, the terror of fat [is] the rationale for a thousand diets'. It might be surmised that almost two decades later, their words have increased relevance with the US Surgeon General locating 'terror within' the 'obese' body (Carmona 2003) rather than a fatphobic culture, or the interactions of bodies and society. Without ignoring biology and naively constructing an alternative social problem, such stigmatizing processes include the medical imposition of a risky or diseased identity on millions of bodies that may actually suffer no ill effects because of their fatness (Campos 2004, Campos *et al*. 2006a, Gaesser 2002).

Of course, the idea of being 'terrified' of fat, or anything else, is antithetical to dominant masculinity (Connell 1995). In everyday life, and depending upon considerations like body size/shape/composition and social circle, men may simply mention they have 'a bit of weight' they want to lose before discussing other mundane matters like the weather or football results. Even so, from a politicized, empirically grounded and critical realist perspective, intentional weight-loss must be understood in a larger society where fatness is being targeted and discredited on an unprecedented scale. Dieting cannot be divorced from this symbolic violence and may even be directly attributed to it. Such violence encircles bodies throughout the life course though it may be especially acute for those subordinated on age hierarchies (just as gender and other social divisions attenuate or amplify the possibility and consequences of sizism). Mike's 13-year-old son dieted after a teacher disparaged his weight in class, with the teacher reiterating a message contemporaneously displayed by the NHS on local anti-obesity posters – a man's 'laughably' large stomach and taut shirt. His son's subsequent 'choice' not only to diet but also to join a slimming club emerged after he expressed suicidal thoughts to his father. Another parent told me a similar story, while a slimming consultant said she observed a quiet and withdrawn boy in her class draw a disturbing picture with the word 'HELL' emblazoned across it (also see Joanisse and Synnott 1999). Hence, I will use militaristic metaphors when critically analysing dieting rather than promote the holy war on fat (Chapters 1 and 2). This analytic move is consonant with a critical realist approach that goes beyond, without leaving out, biomedicine, the biological body and respondents' own meanings and discourses (Williams 2003b).

Using militaristic metaphors to critique militarized medicine, and the broader degradation of fatness it reinforces and legitimates, is useful. This is because men, regardless of the idioms they use to interpret and recount their experiences, do not necessarily escape sizism and 'fall out' from 'friendly fire' (Herndon 2005). Adult male bodies and masculine orientations to the world do not provide an impenetrable 'status shield' (Hochschild 1983) for deflecting anti-fat prejudice and living large. After all, one need only consider opprobrious gendered labels like 'slob' or 'couch potato' that stigmatize men who are said to be 'a real mess' (Watson 2000: 83). During this study many men reported that they had been defined by others, or they self-defined, as 'overweight' (or they used some other discrediting referent, such as 'pregnant' or 'fat bastard'). And, while men talked about mundane, self-initiated and pragmatic bodily concerns that motivated dieting (for example, tighter clothing, wanting to become more mobile), they also sought to lose weight as a matter of psychological, social and even economic survival. That said, in constructing masculinities, these men were not passive victims, just as none reported suffering from a disease called obesity (Chapter 2). As will emerge when exploring how men came to the decision to diet, some talked about being emotionally hurt and discriminated against in diverse contexts (for example, the clinic, the street, at work) but they also expressed scepticism, coolness, indifference and annoyance towards others who treated them as 'fat targets' who should lose weight. Even so, it was under these conditions that dieting had currency. The same could be said for men who were not 'really' fat but felt 'overweight' and misaligned with the embodied meanings of a healthist, fatphobic culture.

Empirically, little is known about men and dieting. During this research, various questions emerged that have not been critically explored in the literature. Thus, what does the word 'diet' mean to men? What is happening in men's lives that makes them want to diet at that time? Given the commonly reported frustrations and disappointments of dieting, what factors are mobilized to sustain this over time? And, if dieting really is an avenue to improved health, appearance and happiness then why is dieting frequently abandoned and weight regained? Finally, given the continuing sexual division of dieting and the idea that dieting is 'not manly' (Watson 2000: 86), how is such action rendered acceptably masculine? This chapter addresses such questions by theorizing from men's bodies while also repudiating the war on obesity and the violence it legitimates in the name of health.

Outlining the embodied meanings of 'diet' and 'dieting'

Before quoting men I will provide some context by connecting with taken-for granted understandings and literature that has empirical and theoretical relevance (for example, with regard to health, weight control, gender and modes of embodiment). Thus, on a mundane level, it is possible to talk about having a diet, going on a diet, being on a diet and modifying one's diet.

Having a diet simply refers to food and drink people consume every day to live. Aside from common starving types (for example, anorexics, neglected children, political prisoners), most people in developed nations have a diet. The nutritional content of somebody's habitual diet is often assumed to manifest itself in the materiality of the body ('you are what you eat') and be more or less (un)healthy. Within dietetic discourses ascriptions of health, illness and disease risk depend upon the amount of fibre, salt and refined sugar in somebody's diet plus other macro- and micro-nutrients, i.e. proteins, carbohydrates, fats, vitamins and minerals. These understandings are also part of an everyday stock-of-knowledge, though, of course, there may well be individual variability in the stock-of-knowledge at hand (Schutz 1962).

Going on and being on a diet convey different meanings. Diet becomes an action or verb rather than a habitual possession or noun. This is about doing rather than having, with such action having a starting point and an intended future-perfect goal. 'Going on' and 'being on a diet' – or 'dieting' for short – refer to out-of-the-ordinary dietary regimens. 'The discourse of dieting' (Chapman 1999) incites people to restrict foodstuffs, usually for a limited period, in order to lose unwanted weight/fat. From an anthropological perspective, dieting is a 'liminal' phase or status passage (Turner 1969). The 'dieter' is betwixt and between an 'undesirable' weight and a 'desirable' weight, a body that supposedly looks 'bad' and one that looks 'good' (or ordinary). 'Normative embodiment' (Watson 2000) is thus prioritized. This is in line with socially constructed body norms and hierarchies that reflect the social value placed on bodily appearance – which is an index of health, attractiveness and moral worth (Featherstone 1991). Of course, some people are always on a diet (Phillip Vannini, personal communication 2007). They are caught in the liminal, which, to extend Turner (1969), means they are always in a limbo state, comprising outsider status, humility, tests and even sexual ambiguity.

Dieting, then, means modifying one's habitual diet with the goal of bringing about observable and measurable reductions in one's weight. This bodywork is aimed at the objectified body, a fleshy body that is rationalized using weighing scales and other technologies (see Chapter 4). While such processes depend on the masculine (a world view that seeks to control, discipline and cut), the targets and executers of this remedial work are often women. 'Dieting', writes Stinson (2001: 4), 'is not a gender-neutral activity. It is the rare woman who has not dieted at some point in her life'. Men in Robertson's (2006) study recognized this when mentioning dieting and why they thought women were more concerned about their health (as appearance) than men. Yet, as will be seen, men contacted during this research also felt it was increasingly acceptable, if not obligatory, for men to attend to their diet and appearance. Also, dietary approaches to weight-loss are masculinized in ways that render them especially relevant for older men or 'really big' men. Dieting may be promoted as a means of feeling healthier and safeguarding or improving the 'visceral' (Watson 2000). And, for the impaired, who cannot fulfil gendered role obligations (for example, work effectively), dieting promises improvements in pragmatic embodiment. That said, success is ultimately evaluated and re-evaluated by how the body looks and how much it weighs.

People also modify their diets without necessarily wanting to lose weight. After all, strength athletes and bodybuilders often manipulate their diets to gain weight (muscle), which is valued bodily capital in their sporting contexts (see Chapter 5). A more mundane and clinically relevant goal is to modify one's habitual diet for *weight management*, while another is to *improve biomedical health and well-being without weight-loss being a necessary condition*. The latter goal informs the Health at Every Size paradigm (Bacon 2006, Robison 2005b). As explained in Chapter 1, weight-loss may occur with this approach, but it may not, with proponents more clearly differentiating between modes of embodiment and refusing to obsess about the normative. In everyday life, dietary modification in order to achieve these goals could be very informal. Somebody is simply more mindful about their dietary intake while making some changes (for example, smaller meals, eating less take-away food and more fresh produce). Hence, they are not on a formal 'diet' or rationalized dietary plan but they watch their habitual diet in order to manage their weight and/or benefit various dimensions of their health. Of course, in Western culture the dominant expectation is that the visibly fat should diet to lose weight and physically 'fit in' with a 'thin' conception of health and attractiveness.

Dieting, in order consistently to lose weight and keep it off, can be a daily struggle. It entails self-denial, surveillance and restriction. 'Crash' diets seek to minimize a sustained sense of sacrifice by promising quick results. Generally, however, the time spent dieting is proportionate to the amount of weight to be lost: bigger losses demand bigger investments in time, energy and resources. This is in a consumer culture where foodstuffs are plentiful and a source of enjoyment, perhaps with other people. To draw from the religious analogy, the abundance and pleasures of 'sinful' foods mean that dieting occurs in the midst of 'temptation' unless the person avoids the profane world of everyday and nightlife. Younger women in Gimlin's (2007b: 418) slimming club ethnography, for instance, reported making 'sacrifices' that 'frequently involved abstaining from social eating and drinking'. Dieting typically entails avoiding or limiting not only one's consumption of alcohol but also fat-laden and/or carbohydrate rich foods. While dieting might alter metabolic health (visceral embodiment) and bodyweight in ways that are welcomed, being on a diet may also undermine experiential embodiment. As noted in Chapter 2, dieting equals a 'bland' life for some men (Chamberlain 2001: 101). The negative emotions of dieting are clearly documented in research among women. Drawing from focus groups, Germov and Williams' (1996) respondents often viewed being on a diet as boring, restrictive, a source of deprivation and guilt. This also compares to Chapman's (1999) study when women discussed so-called 'old' ways of dieting more so than modified diets or 'newer approaches to weight control' where people watch their dietary intake, perhaps permanently.

For many men contacted during this research, the word 'diet' was immediately defined as something people did to lose weight. The definition itself was often concise, though unwelcome ideas about restriction, discipline and irrationality also emerged. Dieting was a 'cutting' exercise – favourite foods and drink were cut in order to cut the body down in size. The word 'diet' was also associated with adopting a healthier lifestyle that might include increased physical activity, and eating more salads and fruit. Several men, who were not slimming club members, immediately stated that alcohol, especially beer, must be restricted or avoided in line with their definition. This sometimes served as a rationale for not dieting and/or following commercial diet programmes (though, as discussed later, slimming clubs promised flexibility but this was limited and compatible with practices that did not fit with the idea of a nutritious diet). To quote typical responses to my question 'How would you define diet?':

> Something you do when you want to lose weight. So obviously you need to cut down on your intake of food and booze. (Howard)

> A diet is not being able to eat specific things, whether it's the carbohydrates, or fats, or proteins, with the specific aim of reducing your weight. (Mike)

> A pal of mine, he's a doctor. I said, 'What is it? If I want to diet, what do I cut out?' He said, 'Well you cut all the things you like'. And it's true. You know? All the things you like, you cut out. (Edward)

> To me it means being strict with yourself. Eating things that you don't normally eat. Eating more fruit, less drink, exercise. That's basically what that means to me. And some people struggle with it. I mean some people do it all their lives and it does nothing for them, and they waste hundreds if not thousands of pounds [sterling]. (Doug)

> I mean, obviously, diet as in just what your daily intake of food is. But I mean, being on a diet is obviously toning down the beer levels and just obviously staying off the late night chips and all the fatty sort of foods. And all the obvious things that are not good for you but obviously taste bloody nice. And obviously sticking more to salads and getting your five fruit or vegetables a day, and that kind of thing. I mean, basically I've cut down a lot but I can never follow things like the Fat Fighter's diet and the points. (Noel)

Sunshine's weight-loss diet was called a 'food optimizing' or 'healthy eating plan'. Other slimming organizations similarly sell 'long-established dieting practices under new descriptions, such as "lifestyle change" or "eating program"' (Heyes 2006: 129). This repackaging is a savvy commercial decision given the common meanings of the D-word. Andy, a recently returned slimming club member, captured this when he said: 'The word in diet is die isn't it? You may as well be dead cos you look forward to your meals don't you, to your grub?' Sunshine's re-definition was also prudent given the goal of recruiting lifetime members, with the modified diet ideally becoming a habitual possession that is instrumental in weight-loss and then weight management. Nonetheless, men from Sunshine often unreflectively talked about being on a diet even when they had just reiterated the organization's rhetoric and claimed they were not on a diet. For all practical purposes, and in line with everyday definitions, they were dieting. They were on a modified and restrictive diet, albeit with the possibility of some improvisation, primarily to lose weight. Some were frank about being on a diet even though others maintained the organization's definition when attempting to render the experience more sustainable:

Field diary, slimming club: Gareth told me that if you follow the club's guidelines then food intake is restricted: 'You're only allowed a small amount of Cornflakes; a small cupful which works out about the same amount as one Weetabix if you crushed it up.' I expressed surprise, adding that I would feel hungry 10 minutes after eating that. Gareth said: 'Well, you can have fruit with it but don't forget that this is a diet.' I asked whether he accepted the club's re-definition of this as an 'eating plan' but he expressed scepticism. I then asked how he would define 'diet'. He paused for a moment, then said: 'When you say "no" to things you'd like.' On the basis of that definition, Gareth felt that he was on a diet though, as observed later, he openly deferred to other people's re-definition when they distanced the 'plan' from dieting.

In sum, diet can be read as a noun ('I have a diet') or verb ('I diet'). If understood as action intended to promote weight-loss, and which thus includes Sunshine's 'food optimizing plan', reference could be made to three distinct phases: going on a diet, being on a diet and aborting the diet. The following is structured around these processes, or, in a broadened sense, dieting careers. Sociologically, a career is not confined to professions but refers to 'any social strand of any person's course through life' (Goffman 1961a: 119).

Going on a diet: Conditions and 'triggers'

Many conditions and triggers render dieting, as with any weight-loss method, meaningful and reportable. Table 3.1, which structures discussion, lists various factors, though separating these out is an analytic move and heuristic since multiple factors were often consequential. Before unpacking these, I will first clarify the distinction between conditions and triggers.

Conditions are general aspects of the social and cultural environment (for example, a consumer culture that valorizes streamlined bodies, public health discourses). These, and other, conditions are part of a stratified reality where experience is embedded and embodied (also Williams 1999). Conditions could promote an 'affinity' to dieting just as poverty could promote a predilection to types of crime (Matza 1969). However, although important, these do not determine social action and are not necessarily personally relevant. Theoretically, conditions could motivate intentional weight-loss for anybody 'exposed' to them, though relying on this 'vertical' explanation would produce an embarrassment of riches. For example, media images of 'bodily perfection' are ubiquitous and over half of men in the UK might be deemed 'too fat' (BBC Online 2007). Dieting is common, but if recent surveys are more or less valid then it is still the case that most men in the UK are not 'trying to be slim' (Crossley 2004: 225).

In clarifying what I mean by conditions, and why I will also explore more specific triggers, it is worth noting the uses and limitations of the *body dissatisfaction* discourse. Dissatisfaction, a conditional experience, is an obvious concern. Richard, a young slimmer from Sunshine, told Gary: 'If I was happy with myself I wouldn't be doing this kind of stuff.' Dissatisfaction is inseparable from the

Table 3.1 Factors relating to men's everyday dieting careers

Conditions and triggers for going on a diet	• General body dissatisfaction in a sizist culture, which is inseparable from the capitalist political economy and masculine domination.
	• The wardrobe effect, i.e. tight clothes.
	• Photographs, for example, being shocked by one's fat, feminized male body.
	• The biomedical health rationale, including: a recent medical, being labelled obese, 'healthy' prejudice, clinical (mis)diagnosis and an unrelenting doctor.
	• Significant females, for example a complaining wife, wishing to 'support' or being 'inspired' by a wife who is dieting.
	• Seasonality and licensed future indulgencies, for example lose weight in advance of Christmas or holiday, the New Year's resolution.
	• Media fuelled moral panic, which is related to obesity epidemic psychology and biographical situation.
	• The quest for longevity and revering youth.
	• Stigma (enacted, courtesy and felt) in various contexts, for example the street and university. Also note: parental pressure, sexualities and men's standing on embodied hierarchies, which relates to: limited dating opportunities, the life-course, changes in the household, lack of confidence when among females and 'body fascism' in gay culture.
	• Sanctioning, such as the wife who refuses to have sex unless her husband loses weight.
	• Special social occasions, for example, a forthcoming wedding or party.
	• Divorce culture and confluent love: the 'endless debut' or an 'interpersonal crisis'.
	• Size discrimination in employment and reduced career opportunities.
	• A disabling built environment and body proxemics.

| Being on and sustaining a (modified) diet | • Size discrimination, stigma and general intolerance.
• Desire to 'keep the peace' with one's wife
• Focusing on the positive, such as expanded social opportunities (which are a correlate of closed opportunities for those labelled fat and unworthy).
• Working in the weight-loss industry.
• Social 'support', 'psychological feedback' or 'covert fat oppression'.
• Picturing the unwanted alternative.
• Following a less arduous 'semi-diet' that, for example, permits one's favourite foods, albeit in smaller quantities.
• Naturalistic considerations, namely diminished appetite with ageing.
• 'Ghost' or 'virtual' slimming club membership.
• Slimming clubs and associated rituals, for example image therapy, mutual 'support', the charismatic consultant, manufactured pain, masculinizing male slimmers and the slimming experience, and various vocabularies of sustainability that are intended to minimize feeling deprived (for example, flexibility talk).
• Feeling healthier, even without weight-loss or while remaining technically overweight or obese. |
| Aborting weight-loss diets | • Hunger.
• Stopping smoking, which may have previously been used to assist with weight-loss.
• Illness, which may be attributed to efficient dieting.
• Monotonous, too restrictive and various side-effects.
• Dissatisfaction with the idea of 'body metamorphosis' and the quest for longevity.
• Sense of deprivation, exacerbated by the specifics of particular diets or the delivery of dietetic advice.
• Looking ill, and other people's negative reactions, for example, 'Have you got cancer?'
• Expense.
• The experience of being on a lengthy and often meandering weight-loss journey, especially the frustrating plateau.
• 'Sunshine stealers', or being made to feel worthless by others ever when seeking to lose weight. |

capitalist political economy (Schwartz 1986). In terms of conditions, it could be posited that body dissatisfaction is reinforced and fostered on a massive scale by the 'health-industrial complex' (Oliver 2006) and 'style' industries (Orbach 2006). Such industries increasingly render men's, women's and children's physicality problematic. Here dissatisfaction *could* be attributed to external 'pressures' that tell people their bodies are 'out of shape' and inadequate (though see Bourdieu 2001: 68).

This was discussed by some men who felt they were living at a time when men were under greater 'pressure' to attend to their bodies. After mentioning TV programmes and 'guy's magazines telling you what is right and wrong' and images of men with 'perfect toned bodies', Noel said: 'I think we've probably had it quite easy in the past, and now it's turned around on us. "You've also got to do this!" Whereas in the past it was completely different.' Trevor offered similar words to Gary, again from the perspective of somebody who was not a slimming club member and who distanced himself from the 'truly' overweight. In offering a gendered account he immediately made a politically astute point, though one that glossed over multiple masculinities and femininities that are inseparable from other divisions such as bodily size, age, sexuality and ethnicity. Trevor felt 'overweight men' were perhaps not treated as 'cruelly' and 'harshly' as women, with women facing greater 'pressure' about their appearance than men and 'tending to diet more often':

> I think we live in a society where we have a massively marketed identity just like the feminine marketed identity. We are sold this through news-papers, through radio. It's promoted through television and through images in the popular press, through fashion, through advertising about what we are supposed to look like. Unfortunately overweight men do not fit into that particular construct of what it means to be accepted.

Danny, a 42-year-old slimming consultant, and a generation older than Noel and Trevor, immediately emphasized health risk before mentioning the obligatory aspects of weight-loss. After appealing to biomedical health, he said: 'I think now men are getting more into the fact that they've got to lose weight because of certain statistics and things'. The 'things' referred to his earlier talk about diseases attri-buted to obesity (extreme levels of fatness) rather than the standard statistical measure of overweight and obesity, the BMI, which he rejected.

Reference to general conditions promoting dissatisfaction in its various embodied guises (for example, not toned enough, too skinny, too fat) resonates with social theory, cultural commentary and emerging studies on men's perceptions of their bodies and health. Thus, Simpson (2005) coined the term 'metrosexual' in 1994 when referring to the hyper-commodification of the typically younger male body (note the proliferation of this, with David Beckham serving as an exemplar). Robertson's (2006: 443) research also cites men's talk where emphasis is given to 'marketing' and its effects on men and women's aestheticized 'body projects' (Shilling 2003). Feminists have long critiqued such processes in relation to women, though there is evidence that men have also been regularly exposed to similar influences in various media throughout the twentieth century (Bell and McNaughton 2007, Schwartz 1986). Focusing on women and paralleling Trevor's talk, Bartky (1990: 40) discusses how the 'fashion–beauty complex' ostensibly celebrates women's bodies but how being bombarded with 'images of perfect female beauty [. . .] remind[s] us constantly that we fail to measure up'. Also, in line with Danny's talk, social theorists discuss how health is rendered thematic for everybody. The role of experts in communicating risk (Beck 1992, Giddens 1991) and the ideology of personal responsibility in the new public health (Petersen and Lupton 1996) are relevant here. However, although important and reflected in men's talk, these are sweeping generalizations that are not grounded in empirical data. Among other things, the above does not say much about how people, as embodied subjects, become dissatisfied or specifically 'concerned' about their weight/fatness and their 'vocabularies of motive' (Mills 1940) for going on a diet.

More concretely, dieting could be attributed to 'triggers', defined as something critical and consequential that brings unwanted weight or fat to the foreground of attention. Life is full of competing priorities and concerns but triggers make weight/fat personally problematic, just as illness and pain disrupt the more or less taken-for-granted status of the body and make it 'dys-appear', i.e. appear in a dysfunctional state (Leder 1990). Within late capitalist and male-dominated societies, dispositions to hate fat are deposited 'like springs, at the deepest level of the body' so that with 'a very weak expenditure of energy' symbolic violence 'does no more than trigger' these embodied dispositions in bodies 'primed for it' through a lifetime of interactions 'informed by the structures of domination' (Bourdieu 2001: 38). Stated more simply, people often do not want to be fat because they have learnt to see it as disgusting and, for men, a threat to their masculinity. Hence, if somebody calls them fat, or if they suddenly see themselves as fat, then this will likely spoil their identity if they do not have an effective counter-definition or account. Trying to slim down is thus a predictable response.

The idea of 'triggers' fits with my appropriation of militaristic metaphors to critique militarized medicine, but this concept is also used in sociological research on illness behaviour and people's decisions to seek medical aid (Bloor 1997, Zola 1973). Offering 'horizontal explanations' by relating particular experiences, observations and events to others (Williams 1999: 808), such studies show that it is disturbances in social living, not physiology, that motivate action. In extending the concept of triggers to dieting, I would maintain that these give 'topical relevance' (Schutz 1970) to unwanted weight, i.e. they make weight or fatness thematic and a largely misrecognized source of social dis-ease. When men's accommodation is broken through triggers, and if this misalignment retains topical relevance, then it makes sense under present socio-cultural conditions to lose weight. Various methods are identifiable (for example, surgery, pharmaceuticals, exercise), though diet is an obvious everyday 'recipe for action' (Schutz 1970). Here conditions, which *could* disrupt men's 'size acceptance', become personally relevant. By recounting these triggers, men also justified contrition – their talk rendered slimming accountable and acceptable as a masculine practice.

Some men talked spontaneously about dieting triggers, though current slimmers were also asked why they wanted to lose weight *at that time*. Several triggers were often cited, ranging from the mundane and seemingly trivial – such as tighter clothing, or what could be termed *the wardrobe effect* – to the unusual and deeply hurtful (see below on comments from family). Triggers had sometimes reoccurred over several years, motivating previously aborted weight-loss attempts that were also discussed. For other men, their weight and thinking about weight-loss only recently became relevant, though that was more common among men who were not 'really' fat even though medicine classed them as such.

A recent medical disrupted Ned's previous size acceptance. Ned, who joined Sunshine with his wife, said he never identified with weight problems but was told by a nurse that he was almost obese. Ned found the word 'obese' deeply prob-lematic, 'which swayed me towards thinking about, you know, weight-loss'. Others said they suddenly realized they were fat when seeing a *photograph* of themselves. This empirically supports Crossley's (2004: 242–3) point that otherwise gradual and imperceptible bodily changes may be disrupted, and awareness of weight-gain triggered, through a shock to habituation. Jim, who disparaged his feminized body that was previously kept 'slim' in the air force, explained:

> I came out of the forces. I'd always been slim. Well, slimmish, round about 12 stone in the forces. And then when I came out and I was giving my baby a bath one day in the living room and my wife took a photograph and I didn't have a top on. And when I looked, the photograph, I looked pregnant and I thought 'Shit, that's actually me, do something about that.' So I just exercised a little bit more and a bit more wary about what I ate. But that's the only time when I'd actually had a photograph and I've thought 'There's something wrong with you bonny lad, you're not pregnant. Do something!'

As one might expect, commonly reported triggers reflected and reproduced the general cultural fear and loathing of fatness. This research thus empirically supports social oppression views and politicized arguments from fat acceptance scholars and activists (for example, Brown and Rothblum 1989). In qualifying my analysis, however, I will make two points. First, it would be misleading to state men rationalized dieting by invoking their 'terror' of fat. One contact, Paul, a slimming club manager working in a largely female domain, said he was 'terrified' of regaining lost weight but other men did not present themselves in this light. Second, and more in response to medical sociologists who have critiqued oppres-sion views within disability studies, I have no intention of 'writing out' biology and ignoring how 'real bodies' in the context of 'real lives' (Williams 1999) exert their presence. Even so, and following the discussion on background conditions, many of my data relate to the dissatisfactions and iniquities of living in a sizist, fatphobic culture – something that is 'in' minds, bodies and society and which hit particular men, in particular ways, in particular circumstances. These conditional experiences constituted 'something critical' (Zola 1973: 679) that triggered dieting, though the personal significance of this emergent reality was subject to perception, interpretation and discursive repackaging. As will be seen, fat oppression took many forms and was not always deemed injurious by men who (critically) consented to (not-so-subtle) 'symbolic violence' (Bourdieu 2001).

Following Danny on health statistics and Ned's reference to a recent medical, much could be said about the *biomedical health rationale*. On one level this draws attention to the problems of the body rather than an oppressive society (Williams 1999). However, the health rationale is inseparable from cultural prejudice (Chapter 1) and prejudice itself may be deemed healthy (Fumento 1997). Wann (1998) explains that health arguments provide a commonly accepted, but thinly veiled, rationale for hatred towards fat people. This also finds expression in clinical practice. Some clinicians are sensitive to the needs of larger people, with Big Joe saying his general practitioner was fantastic, but 'fat bigotry' (Joanisse and Synnott 1999: 58) is a problem in medicine and it may result in clinical misdiagnosis and ill-founded advice. This shared reality, and its relation to dieting, is captured by a joke on a US fat acceptance website: 'If I had a gunshot wound, the doctor would blame me for not losing weight and making myself a smaller target.'

When reporting dieting careers, some men complained that their weight was used as a clinical 'fob off' with weight-loss becoming a prescribed panacea for almost any illness. Dom said his blood pressure increased *after* losing 7 stone, while a doctor blamed his weight and advised him to diet. Dom added, with a sense of hyperbole to underscore his point: 'Every time you walk to the doctors, you can have a blocked up nose, and usually their diagnosis is "well you know you're overweight?"' When discussing sizism, Smith (1990) also refers to clinical misdiagnosis. Though this may still obviously trigger dieting, reflecting the sociological dictum that if people define situations as real then they may be real in their consequences. Thus, Ralph fell ill and was told to diet given the presumed role of his weight in causing a heart attack. He complied but later learnt that the diagnosis was wrong.

As indicated in this and other research on men and dieting (de Souza and Ciclitira 2005), plus historical research (for example, Schwartz 1986), the health rationale was consequential. Jim, quoted above when talking about looking pregnant, was obviously concerned about his appearance and volunteered additional talk about his 'man boobs' which, similar to Watson's (2000) male respondents, threatened masculine identity (also, Longhurst 2005a). However, Jim also accounted for his current commitment to weight-loss by citing his high cholesterol and heart attack – aspects of visceral embodiment that also had repercussions for his pragmatic and experiential embodiment (his ability to work and depression) (Chapter 2). Such talk, alongside his weekly public commitment to slimming, had important identity effects. As discussed in other health research, the chronically ill and physically impaired 'may feel under more obligation to present themselves as moral, virtuous; that is, to be seen to be concerned about their health' (Robertson 2006: 442). However, while real in their consequences, the actual validity of these medically defined triggers is questionable and not always consistent with men's own accounts. As reported in Chapter 2, Jim's heart attack and associated biographical disruption was cited as a cause, not consequence, of his current unwanted weight. Hence, seeking to prevent another heart attack by losing weight could more accurately be read as an act of faith or expression of virtue as well as a situationally fitting assertion of masculine control.

When discussing his dieting career Stan also cited his poor health and what Williams (1999) would call 'the problems of embodiment', though I would add that our interview actually began and ended with Stan talking about clothing and his desire to look presentable. Stan's subsequent invocation of health made sense but, similar to Jim's talk, I would subject his words to theoretical, analytical interpretation. Stan mentioned his angina plus impairment when weighing just over 20 stone and their impact on his pragmatic and experiential embodiment: a reasonable justification for dieting, especially when this culminated in his inability to walk upstairs at home and an accompanying feeling of utter helplessness. However, it emerged later in our interview that his impairment was due to gout in both feet and this was quickly resolved following a change in diet and remaining technically obese. Also, in going beyond Stan's account, there is no scientific proof that fat on the body causes angina or coronary heart disease and losing weight makes unhealthy 'fat bodies' healthy (Campos 2004, Gaesser 2002).

While the validity of other triggers could also be questioned, scepticism when considering the biomedical health rationale should be stressed given the seemingly incontestable invocation of health by obesity warmongers. However, although questionable, it was consequential for triggering and/or justifying men's dieting and cannot be ignored. Indeed, medicalization figured in the masculinization of dieting and the re-packaging of sizism and prejudice in more personally acceptable terms. As with Gareth, a professed attempt to regain mobility after an accident plus future health and longevity were acceptable justifications for going on and sustaining his diet. Certainly, his talk negated any possible associations with vain femininity, paralleling men's rejection of vanity in Gill *et al.*'s (2005) research on men's body projects. And, in openly honouring Gareth's account and the identity he intended projecting, I did not question the continuing relevance of his mobility justification even though he walked without difficulty and reported a recent skiing trip. Perhaps more significantly, Gareth cited other recurring and mutually reinforcing triggers: *an unrelenting doctor* and *a complaining wife* (talk about *significant females* was common, as discussed further below). Interestingly, in remaining circumspect about the health rationale, Gareth also questioned doctors' orders but still complied, with the hope of obtaining some health benefits. Here Gareth questioned anticipatory medicine and the imposition of risk with reference to his physical fitness and 'visceral embodiment' (Watson 2000):

> *Field diary, slimming club*: Gareth explained how he came to be on his diet. He said he fell and hurt his knee and wanted to lose weight because the injury made walking difficult. He also said his wife was complaining about his weight and, although his blood pressure and blood sugar were always fine, 'the doctor kept saying I was too heavy. I've always been fit and healthy. Cholesterol was point 6, so a bit high, but apart from that I've always been OK. But he said my weight would affect my health eventually – eventually,

mmm, when's eventually?' Gareth then said that at 53 he, like other men there, were making changes to improve their health 'because we're all getting on, most of us here are in our 50s, and we all like a beer and we all want to do what we can to live a bit longer and healthier'.

Other men mentioned women in their lives and the pleasures of consumption. *Supporting one's wife who was dieting* was a common and highly normalizing vocabulary of motive, and contrasted with older female slimmers in Gimlin's (2007b) research who downplayed the role of their partners in motivating their diet. Men's talk made sense as a gendered script: it conveyed the message that he was selfless and would not normally have bothered with a traditionally female preoccupation. Other men expressed their own personal investments in dieting, with partners perhaps serving as a source of *inspiration*. Paul, who had been 'big' most of his life and experienced multiple triggers for subsequently aborted diets (including a bigoted doctor), went on a diet shortly after his wife first joined Sunshine. This was at a time of year when people often gain weight, with weight lost in advance providing *a license for future indulgencies*. He said: 'She had such a big weight-loss within the first week I thought "Oh I fancy some of that", you know, get a few pounds off for Christmas.' Here Paul justified his planned gustatory pleasures and anticipated weight-gain with reference to seasonal festivity and the quantifiably reducible body. Others, such as Danny, treated dieting as a 'ticket' for guilt-free pleasure before holidaying. Their words expressed what has been called 'metaphors of the ledger' where people claim to have accrued sufficient credit in order to 'deviate' without remorse (Gimlin 2007a: 53). And in relation to *seasonality* and atonement for 'sins', there was also *the New Year's resolution*.

However, it is important not to be distracted by tinsel (Kassirer and Angell 1998). After all, there is the highly publicized medical and government-backed claim that obesity is a 'health time bomb' (UK Parliament 2004): one's health might be fine now but there is a predicted grim future. *Media fuelled anxiety and moral panic* also shaped some men's dieting talk, with the media not simply informing the public about weight issues but engendering 'alarm and moral panic around the nature of the obesity problem' (Rich and Evans 2005: 342). Similar to Jim's talk in Chapter 2, other men mentioned the media (a background condition for dieting). This is also an aspect of *obesity epidemic psychology*, which is disseminated through channels of mass communication (Strong 1990; Chapter 1). This became personally relevant for some men in the context of *their biographies*, rendering dieting a bittersweet form of hope work.

After mentioning media coverage of the obesity epidemic and 'how we are going to have a nation of heart attack victims in the not too distant future', Tim, aged 55, said to Gary: 'I just hope that I've been able to knock a few more years onto my life by doing this now.' Other aspects of Tim's biography were relevant, with his attempt to improve his health recounted using military metaphors. Thus he sought to 'combat' problems with his vision by getting fit and losing weight and realized his ageing body was no longer 'bullet proof'. Additionally, within the same year there were two deaths in his immediate family and his dog died, rendering mortality thematic. Here death was a 'prison guard' rather than a 'hangman' where '[t]he horror of mortality ha[d] been sliced into thin rashers of fearful, yet curable (or potentially curable) afflictions' (Bauman 2005: 317). Other men recognized this mixture of angst and hope among others at the slimming club, with their talk about other men eclipsing the possible suggestion that they were really talking about their own anxieties. Andy, another slimmer in that age cohort, thought his peers were panicking about how long they had left to live. Here dieting was related to *the quest for longevity and revering youth*:

> I would say they're all panickers in there. The men I've seen have all been roundabout 50 plus, late 40s maybe. But 50 cos that's when they realize: 'Shit!' Finally the alarm bell goes: 'The time's running out. I am gonna die. Look at the state of me!' And it's a grasp of trying to get back their youth I think.

Mike also cited youthfulness when discussing his recent diet. For him, dieting was related to pragmatic embodiment more so than normative embodiment. Mike, who was not from the slimming club but was told to lose 4 stone by his general practitioner else he would die, contested that grim definition and said he was more interested in dieting in order to regain his speed at football. For this 41-year-old, dieting was related to his desire to capture what he called 'the old glories'. In short, Mike presented himself as unperturbed and optimistic after a relatively recent whack. Interestingly, he also volunteered the following comment: 'She [my general practitioner] asked if I smoke or drank. And when I said no I suppose there was nothing really else for her to aim at apart from my weight, which, as I say, I know I need to lose some weight anyway.'

Mike and other men also talked about *stigma*. The obtrusiveness of some men's fatness, what Goffman (1968) calls discredited rather than discreditable stigma, meant that *enacted stigma* was more likely than that reported by people with epilepsy who adopt a policy of non-disclosure (Scambler and Hopkins 1986). And, the safety of this prejudice (Smith 1990), which, like the stigma of epilepsy, is based on ideas of social and cultural unacceptability, meant that stigma was even enacted by social subordinates in contexts where one might not expect discriminatory episodes to occur. When Mike was working as a school mentor, a boy publicly declared 'you aint half got a fat belly', though Mike said he immediately offered a witty comeback rather than dieted.

Larger men from the slimming club often mentioned the stigma trigger. Richard, quoted above when discussing body dissatisfaction, was much larger than Mike. This 18-year-old joined Sunshine with his father. He accounted for this not only given his fear of dying young but also by repeatedly enacted stigma (for example, being told by a stranger that he was occupying too much space on the bus). As reported by others, social proximity did not afford protection, i.e. it was not only strangers but also people at close relational distance who enacted stigma. Bernard, when discussing his dieting career, talked about 'friends' who called him a 'fat bastard' when weighing 26 stone and, after describing an episode of enacted stigma from anonymous teenage boys, said this hurt.

For Al, another really big fella from Sunshine, enacted stigma was the real problem. This was unbearable when he was with his family and loudly subjected to verbal abuse in public from anonymous others: 'There was nothing worse than walking down the street with your family and somebody on the other side of the road shouting out "fat get!" Nothing worse.' Al repeatedly experienced stigma and the explicit or implicit message that he should deny himself food. This was a powerful trigger, with Al ultimately deciding to diet after suffering and then recovering from a mental breakdown. Here sizism, similar to the effects of racism and sexism, resulted in 'psychic alienation' or 'psychological oppression' which 'is to have harsh dominion exercised over your self-esteem' (Bartky 1990: 22). Analytically, Al's talk also parallels men's formulation of a 'psychological suffering' discourse when presenting cosmetic surgery as acceptable (Gill *et al.* 2005). Yet, in contrast to men in that study, Al knew that suffering was socially produced. He was also aware that stigma could discredit his family – what Goffman (1968) calls *courtesy stigma* or stigma by association. If these men were being 'shot at' then the gun in question sometimes took the form of a blunderbuss that was public property. As seen in Dom's account when explaining his current diet, this blunderbuss was also picked up and fired by children, scattering shot that injured innocent parties close to the original mark:

> I'm really doing this [diet] now because of my kids. You know? It's as I say, I wish I'd done it years ago to tell you the truth. I know the sort of stick they can get from school. You know? About me being the size I am. 'Oh your dad's a big fat pig!' All this, that and the other. And 'look at the size of your dad blah, blah, blah'. And it hurts them an all so, and at the end of the day it hurts me as well.

When discussing the pursuit of health as a 'public duty', Edgley and Brissett (1990: 259) state that 'interpersonal strategies of intimidation, harassment and stigmatization, have been commandeered as power vehicles'. However, stigma is not always enacted and, following the reference to psychological oppression, *felt stigma* was also consequential. Scambler and Hopkins (1986) define this as a sense of shame deriving from an often-unarticulated feeling of imperfection, though, in the context of fatness, men demonstrating 'critical reflexivity' (Williams 1999: 809) articulated their awareness that this feeling was socially induced.

Lenny mentioned felt stigma with reference to other people's not-always-spoken evaluations, which interacted with other contingencies that triggered dieting. Lenny attributed his recent diet to a confluence of factors, including: his wife's decision to go on the Atkins diet before their wedding, his mother telling him he had a 'tummy' and a nurse who said he was overweight (a definition he rejected). However, felt stigma also emerged in interaction with embodied hierarchies marked by class, gender and ethnicity. Lenny was a postgraduate student in a university department predominantly attended by White, middle-class English women. He was Black and said he felt stigmatized by what he believed to be his peers' evaluations of his ethnicity and bigness – a level of body mass that was related to his sense of masculinity. Albeit jokingly, Lenny said 'shrinking myself down' (losing another 2 stone after recently losing 7 pounds) would render him 'less conspicuous and intimidating'. Yet, similar to Black American men adopting the 'cool pose' (Duneier 1992), Lenny also distanced himself from this 'niggling thought'. He did not 'fear' enacted stigma as such, even though he said 'there's a lot of stigma attached to being Black, being big'. Survivorship was possible for Lenny because he politicized stigma as a product of racism *and* did not view himself as 'really' fat: a view I shared with him (in clothes he looked like a rugby player). He added that he did not really care if he stayed the same weight.

Various family members also pulled dieting triggers. As seen above, Lenny, aged 33, mentioned his mother's remark about his 'tummy'. Other men also experienced *parental pressure*. Victor, aged 31, also first tried dieting because 'I was getting a little bit of pressure from my mum. Because my weight was about 16 or 17 stone. And my mum kept going on about it. So I thought I'd try slimming.' Cooper (1998) criticizes familial pressure. She notes that family members often believe they are acting with good intentions (the recurrence of the health rationale). However, this is objectionable because it is based on unwarranted assumptions about fatness, health and the effectiveness plus safety of dieting. And, it is not just significant females who pull these sometimes deeply injurious triggers. Paul said his father, who was dying from cancer and on his deathbed, urged him to lose weight. This was for the sake of his health and family. For Paul, this comment was 'like being hit by a sledge hammer', though he accepted this in line with his identity as a responsible family man. He had since lost weight and struggled to maintain most of his 8 stone loss. However, there were irrationalities (see Chapter 4).

Family life, which will be elaborated upon below with further reference to complaining wives and associated concerns (for example, infidelity, courtesy stigma, divorce culture), is enmeshed with *sexualities and men's standing on embodied hierarchies*. These hierarchies are more or less significant for men at particular stages in the life course and the situations they find themselves in. Thus, while Big Joe might have appealed to sexual desirability in the context of nightclub security (Chapter 2), Roy initially dieted 10 years previously because he was subordinated in the heterosexual mate market. This was at a time of life when it is expected men would have had an ongoing relationship with at least one serious partner:

> I was in my mid-20s and, bottom line, I never had a serious partner. I wanted to settle down. I wanted to find the person. And the way I was I think pretty much, not much interest to be fair. And sure enough I slimmed down. I had a few relationships, met the one I'm with now. We've been on for six-and-a-half-year and been fine.

Such hierarchies are embodied in the sense that they not only relate to how the body looks to others, but how the man feels about and sees his body. Harry, in his

40s and a single parent, complained about looking 'flabby' and catching a glimpse of himself in shop windows: 'And it doesn't make me feel good about myself. It makes me feel ugly.' This was defined as a problem at that time because he was planning on going to the Glastonbury festival, where he said there would be lots of sexual opportunities. However, Harry's dieting talk, which he generalized (i.e. he did not consider himself unique), was not just related to casual sex but also *changes in the household* (also see Annandale and Hunt [2000] on how such changes are gendered and related to class, i.e. in Britain it is women encountering material deprivation who are most likely to find themselves living without another adult):

> I think weight is a big issue for many men in their 40s and upwards. There's talk of a mid-life crisis and I think it affects a lot of men, especially if they're single. I mean, one in three households is single, so we're talking a lot of people. And it's especially difficult if your body's gone to pot because it's that much more difficult to meet somebody. (Harry, talking informally to me in a café)

Embodied sexual hierarchies were also significant for men, independent of partnerships careers. Danny, like Harry, was much smaller than Roy but he obviously embodied fatphobia. For Danny, simply feeling unacceptable in mixed-sex interaction was a sufficient motivator for dieting. He talked about first dieting given his *lack of confidence when talking to females* in the office where he worked, with diet seen as a means of becoming more self-assured:

> With me being overweight I thought, well, girls aren't gonna wanna talk to me. They're not gonna wanna look at me cos I thought to myself they'll be thinking inside 'ahh, state of him with the big belly and that, ffff, what a mess'. And that's why I basically lacked confidence. So I thought well, no, I can be confident. All I've gotta do is get into sort of healthy eating and that'll bring on a lot more confidence.

Again, this relates to stigma, which may exact a heavy burden even if other people do not directly enact this (Scambler and Hopkins 1986). Danny's talk also parallels men's narratives about their weight/fat and dieting as broached by Robertson (2006), with some men talking about how they felt their body looked to women and their self-confidence.

This subordination of 'overweight' male bodies, an associated deficit in cultural capital and other emotionally abrasive consequences (for example, isolation, loneliness, feeling of alienation), is also a problem for 'big' gay men (Textor 1999). In the mainstream gay community, stigma, whether enacted or felt, may discredit big men as viable lovers and spoil their identities. Hence, gay men may feel especially compelled to lose weight (Grogan 1999). As commented by Barry, who tried several diets, '*body fascism*' is insidious in mainstream gay culture. This was an original source of dissatisfaction when he first came out as a gay man in his early 20s. Employed as a support worker by a gay men's organization, Barry commented how, for young gay men in particular, 'that pressure is like, you have to have a six pack and be thin'. Barry and his partner were part of the Bear community, which, as mentioned in Chapter 2, accepts and admires 'big' gay men. Nonetheless, he added that stigma was still enacted in Bear nightclubs: 'My partner's quite big and he had somebody say something quite nasty to him on Saturday about the size of his belly. And I was just a bit like [incredulous], well we're in a Bears' club, so!' Barry said his partner was dieting, and, while his diet was not directly attributed to this instance of enacted stigma, men trying to become 'smaller targets' could not always avoid being 'shot at' even when in supposedly friendly territory.

Returning to significant females, it was not only Gareth who mentioned his complaining wife. Nikos, a friend from Greece, immediately said 'my wife was squeezing my balls' when explaining his recent, visible weight-loss (though he then went on to invoke the health rationale, with particular reference to getting older and taking control). Several men from northern England also said they dieted after complaints from their wives – what could be called '*sanctioning*' from a 'dominant' partner (Zola 1973). Stearns (1997) notes a historical record of women 'nagging' their husbands about their weight. Married men, at least in the USA, may be more likely than unmarried men to be 'obese' (Sobal *et al.* 2003) but this does not necessarily mean wives are tolerant (also, Joanisse and Synnott 1999). This is not to criticize women, or gloss over gendered inequalities that disadvantage them. Wives may have accepted the medical case against overweight/ obesity and genuinely be concerned about their husband's health, with UK government health promotion also positioning women as 'trouble shooters' (*cf.* Aphramor 2005). This fits with dominant expectations about women's caring role; as discussed by Skeggs (1997: 109), 'incitements to be a caring person' are inseparable from feminine respectability. However, married men complained about this, echoing Edgley and Brissett's (1999) characterization of other people's health 'concerns' as meddlesome. Andy was slimming and after I asked why he decided to slim down at that particular time he said bluntly: 'Getting nagged. She's giving me earache about my size, and what have you.' The 'what have you' referred to a sex embargo.

When visiting men's homes to interview them, some wives wrongly assumed I would 'help' get their men to lose weight. That included Ralph's wife. By all accounts, his previous wife was even more proactive. This 68-year-old told me his now deceased first wife continually badgered him about his weight and diet: 'With being heavy, my first wife, she'd say, "You're too heavy! Don't eat this, and don't eat that!"' Ralph's brother-in-law, Edward, recounted similar experiences. Here *special occasions*, such as weddings and parties, served as triggers that his wife pulled several months in advance:

> My wife will say I'm overweight. 'If you don't get another suit you better start losing weight', or if you've got a wedding coming up. You know?

'You've got to lose a bit of that.' Oh, we're going away next week. We're going away for some do. And we've been promising before Christmas to go on a diet.

Triggers are an emergent property of social relationships and their possible dissolution. Discussing his own dieting career, Campos (2004) argues that *divorce culture* is adversely affecting how heterosexual men view their bodies. The broader transformation of intimacy is called *confluent love*, with intimate relationships only deemed good until further notice (Giddens 1992). Under such conditions, triggers for dieting include the possibility of separation and divorce. Of course, particular men could gloss over relationship difficulties and present their wife as the guilty partner in such narratives, but I would not dismiss the possibility of separation as a dieting trigger. Fred, an informal contact, reflected on his first diet several years previously, when, aged 35, his wife had an affair with a younger man: 'I had to compete with the fact that he was younger and fitter, and I wasn't in the best shape.'

This is obviously a sensitive issue. And when a woman objects to her partner's weight this may have more to do with 'looksism' (Cooper 1998), and managing courtesy stigma, than a genuine concern for his biomedical health. (It could also be read as a situationally rational response to a public slur on her perceived ability to care for her man and thus her sense of respectable femininity.) Danny, the slimming consultant, who worked closely with several men, provided a lengthy narrative during interviewing about one of his member's reasons for joining the club. This revolved around his wife's embarrassment about being seen with him in public, which culminated in her threatening to leave him. A physical trainer told me a similar story about a man who wanted to lose weight early in the New Year. Campos (2004) calls this '*the endless debut*' where (potentially) single people try to maintain a degree of physical attractiveness or acceptability. Here the occurrence of '*an interpersonal crisis*' (Zola 1973: 683) – the possible or actual ending of a significant, romantic relationship – prompted some men, who may have otherwise accepted their size, to diet. This, of course, is different from saying his weight actually led to the crisis or vice versa, though looksism and 'comfort eating' in response to relationship difficulties do not rule out these possibilities.

Size discrimination in employment and reduced career opportunities also triggered dieting. Aphramor (2006), focusing on women, states employment discrimination is a recurrent problem (also Fikkan and Rothblum 2005). Men also discussed this and, as indicated below, it is not just employers but also co-workers who target big fellas. Mac mentioned his workmates, who acted as 'plate watchers' (Grogan 1999). Rather than saying he was hurt, Mac was like Mitchell (2005), the fat activist quoted in Chapter 2, who was 'pissed off':

Field diary, holiday: Mac told me about the problems of eating 'with the boys' he worked with on the oilrig: 'They all sit there around each other, watching what everyone else eats. If you just have a piece of chicken and salad they're like "Oh! Are you on a diet?" "No." "Well you should be!" Or, if you've got chips on your plate, "Aren't you fat enough?"' Looking peeved, he said: 'You've got to, like, justify yourself.'

Lest one assumes Mac's justifications afforded him protection, much bigger guns were also fired at his body. He said he was instructed to lose weight by his employer's doctor during an annual medical. Mac risked unemployment if he did not comply, and so he went on a diet.

Size discrimination in men's employment is noted in the academic literature. Focusing on the geography of fatness, gendered power and space, Longhurst (2005b) refers to McDowell's (1997) study of male merchant bankers. None of these men were 'obviously overweight' and one man 'frankly admitted' that applicants might not obtain work if they were 'overweight' (McDowell 1997, cited by Longhurst 2005b: 253). Contributors to men's studies note similar oppressive attitudes in relation to masculine business cultures and the need to project efficient masculinity in order to 'pass' as competent (Connell and Wood 2005).

Such discrimination works through the class hierarchy. Fred, who first dieted in a context of confluent love, was a men's health worker. Positioned within and embodying a middle-class habitus, Fred had recently dieted because he was involved in an anti-obesity campaign and thought he would not be taken seriously by health professionals. This was a reasonable and realistic definition of the situation that is also reported in Joanisse and Synnott's (1999) qualitative study, which included men working as health professionals. For Fred, going on a diet was thus tied to his occupational credibility and survival. Roy, who was much larger than Fred, and a manual worker, also discussed size discrimination in employment. Roy, a mechanic, said his past success in job interviews depended on his weight (which, as noted, he sought to lose due to limited interest from potential female partners). Discrimination from potential employers was a primary dieting trigger for other men. The following is from a new recruit at Sunshine. Mark hoped his university degree would benefit his career but he claimed discrimination prevented upward social mobility:

> *Field diary, slimming club*: Mark, a graduate in his 20s, complained: 'Discrimination. It definitely happens. I know I haven't got jobs because of my size. I can't prove it but you just know when people go for the same job and they haven't got as many qualifications but still get it.' Looking peeved, he added: 'I didn't go to uni and get myself into a load of debt for my size to stop me getting a better job than what I've got now.'

Given Mark's admission that he could not 'prove' this, it is worth adding that some authors argue there is 'insufficient evidence' to support claims about discrimination (for example, Dejong and Kleck 1986, cited by Saporta and Halpern 2002: 443). However, Saporta and Halpern (2002: 443) add that a US federal court ruled that an employer 'violated the law by refusing to employ an obese individual [hence] it is clear that not only is such discrimination occurring, but it can also be curbed by the high courts'. A more recent case is cited by Campos (2006: 27), with reference to John McDuffy, an Oregon truck driver weighing over 500 pounds, who was laid off work despite only taking two days' sick leave during one year of employment. McDuffy was awarded $100,000 in non-economic damages.

Finally, for some larger men, *the disabling built environment* was consequential. Geographers call this *'proxemics'* or 'how bodies fit into certain spaces' (McDowell 1999: 4, cited by Longhurst 2005b: 254). Difficulties physically fitting in, when repeatedly experienced, sometimes triggered dieting. Mention was made of cramped aircraft seating, buses, cars, public toilets, amusement parks and other spaces. Consider some words from Al when talking about his experiences in restaurants when weighing over 30 stone. Here he spoke directly to the recurrent problem of anti-fat prejudice and being targeted. Al was not denying himself food at the time of these reported incidents but the social and built environments conveyed the message that he should. Given his disabling experiences, Al was now slimming, but he sounded like a fat activist doing harder repudiation:

> *Field diary, slimming club:* I chatted with Al, who complained about the design of restaurants and discrimination that result in social exclusion. Al said he visited McDonald's with family and friends: 'And I looked at the seating and knew straight away I wouldn't fit in there. I had to stand in the corner and couldn't join the people I'd gone there with which was a bit . . .' The dejected expression on his face said it all. He also said the seating was impossible in a supermarket's cafeteria: 'So, I had to sit at this table which had a big sign over it "For wheelchair users only" and some job's worth, who was actually quite embarrassed, had a word with me after she had a complaint off a customer.' Al believed the customer complained out of prejudice towards fat people: 'Because you're an easy target if you're fat. There's lots of prejudice and nasty people. You can't give Black people a hard time, or gay or disabled people, but you can give a fat person a hard time. Because people automatically think you're a glutton or a lazy fat bastard.'

In sum, various conditions and triggers rendered dieting reasonable if not obligatory among men. These ranged from general body dissatisfaction, reinforced with reference to the biomedical health rationale (especially for older men), to proxemics that were pertinent for much larger men. When discussing these, men presented dieting as a meaningful practice that was intended to allow them to 'fit in' and (critically) reclaim masculinity. Dieting promised men, and sometimes their significant others, the chance to become smaller targets in wartime.

Being on and sustaining a (modified) diet

Going on a diet is one thing. Sustaining it is quite another. Table 3.1 (page 80) provides a summary list of various factors that, either directly or indirectly, sustained men's efforts for at least a short time. Again, this section grounds these themes in data and subjects them to a critical analysis.

Size discrimination, stigma and general intolerance were repeatedly pulled triggers for going on a diet and perhaps sustaining one's diet. After all, a biography of fat oppression can become ingrained in 'the remembered body', or what Connell (1995) calls 'the body inescapable', and intolerance does not necessarily stop just because somebody is dieting. Barry made this clear when talking about his partner who was ridiculed in the Bears' nightclub. Nonetheless, these experiences may be attenuated as weight is lost, with men providing an affirmative response to the question 'Do you feel better?' even when losing relatively little weight. Some men said their wife's complaints ceased, with humour conferring a shared sense of critical yet compliant masculinity. Consider Sean's quip. Expressed in a pre-dominantly male slimming group, this struck a chord with other married men who were 'hen-pecked' or 'under-the-thumb' and dieted in order to *keep the peace*:

> *Field diary, slimming club*: It was announced to the group that Sean had lost a stone in total. Sandy asked him whether he felt better for losing it. He quipped: 'Yeah, I haven't got my wife on my back now.' Several of the men laughed loudly.

Joking aside, some manifestations of fat oppression were deeply injurious. For the remembered male body, which had been labelled fat from boyhood onwards, these ingrained experiences sometimes provided sufficient motivation to sustain dieting. As reported in Hepworth's (1999) study, this could result in male 'anorexia'. Less drastically, remaining on a diet meant following a modified diet for life, as with Sunshine's plan. Paul talked about this, with him seeking to maintain most of his 8 stone loss mainly to avoid stigma. Within a minute of our interview starting he said, 'as I lost the weight, things began to change', adding:

> When you're overweight people treat you very, very differently to when you're not. And I feel, as the weight came off, doors began to open, and opportunities that would never have happened previously happened.

Paul illustrated this by *focusing on the positive*. He talked about his new job as a slimming club manager, which he enjoyed. However, things were obviously better because they were much worse in the past: the interview was peppered with references to extremely hurtful and humiliating size discrimination, which occurred when he weighed over 20 stone. It is also significant that Paul made weight control his life's focus by *working in the weight-loss industry*, a 'province of meaning' that became paramount (Schutz 1970). Slimming and diet were thus central to his occupational identity. This helps to explain the sustainability of his weight-loss and later management through diet. Bernard, Sandy's 'big loser', also became a slimming club employee and this helped him maintain his focus. Here slimming clubs were instrumental in sustaining some men's resolve, but that entailed total commitment to the organization. Of course, most recruits had lives outside the club and, as stated by slimmers who were struggling to lose weight, 'life gets in the way'.

Before focusing on the slimming club and organizational efforts to sustain commitment (while leaving profitable space for failure and repeated attempts by fee-paying members), I will briefly refer to life outside that setting. The vicissitudes of dieting may be especially difficult there given various contingencies or 'temptations', though some motivational factors were mentioned. *Social 'support'* was the most important, comprising welcome feedback and encouraging comments on noticed weight-loss. The word 'support' is in scare quotes because, as indicated by fat activists and others challenging fat oppression (Brown and Rothblum 1989), commenting favourably on weight-loss implies there is something wrong with a larger body and weight-loss should be valued. That, of course, is especially insensitive outside slimming clubs when somebody loses weight unintentionally due to illness, or even terminal illness, with an intended compliment not being experienced as such by the recipient (Brown 1989; also see the next section). Even so, for men intending to lose weight, this was interpreted as encouraging and was welcomed. Ned, who had lost just over a stone, valued what he called 'the *psychological feedback* when people notice' (emphasis added).

Again, this was not simply or even about biomedical health. It was about body image or what Vannini and Waskul (2006: 198) call 'body-ekstasis', which they define as 'a liminal moment in which the qualitative and aesthetic potential of one's body is evaluated and re-evaluated'. This is an interpretive act and perceptual/embodied/emotional experience. It refers to how somebody contingently feels about and perceives their physicality in association with (imagined) others. This is understandable because, at a general level, looks matter in a culture where 'body image' has become increasingly relevant for men and boys (Grogan 1999, Grogan and Richards 2002) and where people endorse this during everyday social interaction. As with Mike's son, who attended a slimming class with his grandmother, familial 'support' and 'feedback' were important – just as enacted stigma from a teacher was important in setting him off on his dieting career. Mike, who was not a slimming club member but had dieted, also valued feedback from co-workers:

> People at work were saying [enthusiastically] 'Eh, you look like you've lost a bit of weight!' And I think that is a big factor in any diet. Is the encouragement you're getting and feedback off other people. That could possibly be the biggest thing. Rather than the weight is that people comment that you look different. So again you're back to this image thing. Our boy used to diet. And he loved the fact he could come to us and say 'I've lost 3 pound, I've lost 5 pound.' The encouragement, I think, kept him going.

For Mike, such 'support' was prioritized though ultimately it did not sustain his or his son's commitment. Hence, this might be transiently positive and enabling but it is understandable why fat acceptance scholars call this '*covert fat oppression*' (Brown 1989: 22, emphasis added). It defines moral worth in relation to an ideal that is unachievable for most people.

Men seeking to lose weight, or manage their weight, without slimming club assistance cited other factors that were intended to sustain their efforts. *Picturing the unwanted alternative* emerged as a theme when Ralph talked about his dietary approach to weight management. He said he intentionally ate smaller portions, with the goal of staying around 17 stone rather than going to about 25 stone. This method suited him because it allowed him to eat his favourite foods, such as chips, bread and butter. He favoured his *less arduous 'semi-diet'* over 'strict' diets because: 'The trouble is, you diet, then you stop. Then you go up. You've just got to change the amount you eat. That's my way of thinking.' *Naturalistic considerations* were also mentioned. Aged 68, Ralph said 'semi-dieting' only became possible with *ageing and a diminished appetite*. This contrasted with his past 'man sized' appetite, which he publicly expressed in an unrestrained way. His humorous talk also drew from militaristic imagery where food was compared to explosives, which he eagerly sought without fearing whether or not his younger body would explode:

> When I was younger I would have never have done it [semi-diet] in a million years. When I was younger we used to go into a restaurant, and if anybody left anything I'd be like: 'Oh, I'll have that' [laughs]. Big mixed grill. If somebody said, 'Oh, I've had enough', then: 'Hey, here!' [he uses hands to signify pushing his imaginary plate forward and laughs] I'd go mine sweeping [more laughter]. That's all gone now.

Brad, aged 16, also said he adopted a restrained approach despite his love of take-away food, especially doner kebabs. Because he hoped to lose weight, he said, albeit tongue-in-cheek, that he was following 'a non-kebab diet'. For men outside slimming clubs who identified with 'weight problems', the idea of reducing or avoiding 'bad' foods (for example, takeouts and fried foods) was more commonly endorsed than going on a 'strict' diet.

A middle ground exists between being and not being a slimming club member, which has a bearing on the sustainability of diets. This is *the 'ghost' or 'virtual' slimming club member*. In this scenario, a woman typically attends the club and her male partner, or perhaps son or grandson, follow her diet outside the group's formal setting. (Another theoretically possible variant is the unintentional virtual dieter who follows a modified diet given the gendered division of household labour; i.e. he simply eats what he is given by the woman of the house and perhaps loses weight.) It could be surmised that ghost or virtual membership would more often appeal to men given the traditional sexual division of dieting and the fact that slimming clubs are still mainly attended by women. Watson's (2000: 86) male respondents, for example, refused to go to slimming clubs when urged by their wives because they felt 'they're just for women' and 'if I went I'd be embarrassed'. When reflecting upon this issue and feminists' interpretations, Bell and McNaughton (2007) make an interesting point that connects back to dieting triggers and associated emotions. They speculate that men may 'feel uncomfortable' about entering slimming classes and their 'limited attendance' cannot simply be read as 'a general lack of anxiety about fatness' (Bell and McNaughton 2007: 116).

Even so, some men, who sought to sustain their weight-loss efforts, valued *slimming clubs and associated rituals*. Arthur, a 'true believer' from Fat Fighters, endorsed group therapy sessions where members shared tips and reaffirmed commitment. Again, such data reiterate the importance attached to social 'support', though this value is contingent since Arthur was offered group support in the past by a nurse but rejected it:

> I had a medical when I was 50. He told me to go and see a nurse. And she said, 'Oh, I want you to come to the diet class.' So I asked what was involved. And she said she'd sit there and talk to a group of us. I said, 'A group therapy thing?' 'Why aye, if ya like. Yes.' I said, 'I don't want to know.' I said that I'd done it before and I said that I don't believe in it. Now I do believe in it. Because I've had that many goes and I've actually said it myself, because I've been asked in class, different views on things. And this woman, this young woman, and I turned round and said to her, 'If you stop coming you will put weight back on. I've been there. I've done it. I've walked the walk.'

Therapy is not specific to Fat Fighters or clinical weight-loss groups. Sunshine also offered therapy. 'Image therapy' is discussed further in Chapter 4 with reference to McDonaldized efficiency or putting customers to work (Ritzer 2004).

Mutual 'support' also emerged at Sunshine when members and consultants chatted among themselves prior to and after therapy. And if somebody lost weight and decided to share this information publicly (most did), then encouraging comments were offered. This was intended to make the slimming experience as supportive as possible. Hence, this had a buffering and even shining effect for slimmers who risked abrasion through contrition (Chapter 2). During fieldwork, the warm sense of community, actively generated by participants, was clearly observable. Bernard progressively lost weight and received extremely favourable feedback. For Bernard there was a progressive emergence of a previously eclipsed male body that had been put in the shadows of stigmatized obesity. Like the sun personified, Bernard emerged from the dark and became an extremely bright, happy and vibrant social body. He also 'supported' others with a radiant enthusiasm. However, other members seldom experienced the big weight-losses that he did with machine-like regularity and they felt frustrated rather than full of life (see next section and Chapter 4). His light might have energized some by example but if their own weight did not melt away then his brilliance effectively cast them in the social shadows. Bernard recognized this and he sometimes attended class wearing heavy motorcycle leathers, which gave him a reason to 'opt out' from the weigh-in. He told me he did this intentionally to give others the opportunity to win slimmer of the week and thus obtain the motivating spotlight.

New members often experienced immediate big losses and were upbeat. In a larger society that demonizes fatness, their weekly meetings offered shared hope and promised salvation. The promised panacea of slenderness may have ultimately been a matter of unsustainable faith but there were many 'positive' (or tolerable) aspects to this experience. Before describing some of these – and, in particular, how *the charismatic consultant* was attuned to masculinity scripts or men's sense of agency as men – the importance of critical judgement should be stressed. This is necessary not least given the reproduction of stigma and efforts within slimming clubs to profit from *manufactured pain*.

Paul condemned Fat Fighters, as noted in Chapter 2, for belittling members. He criticized their 'overweight corner' and what he called 'total humiliation' when presenting Sunshine as superior to their rival (which was actually larger and more economically successful). However, Sunshine consultants were not saints: they still enacted stigma, with the aim of sustaining members' commitment and thus organizational viability and profits. As with other 'meddlesome' trades that are ostensibly about 'care and sensitivity', there was a 'vested interest in human misery' (Edgley and Brissett 1999: 179–80). And if members were getting too comfortable, then pain could always be socially inflicted.

This struck me in Sandy's classes because she often tried to make slimming as pleasant as possible. Sandy, unlike Marjorie Dawes from *Little Britain's* satirical slimming club, was not one of those 'crazy diet-group leaders' (Wann 1998: 26) who offended people at every opportunity. Al said: 'If you've had a bad week you're not made to feel as though you've been a naughty boy.' Sandy knew guilt was counterproductive and she openly responded to her members' confessions of dietary misdemeanours with positive words, for example commending their honesty, acknowledging the pleasure of food and the frustrations of slimming, stating the past was the past and members should think about the future. However, this 'emotional labour' (Hochschild 1983) was intended to sustain members' commitment to a commercial organization that manufactured fatness as a correctable problem. Hence, Sandy unavoidably discredited fatness as an unwanted and even abhorred bodily state.

Props sometimes helped with this staged performance, such as smearing greasy food on a mannequin. Sandy would then ask members to visualize what their bodies would look like if their dietary intake was similarly visible. Other props were also used to convey the message that fat was ugly and unwanted for men and women. Some members, such as Al, jokingly reiterated that definition despite complaining elsewhere about anti-fat prejudice from 'nasty people'. Here a teaspoon of sugar was intended to help an iatrogenic medicine go down, though some men were still left with a bitter taste in their mouth:

> *Field diary, slimming club*: Sandy showed the group a hand-crafted ornament with a joke printed on it. After offering a disclaimer – 'men might not like this one' – she read to the group: 'How do you get rid of 200 pounds of ugly fat in one day?' Immediately, Al replied: 'Divorce him!' People laughed. Ernie, who told me 10 minutes earlier about his divorce, which precipitated unintentional and 'unhealthy' weight-loss, then said quietly to me: 'That's a bit of a coincidence isn't it?' His previous narrative gave expression to lingering emotional pain. This comprised a deep sense of loss, isolation and rejection. The disparagement of men's fatness only compounded his discredited identity. The stigmatization of fatness was also reinforced for the

women with some novelty underwear. Holding a large pair of knickers in one hand with the words 'Big is beautiful' printed on them, and a skimpy thong in the other, Sandy said: 'Now we always say little pickers end up with big knickers, now obviously you want to get into these [thong] instead.' Then, directing similar words at the men, she held up a huge pair of underpants with a picture of a happy man exclaiming 'I can see my feet!'

Stigma is basically socially inflicted pain and slimming club consultants reproduced and capitalized upon this pain, albeit with innumerable sugar-coated justifications. The biomedical rationale was an obvious one, as noted in relation to triggers. Sandy used this in her largely male group when eschewing the idea that slimming was about vanity. Here the sustainability of the 'plan' was claimed to be in men's best interests, albeit without reflecting on how the perpetuation of that message solidified the perceived wrongs of fat.

The ongoing significance and reproduction of pain was starkly illustrated when Sandy offered her group a narrative about how suffering usefully motivates 'life-improving' action. Faced with a member who had lost 4 stone but complained about having a 'hungry head on' and unable to break through a plateau (a point where weight-loss ceases), Sandy replied: 'It's because you're content. Now, you need to hurt bad to get a reaction sometimes.' She continued, with implicit reference to dieting triggers: 'When people walk through that door for the first time they're hurting bad.' She illustrated this with a story about her neighbour's dog that yelped and barked at night. Her neighbour said that it was because the dog was lying on a nail and the dog would get up once it had had enough. For Sandy, maintaining regular weight-loss was analogous to the dog that was in pain but was able to move, thus solving the problem. Of course, the story would not have had the same effect if Sandy had told her neighbour that it would have been more humane to remove the nail.

Sandy also conveyed more 'positive' messages in class. These almost had a magical effect for some men. In order to understand this 'hypnotic power' (Bourdieu 2001: 42) that helps sustain symbolic violence, and a larger system of masculine domination, it is necessary to briefly highlight some themes from interviews with male slimmers. These relate to masculinity scripts and other considerations that transcended specific classes and slimming organizations but which the charismatic consultant was attuned to and drew from in class. Sandy did this when talking up the feasibility of weight-loss despite much contrary evidence. A key theme, related to men's 'active differentiation from the opposite sex' and thus 'the pursuit and exercise of domination' (Bourdieu 2001: 49), was *the masculinization of male slimmers and the slimming experience*. This was important given the traditional feminization of dieting and slimming clubs. Indeed, it was common for men to mention their initial apprehensions about entering a slimming club, with some aborting their journey in the car park several times before entering. The masculinization of slimming and male slimmers included the perpetuation of a naturalized sex dichotomy and gender hierarchy. Men claimed to possess, or they discursively enacted, positive masculine character traits, for example being focused, persevering, innovative, competitive, disciplined and regimented. In becoming 'participants in the war on obesity, rather than its denigrated objects' (Throsby 2007), some claimed they were 'target setters' and hoped they were an 'inspiration' to others. Masculine affirming talk, which was intended to make weight-loss seem achievable even when others were struggling, is reproduced below. Bernard, the sometimes leather-clad motorcyclist, framed his weight-loss as being almost like a road race: this involved competition with other men whom he 'overtook' and 'left in the distance'. Of course, competition is a key aspect of dominant or 'hegemonic masculinity' (Connell 1995), with Bernard's investment in this game or 'illusio' clearly constituting his masculinity and social existence (Bourdieu 2001):

> It's certainly successful as far as I'm concerned. The lad who got me to join, I think is currently sitting at about a 6 stone loss. So I've caught up to him, passed him and left him in the distance. The other lad who joined, he was 33 stone. I think the first week he lost 20 pounds, which is like a stone and a half in his first week. Again he's sitting at about a 6 stone loss. I've caught him, passed him and left him in the distance. And I wish I could – I mean I do speak to them and try and encourage them without being overbearing. And try and motivate them to keep going, and no matter how long it takes just keep at it, keep at it. And I mean the tremendous accomplishments them two guys have made losing 6 stone apiece. And I would love for them to feel how I feel now, you know. But for whatever reasons they're struggling, whatever their reasons are they're struggling.

Men's feasibility talk did not always depend on big and speedy weight-losses (discussed further in Chapter 4). Men also talked up the virtues of the 'plan' itself, though, at least for me, such talk was seldom convincing. Yet, regardless of its validity – the proof of the pudding is in the eating, one might say – this feasibility talk had currency for the slimming club and those reaffirming their commitment during interviewing. Emergent themes included the idea that no great sacrifice was needed; the plan was flexible rather than impossibly rigid; there were no prohibitions; there was a large variety of foods that could be eaten; it was possible to lead a normal, everyday life, or at least have the occasional indulgence; it was not a diet, but a 'food optimizing' plan; or if the narrator conceded they were dieting, then it was reportedly better than all those other quick-fix, illusory, counterproductive and risky diets on the market, etc. These *vocabularies of sustainability were intended to minimize feeling deprived.*

These vocabularies were not necessarily effective even when supported by detailed literature (for example, slimming books). Some men at Sunshine felt deprived even though the organization's vocabulary was elaborate and their 'bible' was a detailed resource. As with John, who had been at Sunshine for five weeks; his wife was the arbiter of the plan and she imposed strict dietary restrictions – no take-away food at the weekend and no meat – and these restrictions made him unhappy. He publicly complained about this during image therapy.

Nonetheless, Sandy sought to show them the 'right path' by espousing some 'biblical truths'. She stated take-away food was permissible so long as it fell within the standard weekly syn allowance. Hence, the following reconnects to the role of the charismatic consultant who masculinized male slimmers, offered vocabularies of sustainability and re-affirmed group commitment:

> *Field diary, slimming club*: Sandy asked John, one of only two men in her first group and who was sat with his wife, how his week had been. He told everyone it had been 'terrible', then said, 'I've lost 3 pounds'. Many in the group laughed, and the woman next to me quipped: 'A terrible week? Yet he's lost 3 pounds! I wish I lost 3 pounds in a bad week.' However, it soon emerged that John was not complaining about his weight-loss; rather, he was feeling deprived: 'I didn't have any takeouts at the weekend. She [wife] wouldn't let me. I'm fed up being a veg man. I want to get stuck into some meat!' This was all said in good humour but John was clearly unhappy. Sandy first congratulated John on his weight-loss to date – 1 stone 3 pounds in five weeks – then said: 'You shouldn't feel deprived. You're allowed 70 syns a week. Fish and chips are about 45. If you miss meat, you can have meat. I often have roast chicken or a big bowl of chicken.' Sandy then turned to the rest of the group: 'Men can be very focused and turn things down even if they have a "face on". They're better at doing that than us.'

Here Sandy eclipsed John's point that it was his wife who stopped him from eating what he wanted. Rather than re-affirming his message that his wife wore the trousers, Sandy presented men in general as having more focus and resolve than women when offered food and even when their imagined refusal of food made them miserable. This talk, which relationally constructed dominant masculinity in order to facilitate the (self-)subordination of specific men and women, worked as such. It framed slimming as an admittedly difficult but achievable, self-directed and masculine activity for John while also helping to negate possible guilt among the larger audience of female slimmers by appealing to an essential, homogenous and subordinated femininity. This contributed to the available repertoire of excuse-accounts for not losing weight, or as much weight as anticipated. This is the safety net mentioned in Chapter 2, helping to ameliorate emotionally abrasive contrition. Negating guilt, even when based on sexist assumptions, was intended to make the 'plan' sustainable for both sexes.

Sandy, a charismatic consultant, could be extremely motivating during image therapy. Even though Andy distanced himself from 'therapy' during interviewing, he still considered these sessions motivating. Recently returning to Sandy's predominantly female class, he said ambivalently, 'It's good for the women but I find it quite boring', then immediately added: 'But believe you me, there's something about it. She does a fantastic job and it keeps me . . . because next week I'm going for the slimmer of the week.' Andy did achieve slimmer of the week on more than one occasion. Field observations from her predominantly male class provide additional thick descriptions of how she positively reframed the slimming experience and re-energized her congregation, at least for the duration of the therapy session. Again, the idea of not feeling deprived was central, alongside essentialist talk about masculine perseverance. She also positioned men as being almost like disciplined soldiers who could focus on their 'target' weight and do what was necessary to achieve that. Of course, a larger social reality exists beyond the therapy session. Thus, if most people eventually abort their efforts this says more about the vicissitudes of the real world than the consultant's skills:

> *Field diary, slimming club*: During image therapy some men said they 'picked' on food in the night because they were busy working in the day and bored in the evening. Sandy drew one of the men into the discussion. He lost 3 stone at the slimming club in the past, stopped coming and gained 1½ stone. He explained that when he was on the plan he could go out for a drink in the evening and rather than have a doner kebab he'd have chicken breast without pitta and lots of salad. After Sandy asked whether he felt deprived he said: 'No, I didn't feel deprived. The guy in the shop thought I was mad but it worked out to be really good value because I got loads of chicken instead of having the bread.' However, after stopping his weight-loss plan, 'I'd get the fried rice and chips. I'd have it nearly every night as it saved washing up!' Sandy, in reiterating the idea that there are no prohibitions, commented 'The white doughy pitta bread is a load of rubbish but you can have it sometimes if you count it as part of your syns.' She then said on a more positive note: 'You guys can really set the pace when you put your mind to it and experience fantastic weight-loss.' She attributed this to men being more 'focused on their target' and not feeling deprived when having lower fat and low carbohydrate alternatives. Gareth, sat next to me, agreed that it was no great sacrifice to cut things out when focusing upon their food optimizing plan. This was discrepant with his other accounts about eating out. To me, Sandy's positive outlook and charisma radiated a warming and energizing glow: she talked up the plan and appealed to men's sense of control, agency and self-determination. It made their modified diet seem doable, at least for the duration of the therapy session.

Finally, some men enthusiastically talked about *feeling healthier*. Respondents in and outside of the slimming club who had modified their diet reported improved energy, mental alertness and improved well-being. This was a case of 'emergent dispositions' rather than 'antecedent predispositions' (Matza 1969), which were related to experiential rather than normative embodiment. These benefits provided additional reasons to 'stick with' the modified diet, i.e. having a diet which was often lower in fats, refined sugars and containing more fruit and vegetables. Importantly, these benefits were independent of weight-loss or were experienced while remaining at a weight that medicine labels overweight or worse. And, for some men, such benefits were more relevant than reducing bodyweight. Barry, who went on a 'healthy' diet because he was suffering from minor illnesses and wondered whether 'living a bit on junk food' was depriving his body of vitamins, said how energized he felt within three weeks, adding: 'it's not so much that I'm on a diet to be thin, because I'm not, cos I wouldn't wanna be actually. I'm quite happy being chunky. I would never want to be thin now.' Extolling the bio-medical health benefits and therapeutic properties of a nutritious diet is evidenced in medical literature. Gaesser (1998), a key contributor to the Health at Every Size paradigm, states that a healthy diet, along with exercise, may resolve medical problems (for example, hyperglycemia, hyperlipidemia and hypertension) without weight-loss or achieving a so-called 'healthy' weight. Fat activists, when expressing softer repudiation, and presenting themselves as responsible and health conscious, also talk about their nutritious diets without endorsing weight-loss (Wann 1998).

Aborting weight-loss diets

'Triggered resolutions' to lose weight are contingent and, like the decision to see the doctor even when symptoms are serious, may be 'aborted by the intrusion of new topical relevances' (Bloor 1997: 61). This section considers the defeas-ibility of dietary approaches to weight-loss (and sometimes the intention to diet), both inside and outside of slimming clubs. As will emerge, men often displayed considerable willpower and were willing to invest much time, energy, hope and money in trying to lose weight. However, there were many reasons why 'success' remained a Holy Grail. Again, Table 3.1 (page 80) offers a summary list.

Some men went on a self-directed diet rather than a commercial diet. I will consider this first before moving specifically to the slimming club. For some of these men, *hunger* was cited as a reason for ending their diet. (Sunshine slimmers were instructed to eat an abundance of low fat foods with a high satiety value, and they did not complain about feeling hungry.) Thus, Adrian simply made a conscious effort to eat less. However, while that appealed to Adrian and others, especially after Christmas, hunger was a problem. The unintended consequence was that dieters could end up eating more than originally intended. What is also clear here is Adrian's display of social fitness, with him underscoring his efforts to 'civilize' his appetite (Mennell 1991) in the midst of plenty:

> At Christmas we eat more than we should and we always do – there's always shortbread or a mince pie on the go at Christmas. By New Year's Eve you're sick of food. I am anyway – 'Mince pie?' – 'No I'm all right.' I really truly am. And then you come to January and you're back at work and you're like 'What am I going to have for my lunch? How can I eat sensibly without overdoing it and counting calories?' So you tend not to take sandwiches because there's bread and that's like high content, if you like. You tend to take a tin of something, a tin of soup. I've gone many a time thinking I'll just have soup today. But come 3 o'clock you're like, 'Oh I'll have a packet of crisps.' Why? I might as well as have had the bread. And I think people do the wrong things out of the good that they think they're doing but they're not at the end of the day.

Adrian's last sentence resonated with other men's talk, with weight-loss at any cost becoming a prized yet unsustainable index of their commitment. Before joining the slimming club, Richard, aged 18, said to Gary: 'I tried starving myself.' Richard remarked that he opted 'for a piece of bread instead of dinner, but obviously that did not work, I just put it straight back on', adding, 'if I didn't eat much in the week then I'd end up pigging out by Wednesday'. While Richard's fast could easily be criticized in terms of the impatience of youth, this indicates the degree to which some younger men desperately wanted to lose weight. It also suggests that the imperative to diet provides rationality for binge eating, as reported in research among women (Burns and Gavey 2004).

Mark, in his 20s, also followed a self-directed crash diet before joining Sunshine. Relying on smoking to regulate his appetite and go from 20 to 17 stone, he said: 'smoking kills your taste buds and that really helped me to lose the weight'. However, while Mark wanted to maintain his loss he did not want to continue smoking. Offering testimony to his willpower and sense of responsibility, Mark said he *stopped smoking* once he reached 17 stone, believing he could 'do anything now' but quickly regained his lost weight. The implication was that he would have kept the weight off if this were naturally possible. Unperturbed, Mark said he took other drastic measures. However, *illness, which could be attributed to efficient dieting*, became an excuse-account for aborting his efforts. After saying he went to the gym every day, lived on water, apples and crispbreads and lost a stone, he remarked, 'but I fell ill after two weeks of doing that'. Viewed historically, this martyring of the self compares to nineteenth century Muscular Christianity, especially the practices of the Grahamites (followers of Sylvester Graham, who invented the cracker) who 'liked nothing more than a hearty meal of honey, apples and cold water' (Smith 1984, cited by Edgley and Brissett 1999: 106). As with Germov and Williams' (1996) research among women and discussed further in Chapter 4, such data also show that dieting can be unhealthy.

Alongside self-directed weight-loss regimens, there are many formalized diets on the market. These are termed 'old' or 'fad' diets in Chapman's (1999) research, which, in contrast to the so-called 'newer healthy eating' approaches, are considered temporary. Chapman (1999: 75) mentions various fad diets, such as the Atkins diet, the grapefruit diet and commercial programmes such as Jenny Craig, NutriSystem and Slim Fast. Some men tried and then aborted various diets, sometimes with formal and informal medical approval. These diets were abandoned because they were *monotonous, too restrictive and had various side - effects*.

The Atkins diet was especially popular several years ago. It was touted as the type of diet that men would like because it consists primarily of meats and other high protein and high fat foods, for example, bacon, steak and eggs. Although several interviewees tried the Atkins diet, none sustained it. The monotony of continually eating meat, the avoidance of carbohydrates and side-effects (for example, lack of energy, bad breath, headaches and pains with internal organs) were often intolerable. Only one man, Mike, said he did not experience side-effects after his doctor advised him to try this diet. However, he did not stay on it for longer than three weeks because he found it difficult avoiding carbohydrates. As stated by two other men:

> I've tried the Atkins diet. That sounds great that, 'Oh you can eat meat and everything.' After a week, oh dear me. It's absolutely terrible. Couldn't face meat. You really get sick of eating meat. You know? You really want to have a loaf of bread or something like that. Bread or some form of carbohydrate. I had terrible headaches. (Dom)

> My God, your breath stinks. And that sounds awful but it was really, it was wrong. And, all right, you can eat all this fatty stuff and what have you, but surely that can't be right. But I was definitely losing weight. But it does have side-effects. (Andy)

Bernard also tried then aborted the Atkins diet. He simply said it was 'crap'. Lenny offered a more elaborate narrative. He tried the Atkins diet partly to 'support' his wife but stopped after three days while she remained on it. Lenny also rejected slimming in general, with reference to what he called '*body metamorphosis*'. He defined this as an agonizing process intended to change the body to suit other people. The following extract, which eschews the idea of fast-food gluttony, also fits with 'self-fulfilment' and a sophisticated 'denial of injury' (Scott and Lyman 1968) account that defines health in qualitative rather than quantitative terms. In short, Lenny maintained that *the quest for longevity* was incomprehensible if it meant feeling ill or depriving oneself of the pleasures of a varied diet:

> All I could smell was bacon and eggs in the morning, which she was eating. And it was just repulsive. I couldn't take it. I just couldn't take it. We used to live on the third floor in a flat. And I used to walk up the steps while I was on the Atkins diet and my body just felt weak. And I said to myself, 'Why am I doing this? My body feels terrible.' I just said, 'Why am I making myself ill, just for my body to look slimmer?' And in the newspaper, the other day, there was this guy who just eats pulses in the morning and afternoon. And he looks ill, and he says that he feels really ill. And that's how I felt. I felt like this is what the Atkins diet was doing to me. It was turning me into this guy here. He was confessing it as well, saying that he feels ill all the time, 'But I will live at least 20 years longer than anybody else on average.' And I was like, 'Well, what's the point of living 20 years unhappy, doing this to your body when you could live for 20 years shorter, happy, enjoying food' [laughs]. I don't understand that. I do not understand this concept of putting your body through agony to change it. And it is this whole idea of meta-morphosis. You know, of the body and what the body really means. To me, I'm not really sure about this metamorphosizing my body to suit other people, if I'm happy with it.

Men also discussed other popular diets that they found unsustainable. For example, mention was made of liquid diets such as Slim Fast and the Cambridge

Diet. These entail drinking shakes as a meal replacement – a practice that has historical, if not biographical, longevity in light of George Cheyne's eighteenth century milk diet and recurring 'liquid diets' from the 1930s onwards (Schwartz 1986: 16, 198). Again, liquid diets were aborted and deemed ineffective. Mitch, who tried the Cambridge Diet before joining Sunshine, said: 'It was these powders and shakes, but it isn't sustainable. As soon as you come off you put the weight back on.' Victor, who did not join a slimming club, used Slim Fast:

> I tried it and I didn't like it. I think probably it was the method of it really. Just having these shakes for breakfast and lunch and then going home and having a meal. That was Slim Fast's basic way of doing a diet. You have a shake for breakfast, a shake for lunch, and then your evening meal. It doesn't work like that. If you have your breakfast, your lunch and an evening meal, that's a proper diet.

Substituting liquids for foods exacerbated *a sense of deprivation* and required considerable willpower. Nonetheless, some men reportedly sustained this over a prolonged period. Dom tried a liquid only diet under the instructions of his local hospital and said he persisted for six months. As can be seen, Dom found the diet extremely monotonous and, with just one type of shake that resembled chocolate, he joked that he now felt nauseous at the sight of chocolate:

> I've tried like the Slim Fast thing but that was through the hospital. What they use is stuff called Modifast. With the Slim Fast there's one of these shakes for breakfast, one for dinner and a healthy evening meal. Well this one from the hospital wasn't. It was a shake for breakfast, dinner and tea. That was it. No food. I didn't have any food over six months. And when I got all this stuff, you didn't have like a strawberry super dooper vanilla flavour. Chocolate. That was the flavour. I got six months' supply of chocolate flavoured Modifast. And oh my God. After six months mind, you put any chocolate bar in front of me and I was physically sick [laughs]. Anything with chocolate in you put near me and I was physically sick. And trying to drink a cold pint of that. Horrible. Well it's supposed to be chocolate flavour, but like the word chocolate, that was about as strong as the resemblance got. You know? What a horrible taste it was. It had a little bit of a chocolaty taste but then all the other chemicals that went in would kick in like, you know, you were gagging you know, arrh. Horrible experience that, a horrible six months.

Because obesity is defined as a massive public health problem, one might assume hospital dieticians would be invaluable. Five other men reported visiting these specialists. Only Ernie said their advice was helpful, though he was quickly silenced when talking with Al and Gareth in the slimming club, both of whom were scathing. During interviewing, Al and Andy said they were treated like 'naughty boys' and, albeit with hyperbole to convey their sense of deprivation, were patronizingly given a list of prohibitions with no alternatives. Their talk is interesting given the presumed centrality of dietetics in combating obesity and the eagerness of this predominantly young, female profession to receive approval from patriarchal medicine (Aphramor and Gingras 2008). The following is from Andy, who wanted to learn about the nutritional content of food for health reasons. After taking the time to visit a hospital, Andy aborted his intention to go on a diet because:

> She wasn't credible at all. I got no advice, good advice on what I could eat. What was good for me, what wasn't good for me. I mean I should know, but I didn't. I mean I've always been fed. Men are fed aren't they? I don't look at the values of packets and things like that. And I don't, I know fatty things are bad for me, but certain foods, I didn't know whether there was cholesterol in them or whatever. And I went for advice. And all I'm told is you can't eat this, you can't eat that, you can't eat this. But nobody said 'This is what you can eat and this is a good alternative' or whatever. Now this is a proper dietician that came to see me, that basically frightened me to death. My life ended that day when she said, 'You can't have this, you can't have that and you can't have the other.' And there was no alternative. And I come out and I thought, stuff it. I'd rather die. I wouldn't like, but it's the way I felt at the time. I can't have that any more? Ever? It was a case of no red meat, no pork, no cream, and skimmed milk for the rest of my life. And my choice was a lettuce leaf. That's all you can have for the rest of your life. A lettuce leaf. Do you know where I'm coming from here? She gave me no good advice whatsoever. The only advice was 'don't do that' and 'you naughty boy'.

Before exploring why men aborted slimming club diets (such as Sunshine's presumably more sustainable 'healthy eating plan'), one last theme is worth noting: *looking ill and other people's negative reactions*. This was relevant regardless of what type of reducing diet men followed. Their talk made sense given the lingering sexual division of dieting, where it is assumed men do not diet. This gendered assumption was implicitly made in Roy's town. Roy talked about when he dieted from 28 stone and reactions from local people who knew and apparently accepted him. As will be seen, he aborted his slimming club diet for other reasons. However, if accepted as valid, such reactions are hardly conducive to dieting:

> Six or seven month into the diet I'd lost a lot of weight, it was visible. I'd lost about 6 to 8 stone. You could see it was coming off us. And everyone was like, 'Oh he's got cancer, he's gonna die. Have you seen him recently? There's gotta be something wrong with him. He's, you know, he's lost loads of weight. He's looking thin. He's looking terrible!' I was like, 'No there's nowt wrong with us' [laughs]. You know? But the rumours spread round. And a friend I hadn't seen for a while bumped into me at the shopping centre. And she's like, 'You're losing weight' [hesitant] 'You've got it like?' I says, 'Got what?' She says, 'Why, cancer.' I says, 'No, I haven't got cancer at all.' 'Well, just

you're looking thin and everybody's, you know, the grapevine, people are on overtime.' I said, 'Well they're wrong.' I says, 'It's called dieting' you know?

Although much smaller than Roy, Edward, who was from the same town, reported similar reactions: 'I lost a stone and a half, 2 stone. And like I say, I mentioned me brother-in-law, they all thought I had cancer. Well I just didn't look right.' Edward's brother-in-law, Ralph, also offered a comparable account when recounting his own dieting experiences. Besides living in neighbouring towns, it is worth noting that Edward and Ralph were senior citizens and they had friends who unintentionally lost weight through illness. One friend was subsequently diagnosed with cancer, while another had food poisoning. The idea that men – and especially older men – who have visibly lost weight are ill is thus easily understood when contextualized. This also resonates with men's justifications for rejecting the BMI.

Sunshine slimming club, as discussed earlier, mobilized various meanings in an attempt to sustain members' weekly attendance. These included an explicit distancing of their approach from dieting – proffering a 'healthy eating discourse' rather than 'the discourse of diet' (Chapman 1999). Even so, many members aborted their efforts to achieve a slimmer and presumably healthier and happier life. There were many reasons for this. To assume it was due to lack of willpower would be a gross distortion of the empirical world and would say more about stigmatizing cultural stereotypes than lived reality.

Illness was a recurrent reason for aborting diets. After all, weight-loss does not simply correlate with improved health even when dieting is framed as healthy eating. Certainly, those on Sunshine's 'plan' were not immune to illness, even when losing a lot of weight. Dom, for example, suffered a heart attack after losing 7 stone. Illness and associated socio-economic circumstances then prohibited his attendance at the slimming club and he began regaining weight. Ernie reflected on Dom's situation shortly after his heart attack. In the following excerpt, Ernie also mentioned another 'big loser' who stopped attending Sunshine because the plan became tedious. This was at a time when men's attendance at the club was waning. As it happened, Dom soon returned to the slimming club, showing considerable perseverance even though this was a financial burden and he was depressed:

> *Field diary, slimming club*: Ernie told me about Dom, who has not been at the club for a few weeks. He said Dom has stopped coming and has gained half a stone: 'Because he's not working after the heart attack he can't afford to come. Well, I mean, it's a lot, £5 for him, and another fiver for his wife. He's finding it difficult.' Later Ernie mentioned that there were a lot fewer men attending the club now, compared to when he first joined six months ago. I only counted five men at the club tonight. Ernie remarked: 'Slowly but surely they're dropping out. I saw Big Tom last week. He lost about 7 stone but stopped coming as he couldn't be bothered with it anymore.'

Illness, expense and monotony were thus reasons for aborting triggered resolutions. Some men stated that maintaining motivation during *a lengthy and often meandering weight-loss journey* was difficult. There were many possible U-turns and 'outside influences' resulting in the 'imposition of new topical relevances' (Bloor 1997: 71) that distracted men's attention and energies. Bernard explained as such, underscoring his own masculine perseverance while voicing proxy excuse-accounts for other men who were struggling at the slimming club:

> I think when you're really overweight, no matter how well you do, you've got a long journey ahead of you. Which is the case I'm in. And the same situation those lads, Dom and Al, are in. To keep your motivation going for long periods of time is very, very difficult. Cos there's times in the past where I've not been motivated, and like tired, and like cannot be bothered. And sick of it. And you just gotta stick with it, go through that and come out the other side and just keep going and then lift yourself up. Outside influences obviously play a part. You might have a bad day at work or there might have been some bother in the family. You might be worrying about something. Something's gone wrong. And you can turn to comfort eating quite easily. You know? So obviously it's easier to keep motivated on a short journey than it is on a long journey.

One aspect of the slimming experience, especially problematic on a long journey, was *the frustrating plateau*. This was mentioned above with Sandy trumpeting the value of pain in sustaining motivation and 'breaking through' this sticking point. Even so, sustaining the regimen with little extra reward was not only frustrating but also expensive. As with Roy, he aborted his diet and eventually regained 11 stone. In contrast to Bernard's talk about comfort eating, Roy stressed that his weight-gain was due to occasional indulgencies – an understandable claim given stereotypes of 'obese' people as gluttonous or sad. Roy also attributed his weight-gain to his economically rational decision to leave the slimming club:

> The reason that I left the weight club, I dropped to 17 . . . my lightest was 17 stone, 17 stone 2. And I stuck at 17 stone 2 for about five or six month. And no matter what I did it wouldn't drop any lower. I could not get below that. And if I had the slightest, I'd say fish and chips or one kebab or bit of pizza, something through the week, like I'd put 4 or 5 pound on. And I would have to really hammer it so hard, virtually eat nothing to get that back off again. And I would still just hit that at 17 stone 2 and would not go any lighter. And I thought, 'Well there's gotta be something wrong' you know? I'd done all I could do. And I proved I could do it. I lost the weight and it just stuck and stuck and stuck and I thought, 'What am I coming here paying £5 a week for to lower your weight?' I left the class and that was it. The line was broken. And that was it. And after that it just crept up and crept up and it's like, 'Oh, it's only a couple of stone to shift, oh it's only 4 stone, oh it's 6 and

oh I'm not even gonna look at the scales anymore.' And I'm back now where I was, 28 stone. But by the same count my life's never been better, so.

Given Roy's reference to positive life circumstances (he was now engaged and had a child), he did not consider himself broken by his experience. Rather, this was proof of his determination and abilities. This presentation of self was a gendered performance and contrasts with the identities presented by middle-class, educated, White women in Chapman's (1999) research – women who, despite various privileges associated with their social location, found it difficult viewing themselves as successful and competent (also see Neckel 1996).

Finally, there was the case of still being shot at and *being made to feel worthless*. Despite trying to lose weight, some slimmers were still discredited. After I explained my astral metaphor to Sandy, and how men like Bernard progressively shined like the previously eclipsed sun, she said 'there are a lot of sunshine stealers out there'. She immediately talked about a doctor who chastised a female slimmer who was technically obese but had lost some weight and reported good metabolic health following a more nutritious diet and exercise. Male slimmers offered similar narratives about '*sunshine stealers*'. Rather than this sustaining the diet there was the common view that if people's self-esteem is undermined then they are likely to abort their efforts. Because men often presented themselves as responsible people who were active rather than passive (with many seeking to sustain their current diet), their talk always related to third parties. As with the following excerpt, there was clear hyperbole. This reaffirmed a shared sense that they were sinned against rather than sinners in a cruel and unforgiving world comprising not-so-subtle symbolic violence:

Field diary, slimming club: While attending Sandy's first class I sat in the church hall and talked with Dom and his wife, who told me about a con-descending cardiac consultant who berated Dom for gaining weight after his heart attack. At the end of the class they left and met Ernie in the car park. Ernie then entered the church hall and sat with me and Gareth. Gareth had also just arrived for the second class. Ernie, unaware that I'd previously talked with Dom, recounted Dom's story about the cardiac consultant. The tone, bluntness and hyperbole of Ernie's words gave the story added dramatic effect. The narrative was much harsher than Dom's version as told directly to me, which did not hold back any punches. Ernie exclaimed, 'After Dom told the doctor he'd given up smoking, the doctor said: "Well, you should have your mouth sewn up so you can't eat either. And tell your wife to stop shopping for food as she's not helping you!"' Gareth, listening to this, expressed his support for Dom: 'Ugh! Never mind that he's already lost 7 stone. Putting only 11 pounds on after losing that amount is pretty good going if you ask me. Nobody can complain at that. If you beat people and undermine their self-esteem it's going to make them want to give up and turn to food.'

In sum, this section explored the defeasibility of diets. Themes ranged from basic biological drives, that is, hunger, to 'sunshine stealers' who were seen to instil feelings of inferiority even if the dieter had adopted a healthier lifestyle, had good metabolic health and/or had already lost a significant amount of weight. Men's talk comprised justifications, as in rejecting the idea of body metamorphosis, as well as excuse-accounts, as in appeals to illness, socially produced depression and comfort eating. In exploring talk from men, who often presented themselves as disciplined or 'good' bodies, the above provides some insight into why the 'enabling moment' (Heyes 2006) of dieting is often transitory.

Conclusion: Dieting as a masculine practice

Feminists, such as Wolf (1991), view dieting as the antithesis of masculinity. There is also evidence from sociological research that men consider dieting unmanly (Watson 2000). However, this chapter explored everyday dieting as an acceptable if not obligatory masculine practice and men's (critical) consent to not-so-subtle symbolic violence. In expanding social scientific knowledge in an empirically, theoretically and politically informed way, I reported and analysed men's views about dieting and their dieting careers.

Attention first focused on the embodied meanings of 'diet' and 'dieting', before exploring conditions and triggers for going on a diet, being on and sustaining a (modified) diet, and aborting weight-loss diets. Admittedly, Sunshine did not call its dietary approach to weight loss 'a diet', but members often talked un-reflectively about being on a diet. And some were frank about being on a diet, especially during interviewing, despite organizational definitions and other members' claims to the contrary. Hence, while 'the discourse of healthy eating' (Chapman 1999) may have helped sustain some men's commitment, and ultimately bolster Sunshine's profits, this 'plan' was viewed here as a diet. This fits with everyday definitions because the goal was weight-loss by changing one's diet, with weight management later becoming relevant for elusive slimmers who reach their 'target weight' and hope to stay there.

Even though the 'sexual division of dieting' (Germov and Williams 1996) persists in the UK, and some men might prefer to emphasise physical activity for weight-loss (Chapter 5), dieting made sense for many big fellas contacted during this research – as it has done for men throughout Western history (Gilman 2004, Huff 2001, Schwartz 1986, Stearns 1997). Dieting made sense as an everyday practice, a game or illusio worth playing (Bourdieu 2001), because 'size acceptance' is not always easy or possible among men (just as it is not among many women and children). Men's status as men did not necessarily 'shield' (Hochschild 1983) them from cultural degradation and assaults upon selfhood, and, indeed, their status as men could be threatened by unwanted feminized (despised) fatness. Hence, dieting was, among other things, a means of reclaiming and enacting masculinity. This is in a field of masculine domination that works on the deepest dispositions of the sexually differentiated and differentiating body (Bourdieu 2001). Besides the aesthetic commodification of typically younger men's bodies,

and relative standing on embodied sexual hierarchies, the everyday inappropriateness of men's 'bigness' was reinforced by medically expressed and ratified
intolerance. During wartime men risked, encountered and perhaps personally
exercised what could sadly be considered 'healthy' prejudice (Fumento 1997). This
was towards bodies that might have otherwise been taken for granted.

Varying in its form and impact, but always conveying the message that fat was
bad and in need of correction, this intolerance was discrediting even when
expressed by people who presumably believed they were 'caring' and acting in
men's best interests. This was clear when talking with really big fellas from
the slimming club who encountered flak that also hit their significant others
(for example, children and wives experiencing courtesy stigma). The idea of 'fat
oppression' (Brown and Rothblum 1989) – a second-order analytical and politicized
construct – was thus useful when interpreting men's dieting careers, though
oppression was subject to perception and discursive repackaging. For example,
when framed as ethical self-care, or a means of accruing credit for licensed future
indulgencies, such action was positively aligned with the future and hardly seemed
oppressive (though men expressing such talk also offered deeply hurtful accounts
that conveyed their sense of socially produced inferiority). Oppression was
also mediated by considerations such as the life course, partnership careers, occupation, self-identity, subcultural/sexual norms, ethnicity and place of residence.
In sum, fat oppression was an emergent, contingent and embodied social process
that worked on bodies that were primed for it given their membership of a fatphobic
society.

Importantly, when analysing men's dieting careers, 'real' flesh and blood bodies
were not ignored. Dimensions of biomedical health, improved mobility, physical
fitness and longevity mattered to men even when they explicitly challenged
biomedicine, clinicians, other people's 'healthy' injunctions and emasculating
actions (i.e. critical events that promoted social disease and which could trigger
dieting). Even if male slimmers reported good biomedical health and physical
fitness, many still wanted to be seen to care about their health – usually defined
in terms of improved mortality risk that was assumed to be associated with a
body made slim – and they expressed faith in dieting as a medically sound practice.
More in line with size acceptance, and similar to Health at Every Size, an expanded
idea of health also justified going on and being on a modified diet for at least
one man outside the slimming club (a man affiliated to a gay subculture, the
Bears, which aims to promote safe space for 'chunky' men). His modified diet,
containing less processed food, was endorsed with appeals to the experiential
and visceral in contradistinction to normative embodiment; i.e. a desire to feel
better through nutrition rather than become thin. Nonetheless, while men's
vocabularies of motive were variously framed (and could not necessarily be
taken at face value), sizism and anti-fat prejudice were recurrent themes. There
was also evidence, as with talk about photographs or glimpses in shop windows,
that fatphobia was embodied, with men becoming the active arbiters of a moralizing
and disciplinary gaze. This was in addition to shots fired by other people in public
and private space, including supposedly friendly territory. Analytically, and to use

Shilling's corporeal realist terminology, it could be said here that bodies are not only the *location* of society (which labels certain bodies as valued or deviant), but also the '*source* for the creation of social life' and the '*means* through which individuals are positioned within and *oriented towards* society' (Shilling 2005: 10–11, emphasis in original).

Understandably, most men quoted above were seeking or had tried to lose weight through diet. However, to follow on from Shilling's (2005) point concerning the multi-dimensional character of bodies and the exercise of bodily agency, it is clear that none of these men could simply be characterized as passive victims or cultural dopes. They demonstrated agency, survivorship, emotionally informed insight and critical reflexivity. Indeed, some men embodying marginalized masculinity (Connell 1995) – especially much larger men who were subordinated by other people – sounding like fat activists who challenge social censure. Even so, their resistance was ultimately constrained: in going from repudiating talk to actual contrition, slimming remained seductive for many big fellas, some of whom had been stigmatized from boyhood onwards, with memory representing a key aspect of 'the body inescapable' (Connell 1995). Fleshy bodies might be intransigent but a displayed commitment to slimming promised bodily alignment and social acceptance. It was the path of least resistance and promised salvation when 'the moral burden of obesity' (Jutel 2005), or the weight of disapproval, loomed large. These men thus displayed an acquiescent version of social fitness by dieting – a conservative everyday strategy that could be transiently therapeutic but was seldom sustainable.

All evidence suggests that diets, similar to physical activity (Miller 1999), are not the answer to 'the obesity problem' (Mann *et al.* 2007). Some people succeed, but, as noted above and discussed further in Chapter 4, most struggle just as people who get to their target weight often continue to struggle. Obviously, stream-lined bodies are socially valued; and bodies that repeatedly try to lose weight are economically valuable for the health-industrial complex. Hence, this complex and its allies mobilize various (dis)crediting meanings as 'power vehicles' when trying to sustain people's commitment. This was observed outside and inside slimming clubs and at the borderlands, as with ghost or virtual member-ship. Nonetheless, despite best intentions and (covertly) oppressive actions, sustainability was elusive for men who were unwilling or unable to make slimming their world.

Rather than assuming attrition was due to individual inferiority, in line with sizist stereotypes, attention focused on men's talk about aborting weight-loss diets. Regardless of which dietary approach was used, there were many reasons why men abandoned their diets or intention to diet. Themes ranged from hunger to ongoing fat oppression and these were consequential, or potentially so, among men who were otherwise seduced by slimming. Because these were recurrent experi-ences and are not peculiar to this study, it is understandable why fat activists claim to offer a more liveable approach. That is, an approach that redefines the problem by challenging fat oppression and the industries that profit from and manufacture this on an unprecedented scale. Of course, that may be easier said than done.

The idea of manufacturing fatness as a correctable problem, and what could be called the 'McDonaldization' (Ritzer 2004) of men's bodies, is explored in the next chapter. As well as considering rationalizing processes and resistances, reference is made to irrationalities or unintended consequences associated with the institutional fight against fat.

4   McDonaldizing men's bodies?

Rationalization, irrationalities and resistances

A counter-intuitive argument

The obesity discourse is saturated with attributions of responsibility and blame. As with the movie *Super Size Me* (Spurlock 2004), the fast-food industry and its products are often blamed. This is reiterated in a popular sociology book that is critical of the fast-food industry and the principles underpinning its massive success. Writing about the irrationalities, or unintended consequences, of a rationalized organization like McDonald's, Ritzer (2004: 145) writes: '[t]here is much talk these days of an obesity epidemic (including children) and many observers place a lot of the blame on the fast-food industry, its foods, and its emphasis on "super-sizing" everything'. Within this type of excuse-account, abstracted, homogenized and objectified 'fat bodies' are passive McDonaldized bodies, the irrational consequence of Western rationalization.

There may be good reasons for critiquing the fast-food industry, independent of its putative role in making people fat. However, Ritzer's (2004) account about obesity causation is sociologically unsatisfying and could even be described as an instance of McDonaldized thinking. This is because he reproduces a simplified, bite-sized and efficient account about medicalized fatness. Nonetheless, as will emerge below, Ritzer's (2004) more general McDonaldization of society thesis may still be used as a reference point when empirically exploring the manufacturing of fatness as a correctable problem. That is, when exploring the idea that fatness is an unwanted bodily state that should be remedied. In the following I will also use Ritzer's (2004) broader thesis when considering whether men's bodies, primarily in the slimming club, were rationalized in practice plus irrationalities and meaningful resistances to these processes. In so doing, I will present a counter-intuitive argument where industries that allegedly cause much obesity, such as McDonald's, are formally compared to organizations in the front line in the war on obesity. First, the idea of rationalization or McDonaldization is worth explaining further.

The McDonaldization of society thesis: An embodied reading

Ritzer (2004: 25) describes his McDonaldization thesis as 'an amplification and extension of Weber's theory of rationalization'. For Weber (1930), processes of formal rationality are a key feature of modernity. Exemplified by the ideal typical bureaucracy, rationalization comprises organizational and rule-bound procedures for seeking the optimum means to a given end. While there are many rationalized institutions, with the army being an obvious example, Ritzer (2004) states that the fast-food restaurant exemplifies rationalization. He summarizes the four basic dimensions of rationalization, and McDonaldization, in the context of twentieth century socio-economic developments. These not only include the creation of the McDonald's chain but also mass produced housing and scientific management through Taylorism and Fordism. Centrally, rationalization entails: efficiency (the ability to perform many simplified tasks quickly and on schedule), calculability (gauging success through large numbers rather than quality), predictability (eliminating surprises) and obviating human judgement (an emphasis upon rules, regulations and controlling structures or technologies). In qualifying his thesis, Ritzer (2004: 19) concedes that 'McDonaldization is not an all-or-nothing process; there are degrees of McDonaldization' and other social processes are also 'transforming contemporary society'.

Even so, Ritzer (2004) maintains that McDonaldization is pervasive and consequential. And, while rationalization may be seductive, there are drawbacks – 'the irrationality of rationality' (Ritzer 2004: 27). A mundane example would be the inefficiencies created by the efficient email system: the speed and minimal effort required to write and send emails often create additional burdens for email recipients. An extremely dehumanizing irrationality, exemplifying the 'dark side' of rationalization, is the Nazi holocaust where technically rational means served the ideological, economic and racist ends of a fascist regime. The holocaust was, of course, a frighteningly efficient form of mass-produced death – the industrialization of genocide – that was only made possible by modernity and rationalized organizational structures (see Bauman 1989). Much of this derives from Weber's (1930) concerns about the 'iron cage of rationality' that is experienced as confining, controlling and spirit-crushing. Though, in the contemporary West, a more appropriate metaphor would perhaps be the 'velvet' or 'rubber' cage. Ritzer (2004: 213) states that a velvet cage is not seen as threatening, it is 'nirvana', while the bars on a rubber cage can be stretched. Other metaphors include the idea that the 'constraining consequences' of modernity compare to a snail's shell that is burdensome but also provides shelter (Smart 1999: 10). One consequence is that rationalization is likely to be surrounded by ambivalence.

Focusing largely on the slimming club, this chapter maintains that the rationalizing principles of the fast-food industry, somewhat ironically, inform contemporary fat fighting. Constructing fatness as a correctable problem entails calculability, efficiency, predictability and technological control. Given the biomedical health rationale for weight-loss and other promised 'benefits' like avoiding stigma (Chapter 3), these rationalizing processes are wrapped in velvet and may be more or less acceptable in everyday life. This is because they are intended to 'help' people (risky bodies, bodies at risk) pursue their supposed best interests. Here promissory bodywork may seduce, rather than simply trap, people who want to be seen to be socially responsible and self-caring. Approaching Ritzer (2004) from the perspective of embodied sociology, the following is predicated on the idea that much of what is done to bodies depends on what bodies do to themselves (Frank 1991). That means people may be more or less complicit in rationalization: lived bodies are not only amenable to McDonaldized production but also self-reproduction. Through slimming, people seek self-improvement, happiness and healthiness in 'epidemic' times. Stated differently, and in using Bourdieu (2001), they seek alignment with the structures of masculine domination that are embodied and reproduced through symbolic violence.

Rationalizing processes may be more or less seductive for those battling with their weight. However, as a double-edged sword intended to cut bodies down in size, rationalization also has unintended consequences that critical or 'corporeal realist' studies must recognize and evaluate (Shilling 2005). As discussed below, there were irrationalities associated with processes intended to McDonaldize lived bodies. There were also observable ground-level resistances to irrationalities and resistances to particular rationalizing processes. This is understandable because the 'raw materials' of McDonaldization are not only claims or ideas about objectified bodies, which are being questioned within nascent critical weight studies (Chapter 1). These 'materials' are lived bodies or active agents who are capable of forming alternative definitions of their corporeal situation. Hence, the following also considers embodied and meaningful resistances to McDonaldization, including what could be called 'expressed distance' or 'secondary adjustment' (Goffman 1961a). This occurs when the man 'holds himself off from fully embracing all the self-implications of his affiliation, allowing some of his disaffection to be seen, even while fulfilling his major obligations' (Goffman 1961a: 161). This concept is useful because 'the idea of "resistance" to disciplinary practices [does not] cover what happens when the iron cage of discipline clunks down on the ground and gets bent' (Connell 1995: 61). When using the idea of 'body-reflexive practices', Connell (1995: 61–2) explains there is space for 'manoeuvre' and perhaps humour in everyday life as people qua bodies interact in ways that energize, play with and perhaps challenge socially imposed meanings and categories.

Finally, I should stress that this chapter offers a partial analysis of rationalizing processes, resistances and irrationalities. Readers will probably be able to think of other processes outside of slimming clubs, and critical contributors have commented on some of these, albeit without using Ritzer (2004). Most notably, there is the simplified and efficient calculation known as the BMI. The official lowering of the BMI threshold for overweight in America in 1998 also manufactures fatness as a massive problem. In this context, Oliver (2006: 5) states that the US public health establishment, rather than McDonald's or Burger King, is 'the most important' source of the 'obesity epidemic'. Men's critical understandings of the BMI, which were often humorous and emotionally infused, were broached in Chapter 2 and are elaborated elsewhere (Monaghan 2007).

Calculability

Ritzer (2004) maintains that Western societies are increasingly quantifiable and calculable. This means there is an emphasis on numerical standards, with quantity becoming a surrogate for quality. Calculability, which works in tandem with other aspects of rationalization, is a recurrent theme in the socially organized fight against fat. Far from being a scientifically neutral undertaking, calculability is a socially embedded process that was also more or less resistible among male slimmers participating in the war on obesity.

Mention was made above of the BMI, which Sunshine reproduced in its handbook but which was largely discredited by male slimmers and consultants. Many other dimensions of calculability were also observed during fieldwork and these were more often accepted and even embraced. Similar to Stinson's (2001) ethnography of a US weight-loss organization, calculability was recurrent. For example, members started each session by getting weighed. This preceded the group 'image therapy' session where members congregated and, under the guidance of the consultant, discussed their quantifiable weight-loss efforts and goals. During therapy, Sandy mentioned successful slimmers from her classes, and classes from around the country, who had lost a specified amount of weight, to the exact half pound. Consultants also reiterated to their classes the importance of calculating their dietary intake when, for example, members lost a significant amount of weight – with weight serving as an efficient and inexpensive proxy for fat. Referring to a new member, who lost 10 pounds within two weeks of joining, Judy told her class: 'If you want results like Oliver then you should weigh and measure!'

All slimmers were advised to calculate their dietary intake, or at least 'keep an eye on the little things that add up'. This is because diet was assumed to manifest itself in the McDonaldized body; that is, a body controlled by calculability that may otherwise signify an 'inappropriate' relationship with food (the obese, fast-food indulging and 'out-of-control' body in sizist McDonaldized accounts). The slimming club handbook, which all members received and were advised to read when first joining, listed numeric values for specified quantities of food and drink as calculated by a dietician. These values were also continually updated and revised, in response to the allegedly changing content and availability of foods on the market. This quantitative information was posted on the organization's website and communicated to members in class.

In recognizing degrees of McDonaldization (Ritzer 2004), it is worth noting Sunshine's dietary approach to weight-loss was not only about numbers but also macro-nutritional content. Permitted items were basically divided according to protein or carbohydrate content (colour coded respectively as red and green) with slimmers focusing on one or another particular food group on any particular day. This so-called 'healthy eating' or 'food optimizing plan' was intended to replace a sustained focus on calories or 'points' as was the case with Fat Fighters. Hence, Sunshine's 'plan' comprised calculability but it was wrapped in velvet and presented as more simple and efficient than Fat Fighter's programme. Tim said this informed his decision to join Sunshine, rather than Fat Fighters: 'My wife's been on Fat Fighter things and it's a point system. It didn't really appeal to me, that counting every morsel I put in me mouth.'

Even so, calculative rationality ran through Sunshine's 'plan' like words through a stick of rock. Members did not count 'points' but they were advised to count 'syns' which were allocated to energy-dense items. Again, these numbers were listed in the club's handbook. Experienced members had little difficulty citing and calculating 'syn' values from memory. As seen with Richie, this was related to feasibility talk, which, following Chapter 3, was intended to minimize feelings of deprivation in a field of gendered power and inequality. Richie's reference to alcohol consumption is also worth flagging as a possible irrationality of rationality (drinking a bottle of vodka in one sitting was compatible with a 'healthy eating plan' that gauged success in terms of weight loss), and this was observed in other men's talk, as elaborated below:

> A guy has up to 15 syns a day. So does a woman but women tend to stick to 10 syns. What syns are: they're simply foods with fat in them, saturated or whatever. So if you ate too much of them it would prevent you from losing weight because it's basically the unhealthy part so to speak. That's what I class it as. But it means for myself, for example – I'm a chocoholic – I can have a two-fingered Kit Kat and a packet of Quaver crisps every day of the week and that's less than my 15 syns. That would be about 13½ to 14 syns. Now I have 15 syns a day. So if I was a drinker at the end of the [working] week I have 75 syns. I can go to the pub and have 75 syns worth of drink; 70 syns is a bottle of vodka. (Richie, speaking to Gary)

Following Judy's previous comment on Oliver's 10 pound weight-loss, consultants also advised members to weigh and measure foodstuffs. Consultants often explicitly directed their recommendations to new members and established members encountering difficulties. However, this was inclusive: it was common for those regularly attending classes to either gain weight or not lose as much weight as anticipated, representing a continual source of personal disappointment and frustration (also discussed below). Faced with this, Sandy publicly advised her congregation: 'if your weight-loss is a bit dodgy you may have to get the kitchen measuring scales and jug out and do a sheet listing what you've eaten'. These utensils were also offered as prizes during a weekly raffle alongside digital pedometers, thereby furthering calculable efforts to rationalize the fleshy body and bodywork.

Calculability was unavoidable, but consultants conceded 'nobody sticks to the plan 100 per cent'. This public admission from Judy was obviously framed by organizational imperatives and the search for profits. Referring to continuously weighing food, rather than counting syns, and in rejecting the idea that theirs was a temporary 'fad' diet, Judy advised her group: 'this is a lifelong commitment and it just wouldn't be normal to weigh your food all the time'. Thus, flexibility, or a more 'relaxed' approach, was 'allowed' and even encouraged by consultants who also had direct personal experience of the vicissitudes of slimming. Similar to their shared orientation to the BMI, this could be typified as a 'rubber cage' or 'velvet cage' – rather than an 'iron cage' – with the intention of 'ameliorating some of the problems associated with McDonaldization' (Ritzer 2004: 215). However, bars were still present and even Sunshine's velvet-covered 'syn' system was impractical and restrictive in everyday life.

During image therapy, members complained that counting syns was particularly problematic in restaurants and during other 'food oriented' social occasions. In contrast to the privatized and individualized pattern of McDonaldized consumption, where 'syn' counters had more direct control over their diets, these events meant that departures from rationalized consumption were practically unavoidable. The flip side of rational quantification was that occasions for pleasant conviviality and commensalism (for example, wedding receptions and Bank holidays) became unwelcome barriers to weight-loss that had to be 'got through' by dedicated slimmers. And, for Tim, relinquishing control when invited to have a meal at a friend's home meant that afterwards he felt 'guilty as sin because I have been good for so many weeks'. Though, as indicated above by Richie, creative accounting and planning enabled some to look forward to social events that revolved around food and alcohol: a rationalized approach to pleasure. Events included parties and drinking practices that are risky from a public health perspective but compatible with slimming. Al told me he would 'save' his weekly syns for house parties where he could drink up to three bottles of wine – with one bottle equalling 25 syns.

Clearly, then, in practice Sunshine's so-called 'healthy eating plan' was not free from the irrationalities of calculative rationality. Also, somewhat confusingly, syn values were contingent. They varied depending on whether items were consumed on 'green' or 'red' days. Some complained about this during interviewing and also about what amounted to the contradictions between a weight-loss diet and a healthy diet. Doug, who recently quit the club, said: 'I could never get my head around the syns part of it. To me if it was good for you, you ate it. If it was bad for you, you didn't.' Others, like Dom, admitted: 'it took me about five or six months to actually get my head around the book and actually follow the plan, but I'm 90 per cent there, you know'. Even Bernard, who was called Sandy's 'star pupil' by a female slimmer, said during interviewing (but not publicly during image therapy) that he considered the system complex. He said '90 per cent of people didn't understand the plan' and attributed many people's limited success or failure to this (though, as explained in Chapter 3, there were many reasons for aborting the plan).

Finally, calculability informed various challenges to McDonaldization – the rationalization of resistance. Thus, some men challenged the attribution of health problems and risk to their weight, implied irresponsibility and 'shameful recognitions' which produce 'defencelessness against the external construction of superiority' and inferiority (Skeggs 1997: 123). Following Chapters 2 and 3, men denied injury by citing quantifiable biomedical criteria while still seeking to lose weight given their expressed wish to 'fit in' socially. That included Dom, who lost about 7 stone, then suffered a heart attack. Still weighing over 20 stone,

Dom openly agreed with Sandy in class that if he had not already lost a significant amount of weight then he would probably be dead. However, Dom told me a week later outside the club that he did not think his weight caused his heart problems, adding that his friend died of a heart attack but weighed just 10½ stone. Dom added that after his mother died of heart failure, all of his family underwent medical tests and he had the lowest cholesterol despite being the heaviest. Furthermore, he said his blood pressure increased after he lost several stone, which he found perplexing. Hinting at the interactions between visceral, normative and experiential embodiment (Watson 2000), Dom thought his hypertension was related to the stresses of moving to his current place of residence. This was a socio-economically deprived area where teenage boys smeared excrement on his car door handles and, as noted in Chapter 3, his young children experienced 'courtesy stigma' (Goffman 1968). I visited Dom at his home. The neighbourhood was oppressive: at least a third of the houses on this council estate were boarded up and await-ing demolition. While I could not confirm Dom's reported metabolic health (calculations such as blood pressure), I would not treat his account simply as a 'sad tale'. To do so would be to give consent, through silence, to larger iniquitous structures (Porter 1993) that work on and through socially located bodies. Contributors to social theory and health (for example, Aphramor 2005, Freund 2006) point to the physiological consequences of stress and social inequality, casting a highly politicized light on Dom's words. Dom also smoked 'at least 20 plus a day' for the past 30 years and, similar to arguments offered in critical weight studies, maintained that smoking is a bigger health risk than adiposity (*cf.* Campos 2004). Smoking is again related to experiences of social inequality (Graham 1995) yet such experiences are often ignored within the personally and politically disappointing war on obesity.

Efficiency

> *Field diary, slimming club*: Using a large collaged roadmap of Britain as a prop, and citing Bernard as an example of somebody on the 'fast track' to weight-loss, Sandy told her group it's possible to 'eat your way slim' by following the plan 100 per cent. However, they could also take a 'scenic route' and lose weight more slowly. She added that the club 'gives' members the tools to take whatever route they preferred. Sandy added, in a light-hearted tone, that if they take the scenic route they may also go for a swim in the sea, meaning their weight-loss journey could be as relaxed as they wanted it to be. Stan quipped to those who were sat nearby, 'I've been deep sea-diving.' Another man joked, 'I've been on a detour to the Caribbean!'

Efficiency entails searching for the optimum means to a given end. For fast-food industries, efficiency comprises streamlined work operations, simplified products and putting customers to work (Ritzer 2004: 43–65). As indicated above and discussed further below, efficiencies, or the idea of efficiency, were recurrent themes during this research alongside resistances and irrationalities that were also turned to profitable ends.

Referring to the 'diet industry' more generally, Ritzer (2004: 49) briefly describes its seductive efficiencies by referring to low-calorie food that is often pre-prepared, freeze-dried and microwaveable. These mass produced items are often sold in supermarkets, with some leading weight-loss organizations producing these items, though Sunshine did not manufacture these. In constructing a sense of superiority in a highly competitive market, female consultants told me such items offered little satiety, were nutritionally suspect and were expensive. In short, these women talked up the irrationalities of efficient rationality in order to distance Sunshine from these foods. Danny adopted a different stance. He favoured ready meals produced by Fat Fighters . He often told his group about those products that were on special offer at local supermarkets, along with scripted commentary on their syn value. This was a no-fuss, or McDonaldized, approach to food preparation, though other men did talk about taking time to prepare food for themselves and their families and, in ennobling the mundane, their chef-like abilities (also, see Bourdieu 2001: 61).

Ritzer (2004) also mentions bestseller diet books that promise efficiencies in time and effort. Bernard purchased cookery books from Sunshine. However, although Bernard was an efficient slimmer, he stressed the importance of variety, not efficiency, when discussing food. It should also be noted that these books were not presented as 'dieting' aides given the organizational rhetoric about food optimizing, with 'quick fix' diets defined as unsustainable and counterproductive – a further example of the irrationality of rationality. Interestingly, this was anticipated, countered and turned to productive ends by consultants. In short, awareness of this irrationality meant that consultants underscored the need for ongoing commitment to the slimming club.

Even so, efficiency talk, if not actual efficiency, was recurrent. Sandy enthusiastically told members about the possibility of speedy weight-loss. During interviewing, male slimmers also mentioned 'speed foods' that reportedly accelerated weight-loss, such as pulses, strawberries and mushrooms. Promised efficiency was also crystallized in Sunshine's literature. After describing the plan as 'a lifestyle, not a life sentence', Sandy showed me promotional pamphlets with glossy pictures of appetizing meals and said: 'That's our Success Express plan. It's the fastest way to lose weight.' Thus, even though members were offered the 'option' of taking the more protracted 'scenic route' (the most common route despite people's best intentions), the widely shared ideal was to lose weight quickly. Efficiency was valued and was publicly commended, and rewarded with the 'slimmer of the week' receiving a basket of fruit, which other members, not the slimming club, supplied at the consultant's request.

As indicated in the above ethnography, material bodies are not infinitely malleable and may be highly intransigent. Certainly, 'big losers' like Bernard consistently lost weight and enjoyed slimming, similar to some women interviewed by Germov and Williams (1996). However, slimming is typically a long and frustrating process. For regular members, the common discrepancy between effort and reward provided the conditions of possibility for moments of ironic comedic laughter. Correspondingly, the idea of efficiency was a narrative resource, especially among consultants, for 'talking up' the possibility of successfully losing weight, promoting hope and 'selling' the plan. This sometimes included talk about the physicality of men's typically larger bodies. Danny explained to my slim research associate that men tend to lose weight faster than women because men are bigger. Such talk, sustained in the face of contrary evidence, was obviously homogenizing and treated men as an undifferentiated mass.

McDonaldized efficiency, or speedy results, may have been the ideal. Nonetheless, some male slimmers warned others about rapid weight-loss, which could occur with Sunshine's plan (especially during the first few weeks). According to their cautionary tales, which implicitly rendered inefficient slimming more acceptable for those struggling to lose weight, increased efficiency equalled increased risk. Stinson (2001: 142) notes that such talk helps to make irrational situations understandable, though there is also scientific evidence that these bodily practices are physiologically risky (Ernsberger and Haskew 1987, Campos 2004). As observed during fieldwork, some men, like Ernie, presented themselves as 'well-informed citizens' rather than 'laymen' with a mere 'recipe knowledge' (Schutz 1964):

> *Field diary, slimming club*: Several men were chatting among themselves. Following news about Dom's recent heart attack, Ernie said that Dom did not 'feel well' after losing weight. Ernie then talked about what he considered the massive and worrying dangers of dramatic weight-loss and 'crash' diets: 'It's dangerous, I don't agree with it. In fact I was reading a book on it, and you need to lose it gradually. Your heart and kidneys lose fat and they need to stabilize, along with your muscles. And it takes time. Now, Dom, he lost 22 pounds in his first week here.' Al, who was listening to this, openly agreed.

The organization of classes was also efficient. At Danny's club, members wishing to bypass the usual queue for the scales, and then quickly leave, were efficiently processed through 'express checking'. However, most slimmers queued to get weighed. Sunshine deliberately manufactured the queue. Paul, an employee, told me Sunshine's success depended on members' mutual 'support' (described as covert fat oppression in Chapter 3). The queue was planned because it provided an opportunity for members to congregate and share weight-loss ideas. That, of course, served to streamline the organization's work operations, with members acting as co-consultants. Also, in order to get weighed, members slowly proceeded past a series of staffed desks (mainly staffed voluntarily by members) displaying weight-loss merchandise. This also relates to Bryman's (1999) ideas on 'Disneyization' and the 'dedifferentiation of consumption', i.e. visitors to one sphere must go through another, which helps to increase profits. This obviously provides fuel for a larger machine that constructs fatness as a correctable problem.

Other features of the slimming class complicated the idea of McDonaldized efficiency. Unlike the McDonald's drive-thru, the group therapy session held after the weigh-in was not intended to be time efficient. Many members welcomed this. At £4.25 per session, they wanted 'to get the most' for their money. Yet, as with McDonald's burgers, value for money was illusory. The ingredients constituting this commoditized experience cost very little for the slimming club. This experience included a sense of 'collective effervescence' (Shilling 2003), or ritually derived energy, which emerged during bodily co-presence in morally significant space. However, this experience was not palatable for all. Some members, whom I observed tapering their last few visits to Judy's class by leaving immediately after being weighed, said the sessions were too long. Doug, who recently stopped attending, along with his wife, said: 'I find that particular slimming club goes on far too long. You shouldn't have to sit there for an hour. I mean, I've been getting home late. And we've both said that's enough. You know? It's, it's barmy.'

Slimming classes, and the slimming experience more generally, were nonetheless organized in a way that was efficient for Sunshine. This relates to bodily labour or 'putting customers to work' (Ritzer 2004: 61), which was intended to streamline fleshy bodies but which was actually about streamlining work operations for a money-making business. This is an important aspect of McDonaldization, and it is the last theme discussed here under efficiency.

Putting customers to work enables the fast-food industry to achieve efficiencies and this process was unashamedly put in motion at the slimming club. Just as McDonald's customers have to undertake much of the work that is done by employees in a traditional restaurant (for example, placing a food order, taking it to the table, disposing of the waste), slimming club consultants sought to put bodies to work albeit under a collective ethos that stressed mutual 'support'. Thus, 'big losers', at the invitation of their consultant, played a leading role in manufacturing fatness as a correctable problem. Sandy would sometimes get regular members, like Bernard and Al, to head the image therapy as part of an interactive question and answer session. For them, this unpaid labour was a source of satisfaction – a concrete manifestation of 'enchanted submission which constitutes the specific effect of symbolic violence' (Bourdieu 2001: 41) not only for women but also men who had been subordinated because of the socially imposed meanings of fatness, meanings called into play through 'body reflexive practice' (Connell 1995: 62). Heading image therapy was defined by these men as an opportunity to 'help' others and 'give something back' to an organization that was 'helping them' to lose a significant amount of weight and reclaim masculinity. Other slimmers, forming the so-called 'social team' (Sandy had 38 members on this team), also provided free labour. This work not only included staffing stalls, which Al did most weeks, but also backstage administrative support and greeting new prospective members. This labour was necessary in Sandy's classes, which sometimes attracted up to 80 people per session. Similar to McDonald's customers, loyalty was as much emotional as rational (Ritzer 2004).

In sum, rather than an all-or-nothing process, efficiency or talk of efficiency was more or less observable but also resistible at Sunshine. Instances ranged from promoting fast-track weight-loss to the very organization of the class, wherein fatness (or, more efficiently, weight) was reproduced as a problem to be corrected by members through bodywork. Efficiency was also intertwined in various ways with other McDonaldizing processes, such as predictability.

Predictability

Predictability 'involves an emphasis on, for example, discipline, systematization, and routines so that things are the same from one time or place to another' (Ritzer 2004: 105). Predictability is part of the socially organized fight against fat. However, while fast-food processing is highly predictable, the McDonaldization of men's bodies was less uniform. Consider two extracts. The first is from an interview with Bernard, who, using Sunshine's online resources, systematically rationalized his body and achieved more or less predictable weight-loss. The second field extract recounts a conversation with Ernie, who regularly attended Sandy's class but was unable to predict whether he would lose weight at the anticipated rate of about 2 pounds per week:

> I go online and put in my weight each week. And I've used that as a motivator, because it also gives you an estimated date when you reach your target weight. So it's something to work towards. And if you have a poor week you see that date drifting away in the distance. And if you have a good week you see it coming closer. So it's a good tool that.

> *Field diary, slimming club.* I asked Ernie, who was queuing to get weighed, if he could predict his weight-loss. Ernie said that he could 'really stick to the plan' during the week and 'do well' with his eating but just lose half a pound rather than the anticipated 2 pounds. He joked and said that in such circumstances 'my bottom lip quivers', meaning he wanted to cry. However, Ernie reasoned that slow weight-loss was healthier, reiterating a comment he made the previous week about how losing weight too quickly is a 'shock to the system'.

As with Ernie, predictability thus included predictably slow weight-loss, a case of rationalized inefficiency. Predictability also included accepting the likelihood of a plateau at some point during the meandering weight-loss journey, which, as stressed by consultants, could be remedied through ongoing discipline and commitment.

Other aspects of predictability were centrally organized and observed in the delivery of the class. Danny said about his training as a consultant: 'the training is exactly the same so whenever you walk into any slimming class it should always be the same'. According to Ritzer (2004: 102–4), McDonaldization is often attractive because things become reassuringly the same. He states that fast-food restaurants, similar to the predictable shopping mall, *aim* to offer safe, pleasant environments devoid of nasty surprises. The same could be said about slimming classes though, following Chapter 3, the overt aim of predictable pleasantness had a covert dark side.

In all the classes researched, there was a standardized focus on the positive. This was the common organizational response to members' often-fraught and frustrating efforts to lose weight. As well as the usual motivational talk from consultants, and what one man called 'happy clappy' rituals (i.e. receiving a round of applause when losing weight), there were awards (for example, shiny stickers) and catchphrases that were more often intended for women (for example, 'little pickers have big knickers'). Here fatphobia and sizism, which could also be highly infantilizing, worked in tandem with sexism and the predictable yet covertly oppressive message that some bodies are less acceptable than others. Of course, all of this was coated with artificial sweetener or, to use Ritzer's (2004) metaphor, the iron cage of rationality was wrapped in velvet. This was also evidenced in the classes' decorative style. All had posters on their walls. These featured 'success' stories (members who had lost a lot of weight, but not necessarily maintained this, as reported in local newspapers), graphs showing some members' weight-loss over time and other motivational paraphernalia that conveyed the message that the system was infallible.

According to Sunshine's centralized, corporately produced, script, those following the plan could expect predictable weight-loss. This was intended to be reassuring and rational. In a fatphobic society, fee-paying slimmers wanted to know they would lose weight, i.e. that 'the game was worth playing' and it was worth playing 'right to the end' (Bourdieu 2001: 74). During the induction session at Judy's class, she assured new arrivals that if they followed the plan 'properly' during their first week: 'I guarantee you'll lose weight. If you don't, you'll get your money back. [As an aside] You'll be the first in 36 years to get your money back though.' This was a standard sales pitch. Danny reiterated this to new members in his class.

While new members often lost 'big numbers' during their first week, there were exceptions. Also, as with Ernie and plenty of other members, the expected loss of 1 to 2 pounds per week thereafter did not always materialize. Weight-gain was also common, laying bare the degree to which the 'illusio' and 'the symbolic capital' slimming promises (Bourdieu 2001: 74) were illusory. Somewhat predictably, many members stopped attending. Heyes (2006) reports similar findings at Weight Watchers. Defaulting members also seldom responded to Sunshine's standard 'support letter', which, in Sandy's larger class, was handled by her administration 'social support' team.

Several men mentioned the predictability of inefficiency, difficulty and 'failure'. Such talk became a resource for displaying their own commitment and character, or 'doing' masculinity in the face of insurmountable odds. Again, even irrationalities associated with slimming were put to situationally rational and rationalizing ends, thus reinforcing the McDonaldization of men's bodies at least for a limited period. Difficulties included not only reaching one's target weight but also maintaining it. As with Gareth's talk, reproduced below, an appeal to the visceral served as an excuse for predictable failure in ways that bypassed fast-food gluttony accounts. Of course, as discussed in Chapter 3, there were many reasons why these men, who may have otherwise been fit and healthy, still sought to lose weight even though they knew failure was common. Predicted health problems, as communicated by one's doctor, were relevant for Gareth. However, unlike Ernie's cautionary tale about Dom, Gareth did not mention how common irrationalities associated with slimming, such as weight fluctuation, may also amplify health risk (Campos 2004):

Field diary, slimming club: Gareth, who was struggling to get below 18 stone, thought it was also difficult to maintain weight-loss. He thought this especially difficult for those losing a lot of weight: 'Take Bernard. If he went on holiday he could put 2 stone on dead easy. Your fat cells are just sitting there waiting for you to take in food containing fat and when you do they soak it up'. Gareth explained that the body has 'brown fat cells' which are there to protect the body from famine: 'You have to get to your target weight and stay there for about three years for your body to say "right, we can shut these down now", otherwise you balloon straight up again with a little extra food'. Gareth thought that of the 'thousands of people who come through the door, only a few get to their target weight and stay there'.

Metaphorically speaking, this was a revolving door. Although attrition was high, some former members, like Ronald, returned. This did not mean he or other slimmers escaped ongoing disappointment. Similar to Puritans, slimmers wanted their hard work to 'payoff in this world' and see 'early results in exchange for their strenuous purity' (Edgley and Brissett 1999: 106). If such results did not materialize in quantifiably tangible ways, then predictable emotions ensued:

Field diary, slimming club: Ronald was disappointed. He didn't lose any weight after re-joining the club last week. Sandy asked the group if they had any tips for him, before quipping: 'Last week one of our members said they should have petrol stations where they fill up for you so you don't have to go inside the shop and face a load of temptation.' Ronald stressed that he could resist temptation: 'I mean, we have a vending machine with chocolate at work and I just walk straight past it.' Johnny, his friend and colleague, confirmed this: 'Yeah, I can vouch for that. He even turns down biscuits.' Ronald complained: 'I expected to lose. It's not fair.' Sandy, trying to make light of this, asked Ronald whether he wanted to hit Liz, who weighed him. Liz interjected with advice on getting through the day without succumbing to the temptation of food. However, Ronald reiterated: 'But I haven't been eating that much food!' Sandy, sensing his obvious agitation, said: 'Right, let's get off his case. Everybody give him a big clap!'

Because the numbers on the scales were not as anticipated, and this was not accompanied by a confession of 'syns' consumed and some form of 'remedial work' (Goffman 1971), there were doubts about Ronald's honesty. Sandy often reframed this with other members during image therapy: 'I'm not calling anybody a liar, not at all. But most slimmers have amnesia. They forget what they had. Honesty is the best policy when trying to lose weight.' Although softening the blow, the message was clear: members, not the predictable system, were at fault. Yet, at other times, Sandy's talk confounded simple predictability (for example, 'different bodies burn off energy differently, everybody is unique'). Importantly, such words were offered when supporting organizational imperatives; for instance, encouraging members to personally tailor the plan to their own needs and expectations rather than expecting the club to do it for them. Hence, McDonaldization remained a flexible process that surrounded/constructed vilified bodies and ultimately served the economic interests of an organization profiting from the war on obesity.

In sum, predictability and talk of predictability were observed at Sunshine. Predictability largely fitted with the social logic and practices of a profit-making organization that promised, but seldom delivered, the valued end product: streamlined bodies. And, while there were irrationalities relative to other aspects of McDonaldization, such as predictably slow weight-loss, and predictable disappointment and attrition, even these could be turned to productive ends among current slimmers seeking to maintain their commitment to McDonaldizing processes.

Technological control

Technology is intertwined with the social construction of fatness as a correctable problem, and presumably has special relevance for men who are culturally associated with what has been called the 'Fordist body, symbolised by mechanical metaphors' (Emslie *et al*. 2001: 227). This element of rationalization, according to Ritzer (2004: 15), entails exerting control over people as a counterfoil to human unpredictability. Various technologies serve as tools for advancing the fight against fat, though there are also resistances and irrationalities.

Information technology (IT) – that is, online computer programmes – were noted above when discussing calculability and predictability. Here technology *facilitated* rather than *replaced* some men's weight-loss efforts. Thus, Bernard still continuously worked on his body; human control was not relinquished to technology. For the weight-loss industry more generally, IT has gendered significance when seeking to expand markets; McDonaldization strategically informs efforts to masculinize and sell the gendered slimming experience. Bell and McNaughton (2007: 116) highlight this with reference to Weight Watchers – 'which has been campaigning directly to men since the 1960s, with little success' – and the promotion of an 'online forum' for Australian men. Men contacted during this research reported similar efforts. As stated by Arthur, from Fat Fighters, his club's IT was marketed to men for predictable reasons. Here rationalization through technology was meant to overcome the disappointments of a disciplinary process that was mainly bought and publicly supported by women:

> I've seen others come along to the club, younger lads and they've tried it. They've dropped by the wayside. I've seen older blokes drop by the wayside. And I think it's because they don't like sitting among the women and doing the same thing as the women. They have a tendency I think to treat it as if

it's a woman's thing, this slimming club. I think Fat Fighters have realized that they're not getting the men through the doors. So they've got a website, and they've got a man's programme on there. And they can do the thing through their computer. They believe men will do it, if they are going to do it, that way.

There were other slimming club technologies, besides IT or the actual dietary plan itself. The primary rationalizing hardware at Sunshine, saturated with ambivalence, was the digital weighing scales. Sunshine's scales were capable of weighing the heaviest of members. That was important for Dom, who weighed about 33 stone when first joining. However, there were irrationalities. Dom confided that when he first learned his weight at Sunshine, 'the floor could've opened up and swallowed me up. I was in two minds whether to go back or not'. His experiences had historical and cross-cultural resonance. Ruppel Shell (2003: 40) states that early twentieth century diet books described the weighing scales as a '"materialized conscience" that weighed not only bodies, but worthiness'. This measurement of worthiness is also explicitly mentioned during recent research among women in Finland who were publicly weighed as schoolgirls and humiliated under an 'authoritative gaze' (Rich *et al.* 2006).

Other men had a problematic relationship with the weighing scales. Paul, who was terrified of regaining previously lost weight, talked about his experiences when using his home scales. To provide additional context, Paul peaked at 21 stone before joining Sandy's club with his wife, Liz. Paul had since lost 8 stone but maintaining most of this loss was a daily struggle that was not helped by 'compulsively' going on the scales and feeling disappointed. After giving the scales to Sandy, Paul said he followed the club's recommendation of only being weighed once a week at the club. Surrendering the scales had symbolic as well as emotional significance. It reasserted the centrality of the organization in weighing unpredictable bodies, on the premise that members may feel 'down' about their daily weight fluctuation and regain weight through 'comfort eating':

I'm a compulsive scale hopper. Because I am terrified of getting to the stage I was before, and it's a real, real fear. I do not want to get that big again. So unbeknown to me, what I've been doing is I've been very, very compulsively getting on the scales two and three times a day. So much to the thing where it was hindering me at maintaining. And I started to gain, because I was so intent on keeping these scales happy. I was falling back into my old habits of being depressed. So I was eating. So yesterday we wrapped our scales up and gave them to Sandy. We haven't got a set of scales now. And that was a big milestone.

Such talk empirically grounds critical theoretical commentary on McDonaldization. Following Ritzer, but also Heidegger on technology as destiny and Simmel on the tyrannizing effects of objective culture, Weinstein and Weinstein (1999: 63) discuss how people may feel 'oppressed' and 'humiliated' by technology but also 'appeal to technology for salvation'.

Biomedical technology, which again is obviously not specific to my slimming club ethnography, should also be mentioned. Biomedicine promises individualized technological 'fixes' for 'the obesity problem'. The biomedical conception of human bodies, drawing from a mechanical metaphor, provides fertile ground for the colonization and control of humans by non-human technology. Of course, medicine also has iatrogenic consequences (Illich 1975), that is, medicine may do more harm than good. The remainder of this section briefly notes the promises and problems of bariatric surgery: a technology, which, according to some research, is much riskier than originally thought, especially for men and older patients (Flum *et al*. 2005).

Bariatric surgery is typically performed on people who, according to the WHO's (1998: 9) criteria, are categorized as 'obese class III' (BMI$\geq$ 40 kg/m^2), though Oliver (2006: 56) states that some bariatric surgeons in the USA will operate on people with a BMI of 32. For somebody who is 5'10" that is just under 16 stone. Bariatric surgery is a McDonaldized intervention since the goal is to permanently control somebody's appetite, behaviour and digestion so that weight-loss becomes much more likely and sustainable. If human unpredictability is the major obstacle to certain, predictable and efficient weight-loss then surgery is a rationalized response that is intended to control the recipient's ability to eat what and when they desire. Mennell's (1991) Eliasian discussion on the 'civilizing of appetite' provides social historical context to what could be called the technological rationalization of appetite. This intervention seems rational if 'obesity is soon to become the leading cause of death' in nations such as the USA and '[c]ase series demonstrate that bariatric surgery can be performed with a low rate of perioperative mortality (0.5%)' (Flum *et al*. 2005: 1903). However, epidemiology does not support claims about obesity per se being a major cause of death (Campos 2004) and until recently perioperative mortality rates were unknown for high-risk patients and the community at large (Flum *et al*. 2005: 1903).

Nobody interviewed for this research had undergone bariatric surgery. However, Jason's sister-in-law did and experienced problems. Jason did not elaborate when speaking with Gary, but he felt other people's faith in biomedicine was quasi-religious: 'people see surgical teams and health interventions as the Holy Grail, the saving'. Roy had faith and he was awaiting bariatric surgery on the NHS. This former slimming club member, as noted in Chapter 3, had previously lost 11 stone but regained it and weighed about 28 stone when I interviewed him. Roy considered himself 'fit for the size of us' but he hoped to gain longevity and mobility by losing weight and keeping it off. Roy's concern to 'do the right thing' corresponded with recent fatherhood and his demonstration of social fitness. Importantly, Roy had to demonstrate to clinicians his worthiness for bariatric surgery by losing weight over six consecutive months with the help of a dietician. Replacing (or augmenting) human with non-human technology, at least for some bodies processed by Britain's publicly funded NHS, is dependent upon the ability to exert self-control.

Roy's decision was situationally rational for him relative to what he deemed a low-risk operation: a position mediated through his interactions with clinicians at a time when clinical certainty about low risk was not medically justified. However, there are resistances and, to employ rationalized criteria, these seem reasonable with reference to Flum *et al.*'s (2005) research. As a caveat, statistical evidence concerning the dangers of weight-loss surgery is equivocal and some procedures appear safer than others (Karen Throsby, personal communication 2007). However, Flum *et al.*'s (2005) study among 16,155 patients reported that men had a 7.5 per cent mortality rate within the first year of surgery, with this figure rising to 11.1 per cent for those aged 65 years or older. That said, even before that research, concerns about weight-loss surgery emerged from 'below' from fat activists. Although fat activists are often very fat and conceivably have the most to gain from surgery, they have offered convincing arguments online when warning others (resisting technological rationalization through IT). Contrary to Ritzer's depiction of the Internet as dehumanizing, virtual communities may help forge alternative and more positive definitions that resist fat oppression and associated stigma (Monaghan 2005b).

Resisting surgery is not only an organized political response from fat activists. Andy, who recently rejoined Sunshine after a previous failed attempt, dismissed surgical weight-loss interventions. His words captured the mood of most respondents:

> I don't think any man alive would go through that. No. I tell a lie. There's some that have it really bad that are stuck, that are 40 stone that type. But the average person, average man, overweight man in Britain, would not go to the extent of having that done

That included male slimmers who would be medically classed as morbidly obese but who nonetheless endorsed cosmetic surgery to remove loose skin associated with substantial yet personally achieved weight-loss. Endorsing human over technological control of diet, rather than rejecting surgery per se, fitted with the meanings, practices and interests promoted in slimming clubs. After all, these organizations profit from a behavioural 'solution' to 'the obesity problem'. Rejecting bariatric surgery also fitted well with the current position of successful slimmers and others who were risk averse. Before becoming a slimmer and weighing 26 stone, Bernard toyed with the idea of surgery after seeing 'something on the tele about a guy who'd had his stomach stapled' but he subsequently rejected this technology after losing a significant amount of weight through diet. Presenting himself as a sage advisor for imagined others, Bernard emphasized the importance of a healthy lifestyle, then remarked: 'I don't think these things [surgery and pharmaceuticals] should be for anybody.' For Dom, procedures surrounding surgery were considered dangerous, alongside other 'after-effects' that were explained to him when he enquired at the hospital. After talking about a 10 per cent mortality risk from anaesthesia, Dom reflected on the possibility of postoperative infections, then laughed, 'Oh, we'll give that a miss then.'

Of course, social location shapes perception. Recipients of bariatric surgery, as explained by Throsby (2007), state this entails discipline and hard work.

Nonetheless, for men contacted during this study, weight-loss surgery was often dismissed as a shortcut. It was also deemed an extreme measure, which, regardless of rationalized risks and benefits, was associated with a qualitatively different and not necessarily better life. Big Joe, who was not slimming, clearly articulated this view. In providing additional context to his words – and the irrationality of another bio-technological 'fix' – it is worth noting that Big Joe was not averse to the idea of slimming, given the hopes and expectations of significant others. He previously attempted losing weight after his mother 'bullied' him to try the drug Orlistat, which impedes dietary fat absorption and is medically endorsed as 'an additional weapon in the war on obesity' (Klein 1999: 1063). However, Oliver (2006: 51) ironically states that Orlistat is more of a cosmetic intervention and is 'no different than eyeliner except for the flatulence'. Big Joe experienced no benefits and learnt about the embarrassing side-effects first-hand after an episode of faecal incontinence in public. He quickly stopped taking Orlistat, saying 'it was the worst thing I ever done'. On types of weight-loss surgery, my contact said the following with reference to people who are made to feel unacceptable because of the social meanings encircling and actively ascribed to their weight. Here Big Joe not only resisted technology with appeals to the 'natural'. He also rejected McDonaldized efficiency while adding that reduced meal sizes equalled a reduced quality of life for people who cannot simply be assumed to be unhealthy because of their size:

> This is where they staple your stomach. Nah. Like I said to the doctor, 'If I want to do it, I'm going to do it.' The natural way. The way it should be done. Not all this quick fix thing. Because at the end of the day if it's a quick fix it's going to have a reverse effect, I think. I mean this thing where they put a band on your stomach to reduce your stomach. I mean, it's a case of, what's your quality of life like after you've had it? You know what I mean? And it's, it's, nah . . . I seen one on MTV, *I Want a New Life* or something like that. And it was some girl that they done. And yeah, the results, fantastic. But you think to yourself that she's now got to go through the rest of her life eating minute little things. And she's not going to enjoy herself. She was one of these people who 'I'm not happy because I'm overweight. I'm depressed.' She's one of these people who were walking around with her head down. But I mean you've got to accept yourself for what you are. Some people are big, some people are small. Some people have got ginger hair [which can be especially stigmatizing for men and boys in England]. You know what I mean? You are what you are. And you've got to accept yourself for what you are. And I mean yeah, in some situations it is very unhealthy for people. But I'm sure that's not the case for everybody.

In sum, technology plays a recurrent and at times irrational role in McDonaldizing fatness as a fixable problem but its meanings were also subject to reinterpretation and resistance (or expressed distance). While for many male slimmers, rationalization was pursued through self-directed and less physically invasive technology – namely, the slimming plan, the effects of which were routinely measured through the weighing scales – for other big men, such as Roy, who had abandoned slimming, bariatric surgery was seductive in the context of his biography. Yet, resistance was still strong among men outside slimming clubs, as evidenced by Big Joe, who, like Roy, was one of my biggest contacts and would be medically labelled morbidly obese.

Conclusion: Resisting McDonaldized accounts and processes

Medicalized fatness is often considered the irrational consequence of Western rationalization. The common narrative is that developed nations are awash with convenience foods that are making everyone fat. Despite the critical edge to his work, Ritzer (2004) draws from this picture when discussing the irrationality of rationality. Such reasoning is itself McDonaldized because it is simplified, efficient and seductive. It is also sociologically unfulfilling and questionable. This type of account reproduces the pejorative (stigmatizing) status of 'obesity' while retrospectively denying human agency. Rather than reiterating such thinking, this chapter critically explored the process of manufacturing fatness as a correctable problem and what that might mean among men in everyday life. Calculability, efficiency, predictability and technological control are the central organizing principles of the fast-food industry (Ritzer 2004) and the above explored the degree to which these work around, on and through men's bodies as part of the current war on obesity.

Using the slimming club ethnography as the main, although by no means exclusive, point of reference leads me to the following conclusion: there are many observable, but not universally accepted and effective, efforts to McDonaldize men's bodies. Certainly, rationalization was a recurrent theme. Whether referring to the weighing and measuring of bodies and foodstuffs or biomedical technologies proposing an efficient means of bypassing human unpredictability, rationalizing principles were clearly evidenced. It may seem counter-intuitive to draw a formal comparison between an industry that allegedly causes much obesity and those seeking to ameliorate it, but, in using qualitative data and the idea of McDonaldization as a reference point, this comparison is justified. McDonaldizing processes are perhaps unsurprising in commercial slimming clubs that promise efficient, rationalized solutions to a public and private problem. Counting 'syns', using online computer facilities and promoting 'fast track' weight-loss, in turn, all reproduce the pejorative status of fatness and the ideology of individual responsibility. However, the slimming club was a critical case for considering the degree to which men's bodies were McDonaldized in practice. After all, objectified bodies are also embodied subjects, capable of resistance – or 'expressed distance' (Goffman 1961a) – and forging alternative definitions of the situation. Interestingly, it was found that even in the slimming club, attempts to uniformly rationalize men's bodies and bodily practices were not always accepted. Even in this engine of anti-fat sentiment and sensibility, people were not passive McDonaldized dopes, just as their bodies could not be standardized like the Big Mac.

Amidst observable and generalized rationalization there were subtle variations, complexities and resistances. Rationalization and resistance (or manoeuvrability, secondary adjustment, ironic commentary) were multi-dimensional and uneven processes, even within a specific fat fighting organization like Sunshine. To be sure, many slimmers embraced rationalization; weight-loss can be a panacea of sorts in a world where 'the obese' are stigmatized as irrational and out-of-control and where triggers work on the dispositions of the embodied habitus (Bourdieu 2001, Chapter 3). The slimming club could be considered a potentially revitalizing cult, promising salvation and rebirth within the broader secular religion of health. However, some observations, which rendered McDonaldizing processes contestable and (un)intentionally resistible, included: the common rejection of the BMI; dismissing 'quick fix' or 'crash' diets (while nonetheless following a modified diet that sometimes resulted in massive and quick weight-loss); limited success in losing weight, or maintaining weight-loss, despite proclaimed intentions and sanctions; eschewing streamlined slimming products, such as ready meals; and rejecting biomedical technologies that promise to make weight-loss much easier. Of course, even resistances like these, which, somewhat paradoxically, sometimes made aspects of rationalization more palatable, were often shaped and constrained by the organizational imperatives of an industry rationally seeking profits. For example, slimming consultants were unlikely to promote bariatric surgery when the economics and ideology of their organization revolved around behavioural change. Slimming clubs also risked alienating and discouraging men if they followed or rigidly imposed the BMI – hardly a wise business move!

This chapter not only explored rationalizing processes and resistances, or attempts to ameliorate some of the worst features of McDonaldization as a 'body reflexive practice' (Connell 1995). Reference was also made to irrationalities, the unintended consequences of rationalization. The focus on irrationalities tallies with critical weight studies and also fits with the concerns of sociology, which has a tradition of interrogating the cold, dark side of Western rationalization. Irrationalities associated with attempts to McDonaldize men's bodies ranged from turning commensality into a guilt-laden obstacle to the reduced quality of life that some men attributed to bariatric surgery. Other irrationalities included: viewing foodstuffs in numerical terms rather than a source of nutrition or pleasure; the compatibility of a 'healthy eating plan' and slimming with practices that would otherwise be considered risky (for example, in relation to alcohol); perpetuating an oversimplified, or misleading, picture of what determines health; feeling ill when rapidly losing weight; gaining weight despite investments in time, energy and money in becoming slimmer; etc.

Given the above, and extending my critical analysis presented in preceding chapters, there is clearly a need to exercise healthy scepticism when researching this field and seeking to promote productive dialogue among those genuinely interested in public health. Certainly, it is extremely problematic to claim dieting is possible and desirable as a collective good. And, even when weight-loss diets are wrapped in velvet and repackaged under a different name, as with Sunshine's plan, achieved slimness often remains a Holy Grail. Efforts to cut the body down in size may also be a Faustian myth given physiological harms and possible early mortality associated not only with dieting, but also pharmaceuticals and surgery (Campos 2004, Flum *et al.* 2005). Even so, and whatever method is used, weight-loss remains a highly valued goal that literally millions of people pursue regardless of the resources needed to do that and possible risks to the physical and social body. This sacrificial action, although critiqued here as an irrationality of rationality, often makes sense for women *and* men who embody fatphobia and seek to avoid being 'shot down' in a society where war has been declared on obesity.

In line with common accounts about obesity causation and correction, dieting is just one part of the equation. There are other everyday efforts to lose weight, framed as individual 'lifestyle choices', which may fit better with men's identities. The next chapter considers men's talk about physical activity, weight-loss and health alongside reference to public health campaigns seeking to fight obesity through physical activity. While talk about such campaigns enabled some men to present a conformist model of masculinity, men also displayed social fitness in other ways. Similar to repudiation, these sometimes entailed challenging the dominant biomedical view concerning the relationships between weight/fat, health, physical activity and personal responsibility.

5 Physical activity and obesity fighting campaigns

Men's critical talk

Physical fitness, social fitness and resistance

Physical activity is officially being touted as a 'kind of medicine' (Gard and Wright 2005: 57) for the 'disease' known as obesity and the epidemic of 'excess' weight. However, as already explained, science provides a soft basis for this rationalized, medicalized prescription. For example, there are serious questions concerning whether populations are in fact more sedentary than in the past. Indeed, as well as doubts about whether people are consuming more calories (UK Parliament 2004) there is empirical uncertainty concerning whether the so-called 'obesity crisis' is actually caused by physical inactivity (Gard 2003, Keith *et al.* 2006). Also, systematic reviews of weight-loss research show that exercise, similar to dieting, is ineffective for losing weight and keeping it off for most people who try (Miller 1999). And, burgeoning critical weight studies, in accord with exercise physiology and the Health at Every Size paradigm, maintain that moderate physical activity may improve metabolic fitness independent of weight-control (Campos 2004, Campos *et al.* 2006b). Chapter 1 stated that there is evidence that cardiorespiratory fitness is more important than fatness or body mass for metabolic health, morbidity and mortality risk (Blair and Brodney 1999, Lee *et al.* 1999). More broadly, these benefits are not distributed equally through populations. Socio-economic status is far more significant for health and illness than 'lifestyle choices' that are indebted to social structure (Marmot 2004, Scambler 2002). And there are more experiential dimensions of health which might be 'ephemeral' but are 'perhaps more crucial' for people than 'biological markers' and 'relative risk' (Edgley and Brissett 1990: 271).

Authoritative public health recommendations to embrace physical activity, in order to lose weight and become healthy by virtue of weight lost, are thus highly questionable on numerous grounds. However, given a complex set of social, cultural, political, economic and historically transmitted reasons (Chapter 1), everyday bodily bigness is routinely discredited as unhealthy fatness. In 'epidemic' times overweight/obesity/fatness must be rationally corrected or, in line with militarized medicine, obliterated. This manufactured intolerance, and the perpetuation of 'shameful recognitions' (Skeggs 1997), is routinely sustained using dichotomous reasoning and violent imagery. As observed within exercise physiology literature, fatness is framed as the 'polar opposite' of fitness, with physical activity constituting 'another weapon in the arsenal with which we [are] attacking obesity' (Gaesser 2002: 48). The media reiterate this strategically offensive message, with men's presumably sedentary and risky bodies also caught within the cross-hair of fat hatred. Referring to men's intra-abdominal obesity, Zimmerman (2006), in association with *Men's Health Magazine*, writes: 'Beyond what you put into your body, the most important thing is what you put out. Exercise remains the best weapon against visceral fat'. Medically and socially valued ends are intertwined with widely approved means. The common mantra for both women and men, if they are to be socially acceptable if not admirable bodies, is 'get fit' and 'fight fat!'

Of course, such injunctions extend beyond obesity science, men's magazines, the fitness industry and slimming clubs (Chapters 3 and 4). Governments also aggressively promote physical activity in neo-liberal societies where individuals are urged to take responsibility for their health and now weight as a 'McDonaldized' (Ritzer 2004) marker of fat and health. This 'top down' exhortation to slim down through physical activity in order to benefit oneself, and also promote the greater good of society, is authoritatively expressed on both sides of the Atlantic. Referring to the Shape Up! America campaign and the Surgeon General's concerns about the nation's physical and fiscal fitness, Herndon (2005: 128) notes that 'being "fit" to be an American means watching one's weight'. The UK government's 'American-inspired philosophy of the "Third Way"' similarly emphasizes individual responsibility (Scambler 2001: 35, 41), with fat fighting becoming a power vehicle for neo-liberalism and depoliticizing healthism. Thus, a government supported organization, Sport England, recently waged war on obesity with its Everyday Sport campaign. This, alongside other anti obesity initiatives, urged people to increase their physical activity in order to help 'kick start the fight against rocketing obesity levels' (Everyday Sport 2004).

This chapter refers to, but also moves beyond, campaigns like Everyday Sport that gave concrete expression to institutional sizism. Theoretically and politically, I will again challenge rationalized/medicalized/militarized discourses that perpetuate fat hatred. Rather than positioning the overweight/obese/fat body as an object to be fought and made compliant, I will extend and complement the analysis presented in earlier chapters by exploring further the social construction of personhood as a gendered practical accomplishment – what Cahill (1998: 135) calls 'the socially defined, publicly visible person'. To this end, empirical attention focuses on men's critical talk about physical activity vis-à-vis slimming, physical fitness, 'health' and the presentation of socially fitting masculine selves/bodies.

While men embodied various versions of social fitness, or situationally appropriate displays of gendered selfhood, this chapter details one common mode of accountability: the justifiably resistant and defiant. Men voicing this did not always resist the idea of embracing physical activity, or more formal exercise, nor did they necessarily reject the importance of health (comprising various dimensions of embodiment, ranging from the visceral to the emotional). Many men were also slimming or had tried to lose weight in the past. However, these men resisted the idea of getting physically active in order to lose weight/fat, or the idea that physical fitness ensures better health or that people routinely disparaged because of the size/weight/shape/composition of their bodies necessarily lack physical fitness and/or can be assumed to be unhealthy. In short, these men challenged streamlined 'health promotion' messages when bolstering masculine identities and resisting not-so-subtle symbolic violence that could discredit them and/or other 'big' people in a field of masculine domination.

Displaying social fitness: Some common types

The idea that people should embrace physical activity to lose weight is ubiquitous. For example, at the time of this study, Sport England, a government-backed organization funded by exchequer and lottery funds, offered a public call to fight obesity with its Everyday Sport campaign. Piloted in north-east England, Everyday Sport implicated sedentary living with the putatively costly obesity epidemic. It urged people to become more active in order to burn calories, improve their health and save the country millions of pounds sterling that could be spent on the educational infrastructure (Everyday Sport 2004). Recommended activities included the everyday, such as walking. These activities were thus differentiated from organized sports and other strenuous physical pursuits or 'exercise'. As explained by Robertson (2006), exercise typically comprises discrete activities, such as going to the gym, which men in his study associated with health and well-being.

Everyday Sport and similar campaigns – for example, a publicized NHS anti-obesity initiative and another project advocating weight-loss for men aged 40 plus – were sometimes broached with respondents. Representing concrete examples of institutional sizism, these campaigns were not given the spotlight (indeed, as the research progressed I came to realize that undue emphasis on these would have been unethical). Rather, depending upon how the interview unfolded, these campaigns were mentioned as part of a more general discussion on men's changing sport's participation, exercise, physical activity, health and weight. Hence, not all of my data on physical activity were generated during a discussion on anti-obesity campaigns, but I will use these data to prompt a rethink of public health discourses that reproduce the idea that 'excess' weight or fatness should be fought through increased energy expenditure.

When reading and re-reading qualitative data on men's talk about physical activity and weight/fat I identified five main discursive framings. I call these: (1) the physical activist and totally compliant; (2) the excusable and partially compliant; (3) the guilty and apologetic; (4) the critically compliant; and (5) the justifiably resistant and defiant. These are summarized in Table 5.1, alongside subtypes. Similar to modes of accountability discussed in Chapter 2, these are ideal types. This means they were not always observed in pure form, with specific individuals sometimes oscillating between discursive positions. For example, somebody 'doing' excusable for their 'failure' to embrace more strenuous exercise,

Table 5.1 A typology of social fitness in relation to physical activity and slimming

---

The physical activist and totally compliant

Physical activity is endorsed as a slimming tool for oneself and/or others. Anti-obesity campaigns are also endorsed. Streamlining bodies through sport, exercise or even moderate physical activity should be encouraged. People should do something, or be encouraged or reminded to do something, about their 'excess' (unhealthy) weight. There are few excuses for not being at or attempting to achieve a 'healthier' if not 'healthy' weight. This position is publicly reproduced by obesity fighting campaigns that focus on the 'energy-out' part of the mechanistic model of bodyweight; i.e. where overweight/obesity is attributed to sedentary lives. Another variant is the totally compliant, where physical activity *and* dietary approaches to weight-loss are endorsed.

The excusable and partially compliant

Physical activity is again endorsed for weight-loss. Narrators relate to, accept or approve of public health campaigns promoting that message for others. However, a discrepancy exists between ideals and actions. The regrettable gap between endorsing physical activity and actually doing it is bridged using excuse-accounts; for example, talk about illness, injury and ageing. Other considerations include work, family life and the possibility of encountering stigma when exercising in public. The keyword here is unable rather than unwilling. Hence, other weight-loss methods, such as dieting, may be endorsed by those identifying with 'weight problems'. This renders narrators partially compliant to the 'energy-in/out' model. Finally, two other subtypes are identifiable: the partially excusable and the totally compliant yet excusable. The former is excusable for a sedentary life rather than 'excess' weight. The latter subtype embraces exercise and dieting but is still unable consistently to lose weight and keep it off despite their best intentions.

The guilty and apologetic

Focusing more on oneself than others, physical activity is endorsed as a tool for shedding unwanted weight, but this is not put into action. Rather than excuse their past and recurrent 'failure' to get active and slim, the guilty and apologetic positively orientate to the future through contrition and prospective aligning actions, i.e. responsibility for their weight 'problem' is accepted and they avow to embrace physical activity in an attempt to address that. Others may be guilty but not apologetic. They accept responsibility for their unwanted weight/fat and acknowledge the value of physical activity as a remedial strategy but they make no amends. Rather, they malign themselves and assent to internalized oppression (for example, call themselves a slob or lazy). A sense of social fitness, and possible attenuation of negative emotions, may still be negotiated through partial compliance (following a modified diet) and perhaps ironic self-deprecating humour.

The critically compliant

There are two main subtypes and both endorse weight-loss: the active critically compliant and the sedentary slimmer. The former, like the physical activist, values physical activity but the presumed role of this in efficiently promoting slimness is rejected. Anti-obesity campaigns are also criticized for promoting this streamlined message. Criticisms include: it is a myth that physical activity promotes weight-loss, massive weight-loss is possible without exercising or the main benefits of physical activity extend beyond weight-loss. The other manifestation of critical compliance is the slimmer who is intentionally sedentary. Unlike the excusable and partially compliant this type is unwilling rather than unable to embrace physical activity, even for reasons extending beyond weight-loss or regulation. Diet rather than physical activity is the route to a slimmer and presumably

continued

Table 5.1 continued

The critically compliant cont.
healthier body. Both manifestations of critical compliance endorse socially approved
ends, a slimmer body, but, for different reasons, resist a commonly prescribed means for
achieving that goal.

The justifiably resistant and defiant
This is about size or fat acceptance, and even admiration though supposedly
'obesogenic' lives may also be justified with or without direct reference to weight or
fat. If weight/fat is discussed, those endorsing physical activity but not weight-loss
could be typified as resistant, while those legitimating sedentary living could be typified
as defiant (though resistance may still be defiantly expressed). Numerous themes are
identifiable. Whether resistant or defiant, exercise is deemed inefficient for slimming;
it may even result in weight-gain. For the resistant, and similar to advocates of Health
at Every Size, physical fitness is prioritized over slimness for biomedical health and
well-being. 'Big' or 'fat' people who are physically fit, active and healthy (for example,
male strength athletes) are often cited. Natural bodily diversity and other dimensions
of physical fitness, such as metabolic and reproductive fitness among sizeable people,
are also mentioned. However, these do not depend on physical activity participation.
More defiant themes include: differentiating health (for example, longevity) from
physical fitness obtained through exercise plus happiness and self-fulfilment through
sedentary living. Obesity fighting campaigns are criticized for being misleading,
authoritative, stigmatizing and unnecessary. In short, this display comprises
justificatory accounts and forms of repudiation, i.e. the pejorative status of what
medicine calls overweight or obesity is challenged wholly or in part, and perhaps
lifestyles are assumed to cause weight-gain, with or without attempts to mitigate
responsibility. Basically, the justifiably resistant challenge contrition and, for the
defiant, healthism more generally.

N.B. These are common ideal types. They are not always embodied in pure form in everyday life,
there are overlaps and specific individuals may offer multiple displays of social fitness.

and lose unwanted weight, could shift to the physical activist discourse by
emphasizing their everyday incidental activities (such as walking rather than using
mechanized transport). There was also overlap, with certain displays providing the
conditions of possibility for others. For example, some men were retrospectively
excusable for not embracing physical activity, but they expressed their intention
to change their sedentary lifestyles and lose weight. Hence, they enacted guilty and
apologetic. Others endorsed the physical activist discourse in relation to themselves
but were justifiably resistant when this message was directed at others, as with
anti-obesity campaigns or initiatives like Everyday Sport that furthered the war on
obesity.

Rather than report data for each ideal type I will focus on the most critical
orientation: the justifiably resistant and defiant. However, other types still challenged institutional sizism and, given the messiness of the empirical world,
some of these types are hinted at below. All make sense and may be interpreted
through a critical lens where the war on obesity is deemed questionable if not
objectionable. Thus, *the physical activist* endorsed the idea of becoming more
active in order to slim down and improve health, contrasting with sizist stereotypes

of the 'overweight' and 'obese' as lazy and unconcerned about health. *The totally compliant* were similar, except they also endorsed diet and exceeded recommendations from those promoting physical activity for weight-loss. *The excusable* had good reasons for not getting physically active and perhaps becoming slim and trim. Again this challenges healthist injunctions and 'lazy assumptions' (Gard 2003: 72). For instance, work demands constrained the physical body, or 'big' people were barred from exercising in public due to stigma and size discrimination (Packer 1989, Savill 2006). *The guilty and apologetic*, who had clearly internalized fat oppression, were not unrepentant sinners; rather, they intended doing something about their unwanted 'weight', thus projecting an acquiescent version of social fitness. And, *the critically compliant* sought to become thinner, with some also embracing exercise, but they saw no value in using the latter to achieve the former (especially when seeking to lose a substantial amount of weight). However, exploring *the justifiably resistant and defiant* contributes most directly to a critical discussion. This mode of accountability, at least in its ideal typical manifestations, challenged the pejorative status of bodies that medicine labels overweight or worse and associated narratives of personal blame and shame. Some of this compares to fat activism, forms of repudiation and the Health at Every Size paradigm, though, as will be observed, there were contrasting themes and some limitations.

The justifiably resistant and defiant

The extract below recounts a conversation I had with a taxi driver. This exchange occurred shortly after media coverage of a university forum I organized, *Expanding the Obesity Debate* (Chapter 1), which challenged the obesity discourse while still accepting the value of physical activity in relation to health (risk). This extract captures some relevant themes characterizing justifiable resistance and defiance, themes that not only resisted the institutional degradation of fatness but also the idea that people should follow 'healthy lifestyles' as a means of ensuring their health and, implicitly, proving moral worth. These and other themes are elaborated in the remainder of this chapter with reference to other qualitative data. What is also noteworthy about this extract is that it shows I am dealing with an ideal type, which is not necessarily embodied in pure form and does not totally deflect fat hatred. Here Patrick was still excusable and experienced 'psychological oppression' (Bartky 1990: 22). Embodying fatphobia, he confessed feeling disgusted with his weight even when repudiating healthist and sizist injunctions. In short, this street-level ethnography highlights ambivalences and contradictions as one man sought to present himself as a socially fitting person:

> *Field diary*: I took a taxi ride. Patrick, my driver, was a big fella. He asked me about my work and I mentioned I was a sociology lecturer with a general research interest in health. Patrick then referred to a newspaper article he recently read. This described a university forum on the obesity debate, which, unbeknown to him, I organized. The article referred to the 'fit and fat' exercise

physiology literature, which challenges the idea that obesity is necessarily risky if accompanied by moderate to good cardiorespiratory fitness, and Patrick mentioned that. He then said he was disgusted with his weight, which was somewhere in the region of 20 stone. As with other excusable and guilty taxi drivers I have met, he blamed some of his 'overweight' on his sedentary job. Being disgusted implied contrition (or the intention, if circumstances permitted, to lose weight), but he changed tack. In short, he resisted the physical activist discourse *and* the critically compliant discourse. His talk included 'non-conforming' cases that challenged the idea that exercise protects health even for slim people with 'healthy lifestyles', and other contradictory evidence. Patrick mentioned three men he knew or had talked with.

The first was a man Patrick gave a taxi ride to, 'and we were talking about weight and health'. Patrick said the man was in his early 40s, 'only' weighing about 11 stone, ran 30 miles a week, had a good diet, never smoked and drank moderately. This man went for a medical, with the doctor reportedly saying: 'You're a heart attack waiting to happen. There's nothing I can tell you to do. You're doing everything you can do!' Continuing with his narrative, Patrick said: 'So, he went for a second opinion, and his sister, who worked at the clinic as a nurse, pointed out several fat people and told him "You have higher cholesterol than them!" ' Second, Patrick described his friend who regularly went to the gym and 'has a potbelly. It's out here and there's nothing he can do to get rid of it. He doesn't look like he goes to the gym all the time.' Third, and more in response to healthism or injunctions to watch one's diet, he cited another friend, aged 90, who eats 'really fatty bacon and goes to the pub every night for a few whiskies and halves of Guinness. And he walks 1½ miles every day, and he is so mentally alert.' Patrick may have initially expressed disgust with his weight. However, he still resisted the obesity discourse and healthism, knowing life is full of contradictory cases.

Before exploring these and other themes, three points should be made. First, I fully recognize that obesity scientists know that good health and longevity are not guaranteed for people at a 'healthy' weight and who follow a 'healthy lifestyle'. This is clearly evidenced by their use of concepts such as relative risk (which is about statistical probability), with people categorized as obese deemed more likely to experience illness and early death as gauged by statistical correlations rather than a proven cause–effect relationship. Yet, everyday renditions of the obesity discourse in the media and public health oversimplify this in ways that may belie people's more sophisticated everyday understandings. The 'official' publicized message is that medicalized fatness is unhealthy and should be fought or, as with the media coverage of the forum I organized, biomedical health need not be poor among people classed as obese if they engage in moderate physical activity. Of course, the real world is much more complex and contradicted when attention shifts from population risks to individual risks.

Second, it was not only men like Patrick, whom medicine might label morbidly obese, who vocalized resistance in response to their feelings of self-disgust. Men of various sizes, who projected more positive identities and did not necessarily see themselves as fat (regardless of BMI), were similar. One explanation is that these men recognized manufactured intolerance when they saw it, including the irrationality of rationalized definitions that equate 'weight' with poor health and fitness. Another is that the obesity discourse is an aspect of healthism, which targets everybody independent of bodyweight or fatness. Resistance, especially in its more defiant forms, was thus not simply a response to fat oppression, though it was often that as well. It was a rejection of the idea that men's moral worth, social fitness and health depended on lifestyle changes that others in authority deemed to be in their best interests.

Third, advocates of the obesity discourse, such as health promoters, might assume that it was 'intransigent' men who mainly expressed resistance and defiance. That is, men who were in 'denial' about their weight, or the risks of obesity, and were not seeking to redress this. Aside from the questionable science and ideology associated with that moralizing stance (Gard and Wright 2005), that assumption is not supported by my data. Resistance and defiance were even expressed by slimmers who were 'doing the right thing' about their unwanted weight, i.e. men who were practically but not discursively compliant. Like gender and the possibility that women may perform masculinities (Annandale 2003), these enactments were not tied to specific bodies. They were fluid. This is understandable and there is no contradiction here. Even slimmers sometimes resented the obligation to lose weight. Also, following Chapter 3, there was the ongoing possibility of being shot at by others (or pulling the trigger oneself, as with internalized oppression), with resistance accounts providing a discursive shield that afforded at least some protection. In short, their words promoted size or fat acceptance even if they did not personally accept their own bodies. More defiantly, they rejected 'health promotion' that amplified and reinforced the socially constructed 'wrongs' of weight/fatness.

Data reporting and analysis is organized under four subheadings: (1) the inefficiency argument, weight-gain and prioritizing physical fitness over slimness, (2) being 'big' and physically fit, (3) differentiating health from physical fitness, and (4) ageing, preferring a more relaxing life and rejecting imposed discipline.

The inefficiency argument, weight-gain and prioritizing physical fitness over slimness

Patrick mentioned his friend who regularly went to the gym but had a potbelly. I have regularly exercised in gyms for 16 years and, based on my observations, I would not simply reject his claim as self-serving rhetoric. Even high-level competition bodybuilders sometimes have 'bellies' during the off-season when increasing their calories and building muscle mass. However, regardless of the validity of Patrick's words, his talk conveyed two clear messages. First, physical activity is not always effective or efficient in promoting weight-loss (a view also expressed by the critically compliant and thus still compatible with slimming). Second, 'big' or 'fat' people may be highly physically active and fit. The second theme is broached below but is elaborated in the next subsection with reference to male strength athletes and 'natural' bodily diversity. Here I will consider what could be called the inefficiency argument plus the possibility of weight-gain through exercise. Similar to the 'fit and fat' exercise physiology literature, which Patrick questioned, I will also flag some men's prioritization of physical fitness over slimness when promoting 'health'.

Patrick was not the only man voicing the inefficiency argument. Mitch, who was in other respects a conformist interested in the 'best' way to lose weight, forcefully expressed this. Reflecting the ambivalences of slimming, Mitch vocalized his resistance when standing close to the slimming club's weighing scales – a rationalized yet potentially irrational 'zone' of 'normative embodiment' (Watson 2000) where bodies were objectified (Chapter 4). His talk was part of a broader discussion where he complained about the social obligation to lose weight even when, as he claimed to be, metabolically fit (he mentioned his blood pressure was good even when his BMI exceeded 30). After denying injury with appeals to visceral embodiment, Mitch added defiantly: 'It's a complete myth that you can lose weight through exercise. It's a total misconception!' This was based upon his previous 6 stone weight-loss, achieved through diet. He reiterated his point about 'misconceptions' after I asked him about Everyday Sport, though, in keeping with active critical compliance and his identity as a slimmer, Mitch underscored the value of diet for weight-loss while adding that he 'exercised' for 'health reasons'. In short, he departed from the ideal type in line with his biographical situation and relevances.

Exercise, particularly in its more strenuous forms, may also result in weight-gain. Paul, similar to Mitch, had lost several stone through diet. He talked about trying to lose weight in the past by exercising in the gym. However, Paul's hunger increased, with him eating more and gaining weight. Although that was an unintended consequence for Paul, weight-gain – with weight becoming an index of muscle, rather than fatness – is the rationale for bodybuilding. Although not exercising with weights, Mitch also buttressed his inefficiency argument when mentioning Arnold Schwarzenegger, who would be inappropriately classed as obese because of his muscularity (Chapter 2). Importantly, Mitch was not suggesting he was muscular like accomplished bodybuilders. Rather, in speaking from his body, Mitch was stating efficient measures and weight-loss prescriptions are irrational not least because all bodies comprise fat and muscle. This rhetoric of legitimization had currency for other men who took the conflation of types of body mass within the efficient obesity discourse (the idea that 'weight' is bad) as their springboard for justifiable resistance. As elaborated below, men who valued physical activity and adopted a fat identity expressed such talk. So too did men who were labelled 'overweight' by others (including health professionals), but rejected that definition when presenting themselves as physically and socially fit.

Ralph, from the fitness centre and reporting an active life, resisted the publicized 'use physical activity to lose weight' message with implicit reference to muscular hypertrophy. Identifying as a 'big, fat lad', this 68-year-old initially accepted the idea of Everyday Sport after I explained it to him. However, after I enquired further and asked whether the weight-loss message was important, he said with regard to more strenuous (meaningful) forms of physical activity: 'No. No [pause] to me, no. I mean, if you haven't got much weight to lose and you start going to the gym, then you put weight on. I think it's the wrong message to give.' Endorsing health promotion, rather than more specific obesity fighting campaigns, Ralph then said 'the message' should be 'get active' in order to improve cardiorespiratory fitness, mobility and well-being rather than lose weight. He rejected the physical activist discourse by prioritizing physical fitness, and other dimensions of healthy embodiment, over slimness. This constituted a form of size acceptance, though he endorsed healthism and was obviously not as defiant as Patrick. This compares with softer repudiation, where fat activists prioritize healthy lifestyles when presenting themselves as good bodies without endorsing weight-loss as a necessary or valued goal. It also compares with the Health at Every Size paradigm, where physical fitness is prioritized over slimness when promoting biomedical health and well-being.

Clearly then, those doing justifiable resistance, in its milder forms, sometimes accepted healthist prescriptions that extended beyond the weight-centred approach to health. Other men maintained that physical activity confers various health benefits independent of weight-loss or achieving what medicine classes as a 'healthy' weight. Indeed, for some men, bodyweight was totally irrelevant. That included Jason who, like Ralph, was not from the slimming club and reported a physically active life. When talking with Gary, Jason said he did not know what his 'ideal weight' was, but, after mentioning exercise, added: 'I think my ideal is probably how fit I am. And I don't think I relate fitness to weight.' Jason claimed that his weight, even when medically discredited, was compatible with, and could be directly attributed to, demanding exercise. What his doctor called 'overweight' was, for Jason, indicative of muscle and a more appropriate muscular (masculine) shape:

> I've done a lot of running in the past. The irony about it is that I tend to put on weight because I tend to – it changes the kind of muscle content and the fat content drops. And it's funny, I remember watching my diet. I went to the doctors for some reason and he said, 'Well, you're kind of a bit overweight.' And I trained and I ate, you know, kind of reasonably well and I went running. I was running 8 miles a day. And I went back to see him and he said, 'Oh, yeah, you've put on a bit more weight.' And I'd put on weight because I'd got more muscle, that's why. It seemed to me about . . . it was based on an idea of weight and not an idea of shape and the two seemed to be quite different. And it was almost the fitter I got, the unhealthier I was on the scales. And it seemed to be kind of rather a crude way of measuring . . . But it wasn't a problem for me.

Although Jason's talk about 'the body inescapable' (Connell 1995) left anti-fat prejudice intact, he still resisted the efficient obesity discourse and its physical activist strand. In short, and as illustrated elsewhere in Jason's interview when he criticized the BMI and government health concerns, he resisted the obesity discourse and messages that could leave people with 'a mental health issue'. Here Jason rejected the idea that most people are overweight or obese – and thus fat, slothful, unhealthy and unfit – and physical activity is a suitable remedy for, rather than a contributor to, this putative problem (*cf.* Monaghan 2007).

Current slimmers, even if unwilling or unable to run 8 miles, also voiced resistance accounts. Arthur challenged sizist assumptions and claimed a level of 'overweight' was acceptable with reference to biomedical health provided it was accompanied by physical fitness obtained through exercise. This reflected his biographical experiences as a young soldier. He said he became extremely physically fit in the past during vigorous army training but his weight stayed constant and he remained overweight on the BMI, a measure he found ludicrous:

> Well, the main benefit of exercise is the cardiopulmonary benefits, as opposed to the weight benefits. You can be a little bit overweight but as long as you've got a healthy heart, and healthy lungs, you're OK. You can be a perfect weight for your health and be in a right bloody mess, because you don't do any exercise.

However, in deviating from the ideal type, Arthur still considered weight-loss beneficial, much in line with his identity as a slimmer. Similar to Patrick's repudiating talk, and consistent with the ideal type, other men offered more challenging accounts. Their talk did not pay lip service to the possible 'weight benefits' of physical activity or any other weight-loss method, with some men also challenging the health benefits ascribed to physical fitness.

Before discussing the fracturing of health and fitness, it is worth exploring further men's resistance talk on the compatibility of 'bigness' or fatness and modes of physical fitness, i.e. anaerobic capacity, or strength, cardiorespiratory, metabolic and even reproductive fitness. As seen below, such talk also included appeals to 'natural' bodily diversity and could be compared to fat activists' accounts that eschew the pathologization of heavier weights and fatness. Again, such talk had important gendered identity effects for narrators who presented themselves as men, or regular fellas, rather than feminized fat targets.

Being 'big' and physically fit: From male strength athletes to 'natural' bodily diversity

Physical fitness comprises various dimensions, though strength and endurance have obvious gendered currency. The combination of anaerobic and aerobic fitness is typically associated with larger male bodies competing in various sports and strength events, with such practices integral to definitions of masculinity. As stated by Connell (1995: 54), 'sport has come to be the leading definer of masculinity in mass culture. Sport provides a continuous display of men's bodies in motion'. When contesting the message 'get physically active to lose weight', some men thus elaborated on a theme touched on above where implicit or explicit reference was made to muscle bulk acquired through exercise. Whether interviewed by Gary or me, men repeatedly mentioned demanding masculine sports and activities even if they did not personally embrace these. In short, men expressed resistance by citing fit, 'big', male bodies that would be medically labelled over-weight or worse. This, of course, reproduced hegemonic masculinity, which, as explained by Robertson (2006: 444), 'continues to be represented in embodied forms based on action and strength'. As seen below, this was also intertwined with other talk, such as the 'natural' diversity of physically fit and healthy bodies, and was also compatible with fat acceptance and even admiration.

Consider some data. Richie talked about male strength athletes when interviewed by my slim research associate. Richie was not an athlete; rather, he was a slimming club member weighing about 20 stone. Unlike Jason, he did not report running 8 miles a night either. Nonetheless, Richie's talk provided 'cover in wartime', a shield behind which he could obtain some protection. Here Richie might have been referring to muscular strength but he also explicitly offered 'fat affirming talk' with his hyperbolic account challenging sizism and anti-fat prejudice. This challenge was mounted even when using the value-laden term 'overweight' (Chapter 1). However, the negativity implied by that term was resisted with appeals to other modes of physical fitness; namely, his metabolic fitness, which he claimed was normal and unrelated to bodyweight:

> If you think an overweight person is unfit, like I say if you look at a lot of your athletes, your rugby players, your weightlifters. I watch the strongest man competition on TV. They pull a big truck. You or I would die as soon as we tried to pull it. And again they say 'a fat person', 'overweight person', and you think he's overweight, he's unfit and yet that overweight person could probably go into a gym or the swimming baths and leave that skinny person standing. You know? I have normal cholesterol and normal blood pressure, even though I'm 4 or 5 stone overweight. And yet somebody who is as thin as yourself could go and get yours checked and you might have high blood pressure and you might have dodgy cholesterol.

Clearly, Richie's reference to metabolic fitness and aerobic fitness – that is, cholesterol, blood pressure and stamina demonstrated by swimmers – could apply to women. His talk compares to 'narratives of resistance' cited in studies of women, fatness and weight (Gimlin 2007b). However, Richie's words also had important masculinizing effects. This was distinctly masculine-validating talk given his appeal to anaerobic fitness, or strength – the strong man who pulls a truck or the rugby player who has aerobic and anaerobic fitness. Here having a male body, even if not physically trained, afforded Richie certain privileges. Similar to men interviewed by Robertson (2006: 446), 'the social meanings invested in his biological sex' enabled him to draw on masculine bodily representations that 'reproduce the idea(l) of male strength and domination'. If the war on obesity is a form of symbolic violence that reproduces masculine domination (Bourdieu 2001) then the masculine habitus also furnishes men with gendered material for their justifiable resistance.

Performing strongmen, weightlifters and rugby players are obvious models of robust masculinity, alongside American footballers and heavyweight boxers. Types of wrestling also reward 'big' male bodies, comprising a spectrum of physiques that cannot easily be placed on a muscular-fat scale. There are, after all, many bodies that vary within and between themselves in terms of organic composition and these are not always easily *determinable* to observers: something well-recognized by bodybuilders who, through habit and exercise, acquire 'ethnophysiological' knowledge comprising finely differentiated ways of looking at bodies (Monaghan 2001). 'The partial indeterminacy of certain objects', writes Bourdieu (2001: 14), also 'authorizes antagonistic interpretations, offering the dominated a possibility of resistance to the effect of symbolic opposition' (also Monaghan 2006). That said, some bodies are obviously fatter than others and are seen as such, but that does not negate the possibility of 'antagonistic interpretations'. For example, Sumo wrestlers' bodies typically comprise a high percentage of fat but they are still physically fit, powerful and carry muscle.

During interviewing, some men resisted the physical activist strand of the obesity discourse by invoking Japanese Sumo. While Sumo has been exported to the West, no respondents actually did Sumo. Nonetheless, that did not stop Big Joe from appealing to Sumo and resisting socially constructed stigma. This interviewee challenged those who publicly perpetuate intolerance by assuming 'massive' men are physically unfit and unhealthy. Again, similar to Richie, Big Joe shielded himself behind these 'really big' men's discursively constructed bodies. This talk emerged at the end of our interview when, after discussing anti-obesity campaigns, I asked if there was anything else he considered important. His differentiation between health and fitness is also salient. It followed his argument that he was healthy even though his physical fitness (aerobic capacity) was not as good as it could have been. I will return to this 'differentiating talk' in the next subsection because it was recurrent. Finally, the word 'overweight' here refers to bodies that medicine deems morbidly obese, thus constituting another form of resistance to offensive medical labels (Chapter 1):

> Well, the main thing is people getting this message across where 'if you're not fit you're not healthy'. And you're being browbeaten into thinking, well, if you're overweight then you're a burden to society and to other people. And not everyone who is overweight is unhealthy, or unfit. I mean you've got these people who perform in sports. Sumo wrestlers. There are some English guys who compete in Sumo wrestling, and they're massive blokes, but they're very, very fit. I mean, look at these Sumo wrestlers in Japan. These guys are massive. I mean, I never realized how big these men were until I went to Madame Tussauds waxworks and they've got a waxwork of some well-known Japanese Sumo wrestler. And you think to yourself, 'well, he is a big

guy', but when you actually see a life-size model of the bloke, you put into perspective what a big guy really is. I mean, this guy was absolutely massive. I mean, he must have been the best part of 7 foot and 40 stone. He was huge. I'm not exaggerating Lee. He had a head on him like that [he indicates using his hands]. And you think to yourself, 'Now he competes in these Sumo wrestling competitions.' In Japan, Sumo wrestlers are treated like royalty. I mean, I mean, it's weird. They treat you like shit over here. But somebody who is big over there is treated like a god.

An obvious rejoinder is that Sumo wrestlers experience health problems and die young. Whether valid or not, that response would miss the point that 'Sumo talk' enabled Big Joe to make his size more liveable. It is also worth noting 'non-conforming' scientific evidence. Gaesser (2002: 124–5) cites a study of Sumo wrestlers with an average BMI of 36 kg/m^2 but who had low levels of visceral fat, which is defined as 'bad' fat, and good metabolic fitness. For Gaesser (2002), this underscores the health benefits of physical activity regardless of obesity. More sociologically, physical fitness, as displayed by really 'big' men, provided some interviewees with a discursive resource for demonstrating social fitness.

In elaborating on the bigness and physical fitness theme, other men appealed to a natural 'body diversity model' (Saguy and Riley 2005). Fat activists expressing softer repudiation use this model. Here somebody could be very physically active and fit, but remain 'big' because that is how nature intended them to be. Correspondingly, whether male or female, it cannot be assumed their fatness is a reliable index of sloth, gluttony or self-imposed risk and pathology. Fatness could even be associated with a sexed/gendered body believed to possess good reproductive, as well as cardiorespiratory, fitness, as seen below when Jason talked about women he knew. Interestingly, what can also be seen here is the 'discursive power' of masculinity 'to operate as an authorizing narrative' for female bodies (Skeggs 1997: 113). Feminists would likely urge a critical reading of men's own terms of reference, though what I would stress here is how this was related to Jason's publicly visible person, i.e. a man who refused to be subordinated by the obesity discourse and institutional sizism.

Jason mentioned two 'quite large, healthy and fit' women he knew 'who would probably be Anglo-Saxon wenches and good, you know, primitive farming stock with childbearing hips, and that's how they were built'. Although recognizing these women would be medically labelled obese and assumed physically unfit, this clashed with his understandings: 'They're both two fit things like, probably in terms of lung capacity and huge stamina.' The social construction of masculinities is relational. This not only concerns the ways in which masculinity 'is constructed in front of and for other men' (Bourdieu 2001: 53), but also how femininity is 'the ultimate legitimator of masculinity' because 'it offers to masculinity the power to impose standards, to make evaluations and confirm validity' (Skeggs 1997: 112). Hence, there is no contradiction when 'big' men displayed their social fitness by citing everyday examples of fleshy, fit femininities that challenged sizism.

Such talk has historical antecedents. Jutel (2005: 113) notes that early twentieth century exercise specialists 'promoted what would today be considered a "sturdy" version of womanhood as the ideal'. While her observation relates to the broader culture and validation of larger women in the not-too-distant past, Jason's talk emerged after discussing his increased physical fitness, weight-gain and his criticism of his doctor, who defined him as 'overweight' and thus, implicitly, unfit, unhealthy and almost woman-like. Of course, obesity fighting campaigns also convey these messages to 'the masses', who are 'traditionally regarded as feminine' (Bourdieu 2001: 79) and suitable targets for masculine domination.

Differentiating health from physical fitness: 'Big' sedentary people can be healthy and happy and slim joggers drop dead

Politically, and in line with harder repudiation (Chapter 2), possessing good physical fitness and embracing physical activity are irrelevant when challenging sizism and obesity warmongering. That said, the idea of health, in its various dimensions, has everyday currency and is obviously not the exclusive entitlement of, or guaranteed for, slim people who embrace 'virtuous habits of life' (Edgley and Brissett 1990: 262). Men voicing justifiable resistance and defiance often appealed to health and, in so doing, displayed social fitness.

At a basic level, 'health' (defined, for example, in terms of longevity) is not assured for those conforming to healthism and/or the culture of slenderness. This was hinted at by Patrick when differentiating normative and pragmatic male embodiment from the visceral, i.e. the slim man who runs 30 miles a week but has high cholesterol and is considered a 'heart attack waiting to happen'. When specifically challenging obesity fighting campaigns, other men also used these norms of cultural intelligibility. In short, they differentiated health from physical fitness – implicitly, good cardiorespiratory fitness obtained through aerobic exercise. They maintained that if 'big' sedentary people already possessed good biomedical health (for example, blood pressure, cholesterol) then they should not be cajoled by external authorities to get slim and presumably healthy through physical activity. Furthermore, men appealed to more ephemeral but obviously important dimensions of health that were differentiated from the visceral; namely, happiness, which is an aspect of 'experiential' embodiment (Watson 2000). However, as a caveat, some men thought happiness was elusive in anti-fat times. Richard, who had experienced enacted stigma from strangers (Chapter 3), said that while 'some people are very happy with being overweight' he added 'I just don't see how they can be nowadays.'

Even so, Big Joe – who identified himself as being 'massively overweight' – maintained that he was healthy and happy, with his self-affirming talk expressing and capturing his 'publicly visible person' (Cahill 1998). Big Joe, in his characteristically assured and defiant style, invoked visceral and experiential embodiment. This corresponded with the idea, intimated in his previously cited words, that physical fitness and slimness are not synonymous with good health and implicitly moral worth. When constructing a sense of functional and healthy masculinity, Big

Joe also appealed to his pragmatic embodiment, i.e. he cited his 'breadwinning' or economically productive body. As with Patrick and other men's talk (see below), Big Joe buttressed his account further by citing the failure of cardiorespiratory fitness to guarantee good health and longevity with reference to slim fitness enthusiasts who drop dead. In effect, these men 'denied injury' (Sykes and Matza 1957), thereby justifying sizeable bodies and possible physical inactivity.

This 'differentiating talk' was recurrent and complemented previously cited accounts that were not always geared toward differentiation (for example, the indeterminacy of a 'big' male body that was more or less muscular or fat). Offered by men who challenged normative health promotion, differentiating talk may be defined as justificatory accounts wherein narrators distinguished dimensions of health (metabolic, experiential, pragmatic) from physical fitness (notably, cardiorespiratory fitness) acquired through exercise.

This rather abstract point may be grounded using qualitative data. Brad criticized anti-obesity campaigns with reference to happiness and health, which were differentiated from physical fitness and were possible regardless of body composition, exercise and dieting. Brad was a self-directed physical activist and sports science student. Reflecting a maturity and reflexivity that went beyond his 16 years, Brad did not extend his own intolerance toward his unwanted weight to other people who were assumed to be fat because of sedentary living. In short, he was defiant by proxy. The following talk emerged after I mentioned the Everyday Sport billboards in the locality. Brad then mentioned an anti-obesity campaign from the NHS, which he had recently seen. This featured cartoon images mocking fatness, illustrating the fat activist complaint that sizism is a 'safe prejudice' (Smith 1990) and Rich *et al.*'s (2006: 184) point that the obesity discourse 'reduces health to a weight issue, and grants authority to publicly monitor, and often humiliate those who are considered "at risk"':

BRAD: I think there's stuff on the Metro [train system], billboards: a picture of a woman with a huge arse. And she's saying 'Does my bum look big in this?' And there's a bloke with a huge belly, and there's stuff written underneath.

LM: What do you think about them?

BRAD: I think for a lot of people they're saying that exercise is what you should be doing. But it is not really something that you should be doing; you shouldn't have to do it. Like, do all this stuff and get fit. It doesn't really matter so long as you're healthy. As long as you were healthy and you were living OK, and everything, I wouldn't say that you have to go off and join a gym, and dieting. As long as you actually are healthy.

LM: So you can actually be big and healthy, as you were saying earlier?

BRAD: Yeah. If somebody says they're happy the way I am, that's like, good for them. They don't have to be doing what these things tell them to do. If a bloke with a huge belly walked up and saw that 'Does my tum look big in this?', they'd think, 'Oh, they're just taking the Mick' [i.e. ridiculing people].

Other men discussed the possibility of being big, healthy, happy and sedentary. This was an obvious rejoinder to the sizist idea that the physically fit and slim have a monopoly on health and well-being. Although generally excusable, Freddy expressed defiance after we perused images from another public health campaign, Idle Eric. (I subsequently decided not to show these images to other men because I did not want to be an agent of symbolic violence and risk causing offence.) Besides making the lazy assumption that older men are physically unfit, the Idle Eric campaign promoted weight-loss using images of young, toned men's bodies: a case of ageism and sizism. Freddy buttressed his differentiating and denial of injury talk with the common 'drop dead' rejoinder (also favoured by sedentary slimmers who were critically compliant) with reference to 'the fellow who brought out jogging'. Whether referring to my own data or other literature, Freddy was not unusual in this thinking. For example, his words correspond with a study on 'lay' perceptions of 'coronary candidacy' (Emslie *et al.* 2001). Also, Edgley (2006: 240) critiques 'fitness and the therapeutic ethic' with reference to James Fixx, the author of *The Complete Book of Running* 'whose life of devotion to health and fitness was cut short when he collapsed and died of a massive coronary while running':

> But I still say that if a person is that age, and he likes to be that size, and he's healthy, he hasn't got heart trouble, and he hasn't got high blood pressure, he hasn't got any trouble, what harm is he doing? You know? What harm is he doing? I mean, look at the fellow who brought out jogging. He dropped dead. So, why jog? So what harm is that bloke doing? He is doing no harm. Because he is happy. He is doing no harm. (Freddy)

Freddy's repeated question about harm deserves an answer. I did not formulate an answer at the time because this was obviously a rhetorical question, my own critical thoughts were emerging and the answer is actually very ugly. However, in making sense of the war on obesity and men's accounts in a world where fatness is often seen as antithetical to health, I would state the following: Idle Eric's fatness, attributed to sloth, offends middle-class sensibilities and deviates from McDonaldized conceptions of health that provide a 'thin' rationale for fat hatred. Such bodies evoke class disdain, misogyny and the fear that men could appear like passive, sickly, vulnerable and disgusting women or indolent working-class slobs (Chapters 1 and 3). Whether intended or not, obesity fighting campaigns target and assault bodies that offend dominant, rationalized/masculinized sensibilities.

In challenging the health rationale for this symbolic violence and reclaiming masculinity, other men similarly reasoned that exercise does not guarantee good health even among types of slim male athletes. Interestingly, tables were turned with the idea of men's sickness used to negate the idea that the narrator's own embodied actions, or corporeality, would necessarily result in sickness. Here, men's talk about unhealthy fitness enthusiasts was structured by gender and the social construction of heart trouble as a man's problem – even though coronary heart disease kills a similar proportion of women as men in the UK (Emslie *et al.*

2001). Famous male athletes suffering from heart trouble were sometimes cited as examples. Similar to one of Emslie *et al.*'s (2001) male interviewees, Arthur mentioned Graeme Souness, a professional footballer. Arthur, who had stressed the 'protective' functions of physical fitness for health, also underscored the fallibility of such thinking. In so doing, this current slimmer, who recently suffered a heart attack after losing weight, sought to neutralize any implication that his heart trouble could simply be attributed to a less active life and, implicitly, his fatness:

> I mean, talk about being active and stuff. You can't go any further than Graeme Souness, for instance. He's had four bypasses him. And you can't get more fit than that, a professional footballer. And even when he became manager he was still on the field coaching. He was still running.

Similarly, consider Noel's talk. He first enacted personally excusable after he stopped attending the fitness centre due to injury, transport difficulties and work demands. His more resistant talk then emerged after I mentioned the 'fit and fat' exercise physiology literature. Echoing Arthur's earlier point that exercise benefited health, Noel felt it was probably 'medically wise' to do some physical activity and follow a nutritious diet, avoid smoking, etc. However, he thought the health benefits of physical activity, in terms of visceral embodiment and longevity, were probable rather than certain. Noel contrasted the idea that 'heart attacks are associated with somebody who is bloody big, they're overweight, and eats pies and drinks pints, and smokes' with the following words:

> A lot of fit people out there have heart attacks. I mean, look at the footballer, he had a heart attack in the World Cup. He just keeled over on the pitch. It was more of a stroke than a heart attack. But again, top of his game. From Cameroon. He just keeled over and died on the football pitch during one of the matches. So, you know?

Relative risk aside, the 'so, you know?' invoked common cultural background expectancies where it is well known and widely agreed that athletic endeavour and 'clean living' do not guarantee protection from an early grave. Through such talk this 29-year-old shielded his experiential body from healthist injunctions associated with anticipatory medicine and, implicitly, his previously expressed concern about his unwanted weight.

While Noel cautiously resisted healthism, Big Joe used these shared understandings to defiantly challenge publicized weight-loss prescriptions and associated sizist assumptions. Big Joe said the following straight after I described the Everyday Sport campaign to him. This extract usefully sums up many of the themes identified in other men's critical accounts, which were geared toward differentiation and the repudiation of normative health promotion:

> You see, to me, that's more of a fitness thing, not necessarily a health thing. But, people are giving you this thing where, you've got fitness and health, and

they only go together. They're not two separate entities. They're saying, if you're not fit, you're not healthy. And I don't think that's right. I personally feel you can be healthy and not very fit. You can be the fittest person in the world but you might not be very healthy. I mean, you hear about these joggers who drop dead. Lads who are playing football who all of a sudden have a massive heart attack and die. Now, that guy is a very fit person, but he obviously wasn't healthy. Because he had a problem. Now, he wasn't overweight, but the way they're making it out to you, it's as if, if you're not fit, you're not healthy. And I think that's wrong. I don't think that's right at all.

Of course, this talk is about the politics of identity and it could be modified from a more critical stance in order to directly challenge the wrongs of instituted fat hatred. In repudiating obesity warmongering, I would slightly change Big Joe's sentence 'the way they're making it out to you, it's as if, if you're not fit, you're not healthy'. I would substitute 'slim' for 'fit'. This is because public health discourses are disseminating the sizist message that if somebody is overweight or obese then they are unhealthy. That, of course, is a questionable and tenuous proposition that might bear no relationship whatsoever to an individual's health, as defined by them and perhaps their clinician (as noted in Chapter 2, Big Joe reported good health following a medical). This is an important point because, following Big Joe and other men quoted above, health is a social construct that includes well-being, happiness and self-fulfilment. These are obviously more qualitative dimensions of health that jar with the rationalized obesity discourse and its emphasis on quantification. Of course, these experiential dimensions of health may also be eroded if people take this symbolic violence to heart, or if others take it as their cue to ridicule people as inappropriately fat and unworthy.

Ageing, preferring a more relaxing life and rejecting imposed discipline

Ageing was a recurrent theme. Patrick, when denying injury by proxy, mentioned his friend who ate fatty food and drank every night but was healthy into his 90s. Although Patrick's talk could be read as a response to healthism in general, rather than sizism and the physical activist discourse in particular, his talk emerged when discussing exercise, unwanted weight and implied health risks. Ageing also emerged above when Freddy criticized the Idle Eric campaign, directed at overweight middle-aged men, with reference to visceral and experiential embodiment. Patrick and Freddy's talk has parallels in the literature. This was broached in Chapter 2 when referring to 'the "Fat Uncle Norman" figure' (Davison *et al.* 1992) who was living testimony of 'the Winston Churchill effect' (Marmot 2004), i.e. the possibility of living a long and healthy life even though 'obese' and following what clinicians would consider an imprudent lifestyle.

When challenging the idea of getting active and physically fit in order to lose weight and become healthy, men talked about age in various ways. While some mentioned relatives and friends who lived a long life, despite their weight and lifestyles (a justification), older men also used the idea of age as an excuse for their 'inappropriate' sedentary living and unwanted weight-gain. That was evidenced in Freddy's interview, with his words shifting from a more critical stance to excusable. Howard, who worked with Freddy and was much lighter, was more consistent and very defiant when discussing Idle Eric. Howard, who reported never trying to lose weight even though acknowledging he was several stone 'overweight' on 'these so-called height–weight charts', said that if he received Idle Eric material through the post he would simply throw it in the bin. Before saying that, his general orientation to physical activity was expressed in the following terms, with this 56-year-old emphasizing ageing and a preference for a more sedentary life:

> Well as you get older, if you don't carry on physical activities – to actually go back to starting again, it hurts dunnit? Aches and pains. But it's just a natural progression isn't it? The older you get the less you want to do. Whereas before it might have been cricket or football, now it's snooker [billiard game]. You don't get out off puff at snooker do you? I mean that's really – and even that, we've not been for ages. I don't like walking.

Analytically, it is worth adding that body size, and how men felt about their weight in association with others, helps to explain this talk. This is because Howard did not experience the psychological oppression and enacted stigma that Freddy, his much larger colleague, did and Howard was less constrained to be seen to agree with the dominant 'fight obesity' message. I would also say something here about research methods and ethics. I interviewed Howard just before Freddy, and it was on the basis of these two men's interviews that I decided not to show Idle Eric or any other 'health promotion' material to other men.

Regardless of whether or not attention was directed at specific obesity fighting campaigns, other men either explicitly or implicitly related ageing to a more relaxing life – lives that would be pathologized as 'obesogenic' by obesity scientists (WHO 1998). In the next excerpt, relaxation was part of the background expectancies of the cultural scene though youthful sporting accomplishments were also flagged – gendered practices that not only imprint on the biological body early in life but also construct a relatively enduring masculine habitus, or sense of agency and value (Bourdieu 2001, Brown 2006). For Mac, as with Howard and other men, a biography of sports participation informed justifiable resistance and defiance. Mac, in his 40s and relaxing on holiday when I met him, certainly moved from the ideal type and found fat acceptance difficult: publicly adopting a fat identity and enacting guilty with regard to his generally sedentary life, Mac also expressed dissatisfaction with his weight and told me he would start exercising after his holiday. However, in the following extract he justified rather than apologized for his lack of exercise plus diet (and implicitly his fatness which he related to his lifestyle). This is what Scott and Lyman (1968) call self-fulfilment, and, in line with harder repudiation, is attuned to the contradictions of human embodiment comprising self-control and abandonment (Chapter 2 and LeBesco 2004):

Field diary, Spanish holiday: Mac was approximately 6 foot tall and, as he told me later, weighed just over 18 stone. He looked like a former rugby player; he was thick-set and carrying, according to him, too much fat around his midsection: 'I'll be the first to say I'm a fat bastard [then chanting] who ate all the pies!' As I learnt, Mac used to be a national Judo champion 'in my youth' but was now much less physically active: 'I've had more comebacks than Gary Glitter. I try to get back into the gym. They've got one at work. I push a few weights and I'm sore for days afterwards, so I give up. And when I get home I prefer to sit in front of the TV with the remote control and a bag of crisps.'

Mac's self-fulfilment account was in response to his initiated focus on his fatness and lack of physical activity rather than anti-obesity campaigns. Men's embodied experiences and understandings – feeling sore from strenuous exercise, not wanting to get 'out of puff' or simply not liking more moderate activity, such as walking – also informed men's rejection of imposed discipline as expressed by particular obesity fighting campaigns. Basically, this was the idea, expressed by Howard, that 'You've got to want to do it yourself haven't you?' His talk was buttressed by his earlier reference to age where becoming sedentary, and perhaps gaining extra weight, was acceptable as part of a 'natural progression' through life. He complained with regard to Idle Eric, and the idea of getting active 'for your health or to lose weight': 'I don't need people to tell me that that's the sort of thing I should be doing. I know I should be doing things to keep myself fit. I don't need – and most people don't need people to tell them'. While there is some discursive alignment here with healthism and fat fighting, Howard still resisted external expectations. This compares to men's adoption of a 'libertarian position based upon bodily autonomy' in Gill *et al*.'s (2005) study on men's body projects and normative masculinity. In their 'elevation of the individual's right to self determination as the only truly ethical position' Gill *et al*.'s (2005: 49) respondents defiantly defended a man's right to undergo cosmetic surgery, which 'required considerable defence against authoritarian and moralistic counter-arguments'.

It was not only older men leading a sedentary life who rejected the authoritative and moralistic obesity discourse. Brad, the young sports science student who was also a gym member, similarly expressed resistance. Again, there was a champ-ioning of the libertarian self, though, unlike Gill *et al*.'s (2005) respondents' talk about cosmetic surgery, there was a clearly defined external authority that men challenged. Immediately after condemning an NHS anti-obesity campaign for equating fatness with poor health and ridiculing fat people, Brad said: 'I don't like things like that. Because I think the idea of getting told that you should be doing stuff is a bit – it's not the sort of place we should be living, getting told what to do.' This followed his argument that 'If you really want to do something like getting fit you should be doing it for your own self, and not doing it just because you're getting it drummed into your head that you've got to keep fit, you've got to look great.' (An admittedly limited resistance account since it assumes one cannot 'look great' and 'keep fit' when at a higher weight.) I mentioned other men's resistances when speaking with Gareth at the slimming club, who endorsed total compliance, i.e. regulating diet and exercising in an attempt to lose weight. He reframed the idea of being 'told' what to do with the idea that these campaigns were simply 'reminding' people of the benefits of exercise. However, it is clear that other men interpreted these campaigns as meddlesome and felt it was unnecessary for them and most people to be 'told' to embrace exercise and lose weight.

Patrick, Howard, Freddy and Mac all led sedentary lives and were not slimming. However, as with Brad, other physically active and 'weight conscious' men still discursively rejected imposed discipline. The final extract is from Edward, aged 73, who was contacted through the fitness centre. He originally joined the centre with the subsequently unrealized goal of losing 2 stone. In the following talk he defiantly challenged a pervasive regulatory apparatus that is concentrated on less privileged socio-economic groups but obviously runs through the social body. Edward's reasoning emerged not in response to Everyday Sport or Idle Eric, but after I told him about a physical activity come anti-obesity initiative, directed at teenage boys, at the same fitness centre he attended. His reply, which again flags ageing, could be seen as a fitting response to those marshalling the war on obesity – an exercise intended to discipline bodies in line with conservative ideas of social fitness. Similar to fat activists who refuse to apologize for their size (Wann 1998), this was a case of 'So what?' Edward's use of the word 'bollocks', similar to Big Joe's use of this gendered expletive at the very start of this book, is also worth highlighting. This was a common emotionally expressive response from White, working-class men who defiantly resisted imposed discipline, regulation and institutional sizism. In short, they strongly objected to corporeal processes, comparable to army training, which subordinate some male bodies on a hierarchy of social and physical fitness:

> The older you get, as far as discipline goes, it goes out the window. You just mentioned a group of lads, keeping fit. When we all went into the forces, we were 18 to 21. And, well, the war just finishing, in the early 1950s, when we joined. So the sergeant majors, and God knows what, really disciplined you. Now then, you came out the forces and eventually some were called up again in the emergency reserve. But because you were those few years older you could handle that sergeant major, 'Oh bollocks to you!' You know? And, 'I've done it all a few year ago. I don't want to start again!' So as far as age goes, the older I get, I mean I – I, you don't want anybody in a sense to be disciplining you, or to tell you what you've got to do all the time. You do your own thing and that's, I don't know, is life, as you go on in life, the older you get. You just decide. You know? You can do what I'm just doing. I'm quite happy with me life and the way I am. You say what the hell, I'm 70 odd! Why should I bloody – I'm enjoying what I'm doing now. What if I am overweight? So what? You know? I think that's the attitude.

Edward's no-nonsense attitude could be considered an appropriate and fitting response to institutional fat hatred. And, while Edward reported good metabolic health as measured by his doctor, as well as a physically active, happy, fulfilling and long life, it could be argued that these should not matter when challenging the war on obesity and the hatred it mandates and incites. Regardless of the actual physical and social fitness of the intended targets, this war proceeds on the basis of lazy, malevolent assumptions (basically, a form of depoliticizing prejudice). These assumptions are sizist and were potentially offensive for big fellas contacted during this research, some of whom felt disgusted with their weight.

Conclusion: Socially, if not physically, fitting masculinities

Physical activity is a central topic when researching men, their understandings of weight-related issues and their presentations of self or 'the publicly visible person' (Cahill 1998). This is central because physical activity, or, more formally, exercise and sport, are 'body-reflexive practices' for constructing masculinities (Connell 1995). Even talk about physical activity among older men, who were not as active or sporty as they once were, had important identity effects. Despite the questionable role of sedentary lifestyles in 'secular trends in obesity' (Keith *et al.* 2006), physical activity is also a central topic because, in line with a masculine sporting metaphor, it is publicly framed as a way of 'tackling' this putative crisis.

When talking with men neither myself nor my research associate set out to generate data to confirm a pre-existing suspicion of obesity fighting and the officially touted role of physical activity, or exercise, in promoting slenderness. The emphasis was on what men thought and how they talked about such issues. When discussing physical activity and its commonly touted role in promoting weight-loss, health and physical fitness, men offered various socially fitting displays that contributed to their sense of 'being in shape' (Watson 2000). These presentations of appropriately gendered selfhood, some of which were highly conservative and conformist, fitted with the embodied identities they sought to project on the social stage. All made sense and although I could have used all of these data to critically engage the obesity discourse (as articulated by various institutions), some displays were more directly challenging than others. Hence, health promoters, and others with a vested interest in fighting obesity, would perhaps be inclined to correct rather than appreciate some of these.

Men's presentations ranged from acquiescent to more critical versions of social fitness, from the physical activist and totally compliant to the justifiably resistant and defiant. These ideal types were summarized in Table 5.1. Data reporting and analysis focused on justifiable resistance and defiance, albeit with some reference to other ideal types that sometimes provided the conditions of possibility for more critical talk. Resistance and defiance basically entailed repudiating the obesity discourse in general and its physical activist strand in particular. This position promoted acceptance of lived bodies that medicine labels overweight, obese or even morbidly obese. Such talk sometimes compared to fat acceptance, activism and Health at Every Size, though there were some limitations. For example, muscle talk in relation to one's own physicality is not the same as promoting fat acceptance for all. Also, men may have justified sedentary and putatively obesogenic lifestyles when defiantly constructing masculinity, though in some instances this depended on biomedical health status (which, for the resistant, might be improved through lifestyle rather than macro-social and economic policies that seek to redress social inequalities and thus health inequalities).

Even so, this was an analytically rich and highly gendered mode of account-ability, comprising numerous themes. These ranged from the inefficiency of physical activity in promoting weight-loss to rejecting imposed discipline. All made sense and were related to the moment-to-moment production of person-hood as a gendered practical accomplishment. Such talk was instrumental in the validation of socially, if not always physically, fitting masculinity and was highly fluid, i.e. it was not tied to specific biographical situations, slimming careers and degrees of bodily bigness. Neither was this only or even about personal stigma management, that is, of attenuating the wrongs of being seen as fat in a fatphobic culture. Regardless of BMI, not all men voicing justifiable resistance and defiance were seen as fat by themselves and/or others. Nonetheless, they challenged healthist injunctions that could fuel the stigma of obesity and further spoil the identities of people deemed fat in everyday life.

The obesity discourse, in discrediting everyday bodily bigness as unhealthy fatness, may be experienced as oppressive and compound the weight of contrition. Yet, there are men out there who identify as 'overweight' and, even though internal-izing fat oppression, are well motivated to challenge institutional sizism. Clearly, men contacted during this research were not passive victims – a position facilitated, no doubt, by the validation of 'bulky' male bodies in masculine sports and perhaps a personal biography of physical activity (including fitness obtained through past military training). None of these men were strength athletes, or currently in the armed forces, but they offered socially fitting responses. These were normal, meaningful and reasonable and they more or less shielded their publicly visible person from symbolic violence, which is very publicly communicated by obesity fighting campaigns.

Of course, within the current social matrix, many men still want to lose weight/fat in order to display a slimmer and presumably more 'fitting' (normative) identity (Robertson 2006, Watson 2000). Whether governments, other organi-zations and health workers should promote this as a public and personal duty is another matter entirely. In line with fat activists, a feminist consciousness and repudiation, I would not endorse such practices and I return to this in the conclud-ing chapter. And for the justifiably resistant and defiant, highly publicized messages and institutional interventions, which assume people's bodies are inadequate, are themselves inadequate. Yet, while there is evidence of healthy scepticism in the population, it should be remembered that this is a gendered practical accomplish-ment. Following Robertson (2006), I would emphasize that different (hierarchical) meanings are invested in differently valued biological bodies. These socially distributed and gendered meanings enable and constrain the possibility of avoiding or attenuating 'intimations of inferiority' (Bartky 1990). Hence, there will be others in the social structure, such as women, who may be less able to resist symbolic violence. I will briefly reflect on this because it points to the broader relevance of this study when challenging the trivialization of sizism within a hierarchical, embodied and thoroughly relational gender order.

Femininity does not provide the same options when challenging the degradation of sizeable bodies as overweight or obese. For example, in the hierarchy of gender, female rugby players and strength athletes do not have the same currency as their male counterparts, as reflected in publicity and economic reward. Male strength athletes are typically credited through naturalized and institutionally embedded schemes of perception, thinking and feeling, but women competing in masculine sports and strength competitions 'often receive a barrage of stigmatization for opposing what is "natural"' (Brown 2006: 178). Drawing from feminist research on the body and the sociology of sport, Connell (1995: 50) explains that 'the disciplinary practices that both teach and constitute sport, are designed to produce gendered bodies'. In this context, masculinity offers certain privileges even for men who do not embody culturally exalted hegemonic masculinity. This is within a gender order where masculinity is defined in contradistinction to femininity and where female bodies literally embody the effects of masculine domination so that feminine softness, weakness and passivity appear to be in the order of things. Bourdieu (2001) explains that masculine domination often disadvantages women from infancy onwards through negative expectations about what they can and cannot do with their bodies. This is inside and outside of sport, with symbolic violence perpetuating hierarchical sexual divisions and '*negative prejudice* against the female' (Bourdieu 2001: 32, emphasis in original) as if these were natural. That said, men, as flesh and blood bodies, cannot avoid masculine domination. Bourdieu (2001: 69) mentions men's height, though men's fatness cannot be ignored – something that carries a heavy stigma since it is often attributed to volitional sedentary lifestyles and, implicitly, feminine passivity. Hence, to return to Patrick, the taxi driver, self-disgust is not always neutralized by big fellas voicing justifiable resistance and defiance. Big boys might not cry, or so the aphorism goes, but internalized fat oppression and the injurious effects of masculine domination were still publicly expressed to me, a professional stranger.

The next chapter concludes the book. The value of exercising healthy scepticism is underscored alongside the empirical, theoretical and political value of 'bringing in' men to critical weight studies. Several policy recommendations are also offered plus some final words on resisting and possibly ending the war on obesity.

6 Conclusion

Social fitness and health at every size

This chapter is divided into four sections. First, the value of exercising healthy scepticism is revisited with reference to preceding chapters, nascent critical weight studies, the Health at Every Size paradigm and fat activism. Second, the empirical, theoretical and political value of 'bringing in' men is discussed. Third, some policy recommendations are outlined. Finally, some words are offered on the possibility of resisting and ending the war on obesity.

Exercising healthy scepticism: A fitting response in wartime

As stated in Chapter 1, we are reportedly witnessing a global obesity epidemic (WHO 1998). It is doubtful whether such claims have much currency in developing nations marred by a historical legacy of European colonization, crippling debt to the developed world, absolute poverty, inequitable land ownership, armed conflict, chronic hunger and real epidemics of contagious diseases that are often fatal because of malnutrition (Young 1997). However, in the developed world, claims about an 'obesity epidemic' do have currency and are widely circulated. Here authoritative declarations of war, and other militaristic talk, are legitimated by the idea that overweight and obesity are ubiquitous. This is evidenced by rhetorical appeals from former US Surgeon Generals, the UK Government, the Chief Medical Officer and agencies like Sport England. Such definitional practices are inseparable from a powerful and profitable 'health-industrial complex' that has done much to construct a massive social problem that should be fought and tackled on an unprecedented scale (Oliver 2006). They are also inseparable from a gender order where symbolic violence perpetuates masculine domination (Bourdieu 2001) and other forms of oppression and social inequality.

While 'the war on fat' has been condemned as 'an outrage to values – of equality, of tolerance, of fairness, and indeed of fundamental decency' (Campos 2004: xvii), there is nothing peculiar about this dissemination of fear, anxiety and moral panic. Late modern societies are risk and body oriented societies where embodied selves have to be reflexively constructed and mobilized amidst continual warnings from experts about danger (Beck 1992, Giddens 1991). Despite scientific uncertainty and controversy, obesity is a fitting metaphorical disease for social dis-ease: the perceived excesses and adverse consequences of rationalizing modernity (Sontag 1978), which also threaten to emasculate men. While the vulnerability of childhood evokes obvious concerns and stimulates action, men's real and imagined fatness is also very publicly targeted as part of a larger disciplinary and instituted project. This was observed in the UK with reference to the Men's Health Forum (MHF 2005), the National Audit Office (NAO 2001) and the British Broadcasting Corporation (BBC Online 2007). Men's and women's health is in many respects similar (Carpenter 2000, Connell 2000) but claiming the majority of men are overweight or obese, and their physiology renders them especially at risk from the putative harms of fatness, fits with the new public health. That is, where men are deemed 'weaker and more physically vulnerable than women' (Petersen and Lupton 1996: 87). The bellicose idea that something should be done to combat this 'crisis' is thus promoted in the name of a 'gender equitable' approach to health.

The invocation of health (risk) rather than beauty or fashion might seem an incontestable rationale for the war on obesity, a war that is presented by respected institutions as vital rather than outrageous. Nonetheless, Chapter 1 reiterated Berger's (1963) point that things are not as they seem. How people understand the world is a product of social definitions and sometimes sharply contrasting interpretations. This is not to deny the importance of biology. Sociologists of the body/embodiment seek cautiously to 'bring in' and debate biology (Williams *et al.* 2003) and I endorse these efforts. There is, to use critical realist terminology, an 'intransitive' reality or 'mind independent world' that human fallible theories attempt to grasp, and biomedical narratives about various diseases may be more or less convincing and useful (Williams 2003b: 52). However, while disease processes may contribute to weight-gain (and embodied social processes, such as medical efforts to improve health, may also have that effect), the idea that there is a real 'chronic disease' called 'obesity' (WHO 1998) is not particularly convincing for many people inside and outside of academia (Chapters 1 and 2).

This book repudiated the war on obesity that surrounds lived bodies and everyday embodied practices. This warmongering, and associated battles, is inseparable from Western cultural prejudice and is seemingly legitimated by solid science. In remaining reflexive about the deeply ingrained nature of anti-fat prejudice, which also finds expression in academic commentary, I presented a more critical and ethnographically rich contribution than other sociologists (for example, Crossley 2004, Giddens 2006) and psychologists (for example, Brownell 2005). Although I have challenged dominant 'background expectancies' (Scott and Lyman 1968, Chapter 2) where fat is bad and in need of correction, I hope I have covered enough ground to at least prompt a reconsideration of the institutional attack on medicalized fatness. While fat fighting often constitutes an aesthetic project, especially for women (Bordo 1993, Seid 1989), militarized medicine also provides heavy ideological and material artillery for this public and private battle. It is thus open to interrogation with a view to improving current institutional practices that are ostensibly intended to improve people's biomedical health and well-being.

As explained in Chapter 1, it is difficult promoting critical thinking or healthy scepticism among those who might authoritatively contribute to the obesity debate and perhaps promote more peaceful relations. Plenty of middle-class commentators, academics, health officials and obesity scientists perpetuate the perceived 'ills' of overweight/obesity/fatness. Many people in everyday life also acquiesce with the view that fat is bad in relation to themselves and others. None of this is to suggest people who are targeted by militarized medicine are passive victims or duped by propaganda. Fat fighting, even among slimmers who are healthy and sceptical, is often situationally rational. Many men are also personally seduced despite the traditional 'sexual division of dieting' (Germov and Williams 1996). To quote Bourdieu (2001: 22), 'the worst humiliation for a man is to be turned into a woman', and talk about looking pregnant, or becoming sickly and frail, obviously justifies his efforts to lose weight (see the next section). Despite scientific evidence that moderate 'overweight' and 'obesity' may benefit biomedical health, fatness is made into a problem by and for many people.

If fat is defined as a real problem then it will have real consequences in terms of how people relate to themselves and others, with possibly deleterious effects on health and well-being. Streamlining the body, for those who have the resources, might be risky and largely ineffective but it is an eminently sensible 'body project' (Shilling 2003) in late modernity. This is because the consequences of being seen to 'fail' can be high indeed. That, however, underscores the importance of exercising healthy scepticism in informed academic studies. Despite the seductions of slimming, a theme running through this book is that the institutional attack on fat is highly questionable if not objectionable. Although we are authoritatively told there is an obesity epidemic, and most people should lose weight, such claims are highly uncertain and may do more harm than good (Gard and Wright 2005, Rich and Evans 2005). Of course, such a statement might seem heretical to 'true believers' but this book connects with a growing critical literature. This is from a range of disciplines and it is reaching a critical mass (for example, Aphramor 2005, Burns and Gavey 2004, Campos 2004, Campos *et al.* 2006a, b, Carryer 2001, Cohen *et al.* 2005, Evans *et al.* forthcoming, Gaesser 2002, Gard 2003, Herndon 2005, Jutel 2005, LeBesco 2004, Mayer 2004, Miller 1999, Oliver 2006).

This literature sometimes draws from or extends the Health at Every Size paradigm (Robison 1999, 2005a, b). This clinically relevant approach is not a substitute for tackling socio-economic inequalities and reducing the social gradient in health (Marmot 2004). Nonetheless, it has pragmatic value, it is inclusive and it has depth, with proponents looking beyond normative embodiment (size, shape, weight, appearance) as a criterion for success. Instead of obsessing about and profiting from a culturally prescribed image of health, this paradigm is formulated on the basis of evidence of what works and with a genuine concern for people's biomedical health and well-being. Basic themes include the acceptance of 'natural' bodily diversity, the view that dieting is ineffective and risky, and a more rounded appreciation of what affects health (social, emotional, physical factors, etc.). People's weight might change with this approach, but it might not, with contributors such as Gaesser (2002: xxiv) stating 'the roads to good health are wide enough for everyone'. In my view this is a significant improvement on biomedical reductionism and the weight-centred approach to health.

As a caveat, it should be clear from preceding chapters that I have no intention of proscribing and prescribing ways of living for everyday people who are making their way in the real world. In my view it is not the place of sociology to deny people the right to try to lose weight/fat or, for that matter, preach the merits of healthy lifestyles. However, in seeking to interpret everyday life, critically evaluate and perhaps improve institutional practices, it seems to me that intentional weight-loss is primarily an exercise in social not metabolic fitness. It is about fitting in with a society where 'fat' does not 'fit in' with the favoured view. This is a conclusion I have reached even when researching men who often masculinized slimming through medicalization (Chapter 3). Such action is socially logical in developed nations, but, crucially, this does not have to be aggressively promoted by militarized medicine on a massive scale. The fashion or 'style industries' (Orbach 2006) obviously constitute a 'multi-billion dollar industry which not only capitalizes on male as well as female insecurity, but also actively fosters them' (Annandale 2003: 89). However, it is disturbing to see that medicine is also implicated, given its ties with big business and highly profitable pharmaceutical companies (Angell 2004, Conrad 2004, Kassirer 2005). This, of course, would come as no surprise to theorists of modernity and advocates of corporeal realism where it is maintained that 'the money economy' is thoroughly implicated in the 'rationalization of life' and the constitution of gendered and feeling bodies in ways that may undermine human potentiality (Shilling 2005: 34).

As discussed in the opening chapter, political economic forces are powerful. They constrain critical discussion alongside other considerations like healthism, obesity epidemic psychology, class disdain and religiosity. As made clear throughout this book, gender is also central because it is inscribed in the whole social order and bodies co-constituting that order. Western culture comprises an 'androcentric unconscious' that is embodied and at the heart of social interaction (Bourdieu 2001). Social games that construct sexually differentiated and differentiating bodies are often taken seriously, with slimming constituting a 'truth game' (Frank 1991, Chapter 2). However, if biomedical health is the *real* rationale here – as measured by metabolic fitness and other markers like cardiorespiratory fitness, morbidity and mortality risk (for example, Blair and Brodney 1999) – then Health at Every Size makes sense.

Based on my reading, this paradigm enables people to avoid the common frustrations and irrationalities associated with practices intended to cut bodies down in size. This approach eschews aesthetic commodification, irrational rationalization and aggressive militarization. It would be promising if this paradigm informed institutional practice, or at least prompted collaborative, rather than combative, discussion among groups who are genuinely concerned about people's biomedical health and well-being. This fits with my stated intention to advance critically informed, and productive, dialogue in ways that are attuned to the biological and social. This is consonant with an embodied approach to sociology, as evidenced by key body theorists such as Shilling (2003). There is also nothing more practical than a good theory and the above also fits with the concerns of health professionals and contributors to the obesity debate who thoughtfully challenge and go beyond militarized medicine.

Rather than warmongering from above, then, I concur with sociologically imaginative health professionals when stating there is a need to promote peace if not peace of mind. This is in the context of public health discourses and clinician patient interactions (Bacon 2006). Certainly, there are international differences in healthcare contexts and healthy scepticism may be more difficult for US clinicians than those in nations such as Britain, given the aggressive and inter-ventionist nature of US medicine. However, it is clear that health professionals in various nations do not always consider militarized medicine helpful. As remarked by Aphramor and Gingras (2007: 170), in their role as dieticians in Britain and Canada: 'how a militaristic approach is going to help anyone make peace with their bodies or food is unclear'.

In underscoring the value of healthy scepticism in academic and policy discussions I would add that it is also unclear how militarized medicine and obesity warmongering are going to (a) enable contributors to talk with, rather than past, each other and (b) foster cohesive social relations when they provide people and organizations with a license to take shots at others – including shots fired in the targets' supposed best interests (Chapter 3). After all, telling most men they are 'too fat' and 'are denting their seats' (BBC Online 2007), their waists are 'hazardous' (MHF 2005), or men with a 'potbelly' are pregnant (Schauss 2006), hardly smacks of a responsible and caring approach to health. It is not much different from saying diets fail because people lack willpower (Chapter 3). Such moralizing and empirically unsubstantiated claims nonetheless provide a clear index of institutional sizism, which is deemed acceptable even among those who ostensibly care. Whether intended or not, these definitional practices further the war on female and feminized (despised) fatness regardless of the targets' biological sex. It pathologizes fatness and assaults people deemed fat for sup-posedly being lazy, gluttonous, ugly, immoral, costly and culpable for all the ills that befall them (or, if we are referring to children, it is mothers who usually get flak). This metaphorical war clearly does not invent fat hatred but, as with real war, it is 'an enormous amplification' of the prejudices and cruelties already present in society (Berger 1997: 171).

As a reflexive discipline with an ethical base and critical outlook (Stanley 2005), sociology should challenge this symbolic violence. Even when entering a slimming club that profits from fat fighting, I had no intention of validating anti-fat prejudice and joining the search for a magic bullet. There are already plenty of industries and entrepreneurs doing that, with their actions reproducing stigma. Stigma is an emergent product of social relations, definitions and structures, not the supposed intrinsic 'ills' of weight/fat, and the obesity industry is far from innocent in reinforcing and manufacturing this. Indeed, manufacturing is an apt descriptor because industries in the front line in the war on obesity are compar-able to the frequently condemned fast-food industry (Chapter 4). Scepticism, then, should be viewed as healthy. This is a politically crucial point, with this book also *critically* drawing from and extending fat acceptance scholarship and activism (for example, Brown and Rothblum 1989, Cooper 1998). Such work deserves wider recognition because it has long challenged fat oppression as sexist and harmful to public health (Freespirit and Aldebaran 1973).

Reservations within medical sociology about 'social oppression' views notwithstanding, the value of fat activism in formulating different, more humanistic and potentially transformative knowledge should be underscored. As with Health at Every Size, this movement significantly predates the new wave of academic studies that challenge the war on obesity, and, as explained in Chapter 2, strands of fat activism informed this study. Like disability activists, fat activists often flex their sociological imaginations by focusing on social, cultural, economic and political factors that result in exclusion, marginalization, reduced life chances and compromised health (especially for women who are 'really' fat). This appealed to my sociological sensibilities and was useful when critically interpreting data (for example, viewing efforts to 'support' slimming as a covert form of oppression that bites back when diets are aborted). Pragmatically, fat activism also offers participants the promise of 'identity reconstruction' (Williams 1999). This makes sense in a society that routinely shames and blames those who are seen as fat in everyday life. Identity reconstruction is intended to make fatness more liveable and possibly a source of pride (Cooper 1998). Hence, fat activism may be seductive for different people on various levels, though caveats are required.

When drawing from fat activism I continued exercising critical judgement. Certainly, fat activism is a diverse field of debate and I critiqued some arguments that also find expression in academic and popular accounts (for example, appeals to addiction and blaming fast-food industries) (Chapters 2 and 4). What LeBesco (2004) calls 'the will to innocence' was not always accepted if such claims were sociologically unimaginative. I also recognized that some fat activists (for example, Cooper 1998), and potential feminist recruits (S. Murray 2005), are themselves critically reflexive. Thus, S. Murray (2005) makes clear that identity and fatphobia are embodied and efforts to feel proud about one's fatness may actually be more difficult than trying to become and remain slim. Hence, fat acceptance might sound like a good idea for those who risk social censure but ideas are not simply the property of free-floating minds that are separate from bodies and society (Williams and Bendelow 1998). Also, Cooper (1998: 182) states that some fat activists are themselves prejudiced (for example, towards thin people, smaller or much larger fat people and people with eating disorders), which contradicts the goal of attempting to 'free everyone from body hatred'. By the same token, I would question fat activists if they condemn people for slimming. An individualized 'solution' is problematic but it is understandable and perhaps personally necessary under present social conditions. Given the fluidity of bodily alignment and accounts (Chapter 2), I would add that slimming does not preclude people from challenging fat hatred, the realities of size discrimination and the supposed effectiveness or desirability of 'cures' (Chapters 3, 4 and 5).

In remaining critical I also took a leaf from medical sociologists when discussing social oppression views on disability (Williams 1999). Thus, given parallels with the social model of disability – which has been recommended to fat activists, if not always explicitly used (Cooper 1997, LeBesco 2004, Chapter 2) – I accepted the critical realist point that 'real bodies' exert their presence in the context of 'real lives' and impairment and illness cannot be ignored (Williams 1999). Fatness, like disability (Shakespeare 2006), cannot be reduced to oppression and the definitional workings of a prejudiced society. Yet, I still think fat activists are right to emphasize the *social relational* aspects of their disabling experiences over the 'real limitations' of their corporeality. After all, most people encountering size discrimination and compromised living are not necessarily physically impaired or ill and even if they are one cannot simply assume it is because of their fatness, which is somehow abstracted from an iniquitous society that works around, on and through real bodies (Chapters 1 and 2).

If approached cautiously and reflectively fat activism thus has its uses, though, like disability activism (Oliver 2004), it does not do the work of sociology. This is understandable because fat activism is a pragmatic project that has less to do with contributing to social scientific knowledge and more to do with making life better for people who are seen as fat and identify as fat. That said, the fat activists' pragmatic motive could also be critiqued. This, I want to stress, is not simply for the sake of criticism; rather, I want to maintain that aspects of fat activism have broader value and this extends beyond the interests of 'fat people'. It is also to place fat activists' political hopefulness within a critical realist and interactionist framework that recognizes the limitations of fat politics in a field of social inequality and domination.

Thus, to extend insights from Goffman (1968), it should be recognized that fat activism may have the unfortunate effect of consolidating a public perception of 'fat people' as constituting a real, stigmatized group. Stated differently, 'the symbolic strategies' of those dominated by masculine domination, rather than subverting existing social relations of domination, 'have the effect of confirming the dominant [negative] representation' (Bourdieu 2001: 32). It is unsurprising, then, that people advocating the fight against obesity often do so by stating obese people are stigmatized, thus offering a circular line of reasoning that reinforces rather than challenges symbolic violence. Fat oppression is a real, emergent process that should be taken seriously and condemned (Chapter 3). However, the fat activists' argument that 'fat people' are a socially oppressed group, who experience discrimination and hatred solely because of their body size, is an essentialist position that is politically limited and limiting. This is problematic not only for confirming prejudices that could intensify rather than end obesity warmongering. It is problematic because public health officials – in blurring dichotomies such as normal/deviant, us/them, majority/minority – seek to democratize fatness. After all, most people in developed nations are supposed to be fat! This symbolic violence, which reproduces a corporeal version of 'healthism' (Crawford 1980) that hits the visibly fat hardest, rationalizes various injustices that are inseparable from other embodied social divisions like class, gender, ethnicity and ability. Even if fat oppression disappeared tomorrow, these divisions and associated inequalities in life chances would persist because they are part of the very fabric, structure and organization of Western societies. For me, this means aspects of fat activist thinking, when used as a sociological resource, have broad but not exclusive and exhaustive relevance (for example, when critically interpreting weight concerns among people in everyday life, when politicizing fatness and repudiating obesity warmongering as directed at everyone). In short, fat activism is not synonymous with sociology but it may inform it in ways that go beyond activists' intentions. Rather than being parasitic, I hope fat activists can also learn from sociology in ways that benefit their efforts to promote social change and a more equitable society. This, I would stress, should be a more just society for everybody regardless of where or if people fall on a crude fat/thin dichotomy.

Despite my goal of promoting productive dialogue among a range of parties, and the ground I have covered to facilitate this, I know not all audiences will be receptive (Chapter 1). These include people who are most heavily invested in the status quo and perhaps some sociologists who rightly claim 'fat is a sociological issue' but nonetheless misrepresent fat politics with comments like '[w]hatever the protestations of the representatives of "fat politics", obesity is not defined as a bodily ideal in late modern societies' (Crossley 2004: 228). Certainly, I do not naively draw from fat activism, believing this book will be enthusiastically welcomed by most obesity researchers and anti-fat campaigners (a proportion of whom not only believe they are right, but who are also righteous in what they believe is right for everybody else). Unsurprisingly, biomedical experts and researchers working within, and deriving income and status from, 'the health-industrial complex' (Oliver 2006) dismiss fat activism. Accepting fatness, or trying to develop better self-esteem by taking pride in one's fatness, is anything but socially fitting according to the dominant biomedical view. Within the typically polarized obesity debate there are efforts to discredit politicized interpretations (Saguy and Riley 2005), much in line with the cut and thrust of masculinist, militarized medicine. Yet, while productive dialogue is theoretically possible, if the activists' political, experiential and corporeally grounded knowledges are dismissed or misrepresented then hostilities will persist. I am not a fat activist but I can see there is much ammunition to enable them to fight back. And, with warnings from dieticians about possible litigation from patients in the absence of informed consent (Aphramor 2005), plus the awarding of substantial damages to people encountering size discrimination in other contexts (Campos 2006), there are good pecuniary as well as humanistic and clinical motives to take heed (Chapters 1 and 3).

In short, an affinity exists between fat activism, academic work and clinical practice. A growing coalition is providing a critically informed response to the obesity discourse and oppressive systems of meaning and practice. Rather than proponents of the obesity discourse simply rejecting alternative ways of thinking and acting, one is likely to witness defensive moves, countermoves and even incorporation for the purposes of containment. Indeed, as mentioned by Aphramor and Gingras (2007: 160), Health at Every Size is now being interpreted within mainstream dietetics through the lens of anti-fat bias so that it becomes a 'blunder-buss' where weight-loss is still endorsed. This continued recommendation is offered, in part, given the stigma of obesity. This resistance to a more rounded understanding thus underscores the real world relevance of repudiating the war on obesity and authoritative messages and practices that tell millions of people their bodies are inadequate.

As explained in Chapter 2, repudiating discourses vary. Softer versions attempt to mitigate individual responsibility for fatness, while challenging its pejorative status. This is not the same as rejecting biomedical health (notably, metabolic fitness) and the value of adopting 'healthy lifestyles' should socio-economic circumstances permit this. However, and for good reasons, this discourse refuses to treat health and slenderness as synonymous and weight-loss as necessary in order to lead a healthy life or life worth living. The Health at Every Size paradigm is again relevant here. Harder versions are more attuned to the contradictions of human embodiment and are not dependent on mitigating personal responsibility or proving moral worth by capitulating to healthism. As observed during this study, men, who were not fat activists also expressed such understandings. Their views are summarized in the next section when discussing the empirical, theoretical and political value of 'bringing in' men. Harder repudiation also explicitly informs my thinking in the penultimate section on policy recommendations. In so doing, lifestyle is relegated under social structure in matters of health and illness – a harder but more sociologically warranted move than that taken by other critical contributors (Campos *et al.* 2006b, Gaesser 2002). This is necessary because social structural inequalities have the biggest impact on population health (Marmot 2004, Scambler 2002). It is also necessary because the idea of health goes beyond biology and statistical risk and involves questions about how people wish to live and relate to each other in a broader interpretive community.

Finally, I recognize that whether most people researching and working in this area are willing or able to publicly exercise healthy scepticism is itself questionable, even outside the USA. After all, there is the risk of being accused of 'organizational insubordination' and 'professional irresponsibility' even when efforts to engage colleagues and the public are extremely well researched (Aphramor and Gingras 2007: 165). Fitzpatrick (2001) makes a related point in relation to many clinicians in Britain who have private reservations about public health promotion but dare not express these through fear of repercussions. However, barriers are not only, always or necessarily about government commitments, medical vested interests, profits, careers or (mis)perceived efficiencies in tackling obesity at a population level. There are also quasi-religious, personally therapeutic and highly emotive investments in sustaining the largely individualized fight against fat. And, as evidenced by the popularity of slimming, people often align themselves, however fleetingly, with the dominant view where fat is bad and in need of correction. Why should we expect any different? If fatness is routinely discredited, and weight-loss is framed as ethical self-care (Heyes 2006), then people will try to align their maligned bodies in socially expected ways. And they will do this even if remedial work is risky, expensive, frustrating and largely unsuccessful. Publicly challenging received 'truths' and adopting a more tolerant and accepting, rather than aggressively masculine, approach is difficult during wartime. Going somewhat further and advocating pride, liberation and civil rights (Wann 1998) is also extremely difficult, if not impossible, for some people who conceivably have much to gain from 'doing politics' (S. Murray 2005). Yet, as evidenced by critical weight studies, feminisms, fat activism and the Health at Every Size paradigm, there are dissenting voices. Critically drawing from and contributing to these, I would stress the value of incorporating social structural concerns, an understanding of sexed/gendered embodiment and qualitative data from everyday people who may accept and reproduce but also resist and challenge the dominant biomedical narrative.

'Bringing in' men: Empirical, theoretical and political gains

By 'bringing in' men and exploring their views, this book offered empirical data on an under-researched topic, used and expanded social theory and contributed to politicized thinking that challenges the degradation of lived bodies. This section elaborates on these interrelated points, thus providing a summary and synthesis of this book's various contributions.

Sociological research on men's body projects and identity construction has been criticized for largely excluding men's voices (Gill *et al.* 2005), while Bell and McNaughton (2007) bemoan the lack of gender aware research on men and the war on fat. During this study the aim was to generate data on men's understandings about issues that could be related to, if not always directly about, weight or fatness. More formally, I also wanted to subject these data to a sociologically imaginative analysis that was appreciative of men's presentations of self but also critical of authoritative warmongering and 'the obesity discourse' (Rich and Evans 2005), i.e. institutional messages, dominated by medicine, that tell people their bodies are inadequate because of their real or imagined fatness. Many questions were thus posed. For example, how do men, regardless of whether or not they consider themselves overweight or obese, talk about their lives as flesh and blood bodies? What do men have to say about health and fitness, which might include body size/weight/shape/composition but also other modalities of embodiment such as the pragmatic, visceral and experiential (Watson 2000)? How do men talk about diets and, if weight-loss and dieting are personally relevant, how do they arrive at the decision to go on a diet? Why are dietary approaches to weight-loss often aborted? How do male slimmers negotiate masculinities given the pathologization and feminization of fatness and 'the sexual division of dieting' (Germov and Williams 1996)? What do men think of government-backed campaigns that promote physical activity in order to fight obesity? In addressing such questions, and in theorizing from men's bodies, this study has offered a timely contribution to the literature. If weight/fat is being defined as a worrying masculine issue, by various agencies and advocates of men's health, then it is incumbent to critically explore what this might mean in relation to men's definitions, identities, 'body-reflexive practices' (Connell 1995) and 'modalities of embodiment' (Watson 2000).

Empirical chapters reported men's views and subjected these to a theoretically informed and politically attuned interpretation. This was a case of including, but also going beyond, respondents' meanings and discourses (Williams 2003b), with sociologists such as Bourdieu (2001), Connell (1995), Watson (2000) and Ritzer (2004) providing theoretical purchase on empirical data. As seen with reference to modalities of embodiment, Watson (2000) was useful when exploring how male bodies are lived, experienced and visualized, while Ritzer (2004), following Weber (1930), sensitized me to rationalizing or McDonaldizing processes. And, while Bourdieu (2001) offers concepts such as symbolic violence that make sense of masculine domination and sexual differentiation, Connell (1995, 2000) offers complementary theorizing on the relational construction of plural masculinities, bodily agency and social justice. Drawing from such work in a sometimes critical way (for example, symbolic violence is not always subtle, claims about fast-food and obesity are themselves McDonaldized), this research explored how men, who risked subordination in wartime, constructed masculinities. These embodied constructions were ongoing practical accomplishments among men who presented themselves as everyday fellas, rather than deviant and woman-like.

Before summarizing empirical themes I should stress that this study is partial. Space permitting, much more could have been said, for example, about men's immediate strategies for partially or totally eclipsing discredited corporeality: an exercise in embodied sociology that would have conceptual and political value. Conceptually, this would have enabled me to develop the astral metaphor, used in Chapters 2 and 3, to understand how relational bodies generate social warmth, heat or are placed in the shadows. This would have political value because it would show the various means by which men *as* men 'shined' or blended with others in social space. These means of 'doing' masculinity are inseparable from gendered power that valorizes different aspects of fe/male embodiment/bodies; note, for instance, the common emphasis on transient female beauty in the 'economy of symbolic goods' (Bourdieu 2001). Substantive themes that deserve attention include: looking beyond the physical body and projecting confidence (i.e. men's talk about the importance of who you are, rather than what you are); being jolly and humorous as a means of aligning with, or disarming, other people; using physical violence as a situationally fitting, though qualified, response to redress masculinity challenges; the meanings of grooming, clothing and other props; and, maintaining women are under much more 'pressure' to attend to their appearance and lose weight.

Even so, this book has still offered a detailed and appreciative understanding of what it might mean for men to live at a time when their bodily 'bigness' is authoritatively maligned and ridiculed as unhealthy fatness. As might be expected from a qualitative study, men's views reflected the richness of everyday life. Their positions ranged from acquiescence with fat fighting as a personal and publicly endorsed bodily practice (an obvious route to demonstrating social fitness) to justifiable resistance and defiance, or, more usually, a complex mixture of conformity and resistance. This nuanced picture challenges simplistic accounts that portray men as unconcerned about their health and well-being.

Of course, for men who might identify with 'weight problems', negotiating identities is not dependent on weight-loss. The possibility of bodily alignment through 'accounts' (Scott and Lyman 1968), which bridge the gap between (in)actions and expectations, meant that even if weight or fat was personally problematic it was possible to negotiate identities in ways that were more or less successful. Such accounts, inseparable from interactions, institutions and gender (West and Zimmerman 2002), drew from a socially shared 'stock-of-knowledge' (Schutz 1962). Men's accounts typically comprised excuses (for example, working long hours or physical injury) and justifications (for example, the love of beer and socializing in the pub). However, as seen with medicalized excuse-accounts, which ostensibly mitigate personal responsibility, these aligning actions do not necessarily negate the cultural 'suspicion' that 'fat people' are still 'their own worst enemies' (Edgley and Brissett 1990: 262; Chapter 2). Hence, attempts to lose 'weight' (implicitly or explicitly fat) made sense for big fellas even though, as many asserted, women are under more 'pressure' to be slim. While various techniques promise a slimmer body, diet, or what has been called 'healthy eating' (Chapman 1999), is an everyday 'recipe for action' (Schutz 1970) inside and outside of slimming clubs. In contrast to some feminist accounts, such action cannot be considered the antithesis of masculinity (Wolf 1991), if, indeed, it ever could be seen in such terms (Huff 2001, Schwartz 1986, Stearns 1997).

Men participating in this study often wanted to lose weight through diet and enacted contrition (Chapter 2). However, to cite a sociological truism, they did not act under conditions of their own choosing. Rather, they acted under historically transmitted conditions that were directly encountered. These conditions, although not determining social action, are sociologically relevant. In an age of abundance, there is the taken-for-granted view, if not obligation, that competent men should display rationality, efficiency and control over their fleshy bodies. There may be greater latitude for men than women to resist the culture of slenderness. As noted when discussing justifications, being an adult male means having a physical presence in the world (Connell 1995, Morgan 1993): extra bulk, regardless of whether it is muscle or fat, is related to the space-occupying dimensions of male bodies and gendered power (Klein 1996). However, there are degrees of bodily bigness/fatness and associated judgements cannot be divorced from streamlined bodily aesthetics, biomedical health (risk) and dominant ideas of social fitness. Hence, slimming has currency for many big fellas as a means of aligning themselves with gendered body norms, the imperative of health, other people and their own socially acquired schemes of perception, thinking and feeling.

Some men mentioned the importance of masculine bodily aesthetics, or not wishing to be abjectly associated with the feminine (look pregnant or have 'man boobs'). In Watson's (2000: 118–19) schema, their attention shifted to 'normative embodiment' with 'soft edges' seen and felt to threaten gendered bodily boundaries and manhood (also Longhurst 2005a). Such concerns – perhaps prompted by photographs, a glimpse in a shop window, forthcoming social occasions or other people's comments – were not confined to younger men. Middle-aged men, both inside and outside of slimming clubs, also expressed dissatisfaction with their bodies. This is in a larger consumer culture that valorizes the image of youth for women and men (Featherstone 1991, Grogan 1999), with the 'hard edged' contours of an athletically muscular male physique symbolizing power and sexual currency. While men who identified as heterosexual felt they were living at a time when there was more 'pressure' to look trim, this was deemed especially relevant in the mainstream gay community. That said, power meets resistance (Foucault 1978) and, for 'big' gay men, the Bear subculture provided some relief from what one man called 'body fascism' (Chapters 2 and 3; also, Monaghan 2005b).

More broadly, intolerance towards men's real or imagined fatness is intensified in late modernity given the socially defined risks of overweight and obesity and the obligation to do something about this – a case of what Edgley and Brissett (1990) term 'Health Fascism'. Regardless of the rights or wrongs of this, it is clear that illness, disease and implied vulnerability are an affront to masculinity (Shriver and Waskul 2006, Chapter 2). During this research, an appeal to biomedical health (risk) – usually the idea of promoting longevity in the absence of health problems and perhaps the presence of good metabolic health – was more often emphasized in a sample largely comprising middle-aged male slimmers self-presenting as heterosexual. Besides eschewing the idea of female vanity, health talk made sense amidst highly publicized claims about an obesity crisis. As stated by LeBesco (2004: 29), 'the predominant discourse about fat . . . is a medical one that pathologically constructs fat bodies as "obese"' and it is hardly surprising that medicalization figured in the masculinization and justification of men's slimming. However, even when biomedical health formed the 'meat' of an interview, so to speak, this was sometimes sandwiched and often garnished with aesthetic concerns. Also, without prompting, men often questioned the health rationale for slimming, though they still endorsed health when displaying an acquiescent version of social fitness.

Although questionable, the idea of health was a situationally rational, if ultimately irrational, justification for (repeated) dieting in the context of men's own biographies. Talk does not simply provide a transparent window on the world (Silverman 2001) but dieting careers made sense with reference to multiple 'triggers' (Zola 1973). Triggering deposited dispositions within the masculine habitus (Bourdieu 2001), these critical events made his weight 'topically relevant' (Schutz 1970). Although many and varied, triggers gave concrete expression to the Western cultural fear and loathing of fatness that is 'in' minds, bodies and society. While triggers were sometimes harsh and hurtful, especially when pulled by other people, sugar-coated rationales were forthcoming (notably, health concerns). Hence, triggers were more or less acceptable among men (critically) consenting to symbolic violence.

Triggers were an emergent property of social relations and self-body relations within a larger gender order. Similar to Germov and Williams (1996), Stinson (2001) describes dieting as a gendered practice (common among women) and, empirically, it is worth noting that men's diets were often mediated through their relationships with women who were dieting (Chapter 3). Health promoters would probably welcome this but there is a darker side. In a context of healthism, obesity epidemic psychology and 'courtesy stigma' (Goffman 1968), the meanings constituting male obesity could discredit women who are assumed to care for their men as a conventional route to respectability (Skeggs 1997). From the perspective of some men, their women were nagging, but women's complaints made sense just as men's diets were situationally rational and geared to the practical logic of everyday life. While single men might have enacted contrition because they felt they did not have the requisite bodily capital 'to get laid' or meet a romantic partner, married men's efforts to lose weight through diet (or any other means) made sense given their desire to keep the peace, perhaps keep their sex lives and even their relationships in a context of 'confluent love' (Giddens 1992).

These symbolic interactions and associated 'body projects' (Shilling 2003) gave expression to and reproduced a much larger and consequential reality that is well recognized by many feminists and female fat activists. This is a world where one's value as a person is inseparable from how one's body is seen through masculine eyes or categories (Bourdieu 2001). Critically, it was observed that dieting was frequently triggered by size discrimination or stigmatizing 'fat oppression' (Brown and Rothblum 1989). Fat oppression was an emergent and embodied reality and there were many smoking guns. These included clinical misdiagnosis, discrimination in employment, name-calling and generally being put down or feeling down. As with studies on stigma and health (for example, Scambler and Hopkins 1986), these processes discredited people and 'spoilt identities' (Goffman 1968) though there was more, such as the real impact on earning capacity. Fat oppression was especially problematic for 'really' big fellas from the slimming club, though much smaller men, who were contacted outside of slimming clubs and identified with 'weight problems', also talked about being targeted by others. Reference was made to sniping comments from 'friends' or strangers and 'advice' from parents. Some also talked about feeling ugly, their lack of confidence and poor self-esteem because of how they imagined their bodies looked to others.

In such a context, some of these men felt hurt though they demonstrated survivorship. Sociologically, gender differences should not be exaggerated (Carpenter 2000, Connell 2000) but masculinity offered certain privileges that apparently outweighed those associated with social class. Largely from working-class backgrounds, these men demonstrated more resilience than women in Chapman's (1999) research who had economic and cultural capital but were unable successfully to lose weight and see themselves as competent. Even if men aborted their diets and/or embodied fatphobia (for example, felt disgusted, reiterated sizist stereotypes, felt terrified about regaining lost weight), none presented themselves as emotionally broken, failed or 'devastated' bodies during interviewing or publicly in other contexts (though some men felt broken in the past due to mental health problems associated with oppressive social circumstances, or chronic illness such as heart problems that preceded and precipitated unwanted weight-gain). In terms of survivorship, dieting enabled men to reclaim masculinity regardless of its outcome in making their bodies smaller. Men also immediately displayed survivorship in response to fat oppression. This was through coolness, indifference and half-hearted compliance. Others were more obviously peeved about social censure and sounded like fat activists. I will say more below about emotions and gendered politics. However, by empirically exploring and challenging the effects of sizism and fatphobia among men, this study supports and extends critical weight studies that focus on women and girls (for example, Burns and Gavey 2004, Carryer 2001, Cooper 1998, Evans *et al.* forthcoming, Rich *et al.* 2006).

Of course, not all men contacted during this research identified with 'weight problems' even if they would be medically labelled overweight or worse. Such men were included given my research interest in men's health more generally and their views about issues that could be related to, if not always directly about, weight/fat. Including such men was important not least because most men do not attend slimming clubs and, regardless of their BMI, would not necessarily accept the idea that they are 'too heavy' and should lose weight. Yet, in a sample that was purposely selected to reflect the personal rather than research-imposed relevance of unwanted weight (an ethical but also theoretically important decision), many men identified as 'overweight' and sought to 'fight fat' with institutional 'support'. Understandably then, many empirical aspects of this research do not fundamentally challenge medicalized meanings that oblige people to take arms in the war on obesity. This is an important point in a study that is critical of the institutional attack on fat and the battles it mandates or incites. In short, I have not gone out of my way to include men who fundamentally disagreed with the cultural degradation of fatness. By purposively selecting and including men who publicly identified with 'weight problems' and sought to slim down, I was able to empirically explore whether fat fighting really was acceptable among people personally invested in this.

This study thus constituted a critical case when researching the acceptability or otherwise of intentional weight-loss. Interestingly, even when men publicly and recurrently sought to slim down, compliance usually only went so far. There was movement away from the ideal type, the stylized slimmer who fully embraces contrition and seeks forgiveness for their 'sins' (Chapter 2). Thus, biomedical health might have been a common 'vocabulary of motive' (Mills 1940) for slimming but few men within and beyond slimming clubs accepted the medicalized claim that they should achieve a putatively 'healthy' weight as defined by the BMI. This index was often considered ridiculous, even though endorsing it could enable men to present a 'responsible' image of themselves as knowledgeable about official definitions and keen to comply. Here a supposedly 'healthy' BMI was considered highly restrictive (a case of looking and feeling ill), with men's talk constituting 'secondary adjustment' to, or 'expressed distance' from (Goffman 1961a), slimming, i.e. fulfilling major obligations while expressing a certain degree of disaffection. While policy concerns are discussed in the next section, it should be clear from what has already been said that men's disaffection should not be rejected by health promoters and taken as a cue for reinvigorated anti-obesity campaigns.

In entering a slimming club and exploring men's weight-loss efforts, other social processes were also explored. These processes, rather than specific individuals, were critiqued if they sustained institutional sizism, fatphobia and body dis-satisfaction. Thus, Chapters 3 and 4 discussed various 'irrationalities' (Ritzer 2004), or unintended consequences, associated with slimming as experienced by men and interpreted by me through a repudiating lens. Empirically, the aim was to place readers in the slimming life world that sustains various irrationalities that account for the justifiable and excusable abandonment of weight-loss diets. These irrationalities, which had variable significance for different men, and have also been documented in critical weight literature, and research on women and dieting (for example, Aphramor 2005, Heyes 2006, Stinson 2001), included: feeling or being made to feel guilty; viewing social events that included eating as obstacles rather than occasions for pleasant conviviality; the compatibility of weight-loss diets with diets that would not be considered nutritious; hunger; smoking; illness that may be precipitated by rapid weight-loss; frustration about not losing weight, or as much weight as hoped; weight fluctuation, which may adversely impact upon biomedical and psychosocial health; the 'double edged' nature of 'support' (i.e. reaffirming the importance of slenderness, which is seldom achieved); doubts about one's honesty; living in a state of intense fear about regaining previously lost weight; and so on. Slimming consultants also played a central role. I would not compare them to the 'pleasantly' offensive Marjorie Dawes in the BBC comedy *Little Britain*, not least because men were often emotionally attached to charismatic consultants who assuaged guilt and bolstered their masculinity. Yet, manufacturing and capitalizing on pain was part of their work even when they honoured members' expressed distance (for example, agreeing the BMI is 'ridiculous').

This did not mean slimming was always unpleasant or devoid of laughter. Religious asceticism, as observed in studies of dieting women (for example, Stinson 2001) and during this study, did not mean slimming was necessarily a cold monastery or 'iron cage' (Ritzer 2004). For successful slimmers, or those who lost weight quickly in the early stages of their dieting career, there was a sense of empowerment and pleasure as expressed among other slimmers (who were often struggling) (Chapters 3 and 4). 'Collective effervescence' (Shilling 2003), or socially generated emotional warmth and solidarity, was observed at Sunshine – a commercial space, metaphorically wrapped in velvet (Ritzer 2004), that was intended to be predictably pleasant for fee-paying members. Given the common discrepancy between effort and reward, male slimmers also joked about their dietary and bodily deviations when enacting 'role distance' (Goffman 1961b). Restated, these men did not take slimming, and its common frustrations, too seriously and definitive of self, at least in terms of their 'publicly visible person' (Cahill 1998) (Chapters 2 and 4). Although oppression was always on the horizon and could become thematic at any stage, some men at Sunshine humorously enacted what I termed unperturbed and hen-pecked masculinities. These displays were especially common in Sandy's predominantly male group. That said, joking also reproduced fatphobia and enacted stigma. For instance, slimming consultants sought to motivate members and sometimes used props that reproduced the idea that fatness was ugly (Chapter 4).

Stepping outside of the slimming club, some men also expressed distance when talking about physical activity – action touted within public health as an efficient tool to achieve 'healthy' weight-loss (Chapter 5). Scientific evidence supporting the sloth narrative, where fatness is caused by sedentary living, is uncertain and equivocal (Gard 2003, Keith *et al.* 2006). However, sport, exercise and physical activity are definers of masculinity and deserved attention even if men did not personally embrace these as 'body-reflexive practices' (Connell 1995) or 'body projects' (Shilling 2003). Various modes of accountability were identified. Analytically, all provided material for challenging the war on obesity and were expressed by men when presenting themselves as socially, if not physically, fit. These enactments ranged from acquiescent to justifiably resistant and defiant. The latter 'display of perspective' (Silverman 2001) was explored in detail, though as an ideal type, this did not always buffer men from 'psychological oppression' and 'intimations of inferiority' (Bartky 1990). This was mediated by various contingencies, notably body size, shape, weight or composition and how men felt about their corporeality in association with other people.

Regardless of whether men were slimming, justifiable resistance and defiance meshed with size or fat acceptance and even affirmation. It comprised numerous themes and fitted various life situations, though some arguments did not fundamentally challenge 'the status quo of symbolic domination' but instead 'merely [sought] accommodation within the prevailing symbolic order' (Brown 2006: 180). This was seen when men's talk was more obviously about muscle than fat, with the former implicitly associated with valued masculinity and the latter with devalued femininity. Nonetheless, explicit reference was made to the fat, physically fit and/or healthy alongside the inefficiency of physical activity for weight-loss (a view also expressed by the critically compliant and thus compatible with slimming). Other men rejected healthism more generally, which subsumes obesity fighting under a larger depoliticizing neo-liberal project where individuals are obliged to 'do the right thing' by getting physically fit. Here respondents challenged health promoters' projection of sizist messages that compounded and confounded health, fitness and weight in ways that belied these men's more sophisticated and sometimes indignant understandings. Again, masculinity was enacted and buffered through such talk, with gender and other 'big' men's discursively constructed bodies providing a 'status shield' (Hochschild 1983) behind which narrators could obtain some protection during wartime.

Regardless of men's own physical activity participation, such talk was about negotiating masculine identities, as explained using the sociology of 'accounts' (Scott and Lyman 1968, Chapter 2) and the person (Cahill 1998). When men voiced self-fulfilment accounts, this was also about resisting imposed discipline; that is, carving out a space to please oneself as these men saw fit and indulging self-defined pleasures that may or may not have resulted in weight-gain. These pleasures included regularly sitting on the couch, and perhaps eating calorific foods, instead of suffering the aches and pains associated with strenuous exercise – distinct, formal and organized pursuits that are deemed 'properly masculine' and which young men often embrace despite possible bodily damage (Connell 1995). No doubt, anti-obesity campaigners would condemn sedentary pleasures as 'obeso-genic' (WHO 1998) – ways of living that, in earlier times, were the preserve of 'the aristocratic leisure classes' (Edgley and Brissett 1990). Yet, if attention focuses on measurable biomedical health, rather than the image of health and behaviour assumed to affect weight, then it is worth stressing that mortality and morbidity risk largely extend beyond lifestyles. Social factors are much more significant, such as status, autonomy, class relations and stress (Aphramor 2005, Chandola *et al.* 2006, Marmot 2004, Scambler 2001). Given this, and the possibility of pleasure and relaxation through 'transgression', I would honour men's justifications.

As can be seen, empirically grounded discussion was theoretically informed just as this research informs social theory. Theory helped me take a stance on matters ranging from men's everyday negotiation or enactment of gendered meanings, practices, identities and personhood to macro-social influences on health, health inequalities and 'socially constructed embodiment' (Freund 2006). Recognizing the interplay of the micro and macro – the salience of personal biography in a broader social and historical scene – this book offered a sociologically imaginative account of the so-called obesity crisis as a public issue and sometimes private trouble (Mills 1970). As well as drawing from sociologists such as Bourdieu (2001), Connell (1995), Watson (2000) and Ritzer (2004), I remained heavily indebted to interactionist or interpretive sociology. Thus, concepts like 'accounts' (Scott and Lyman 1968), 'expressed distance' (Goffman 1961a), 'epidemic psychology' (Strong 1990), 'triggers' (Zola 1973) and 'status shield' (Hochschild 1983) were taken from interactionism. Edgley and Brissett's (1990, 1999) symbolic interactionist work on meddling was also useful. Reflecting the sociologically imaginative call to explore the relations between personal biography, social structure and history, such writing is also attuned to how the past shapes the present (for example, the role of Puritanism in the USA as an antecedent for many health crusades). This type of sociology is valuable and informs other recent qualitative research on body matters (Waskul and Vannini 2006). Such research grounds and expands social theorizing on the body – theorizing that is often abstract and sterile. Similarly, I hope that this book furthers efforts within sociology to empirically ground, re-read and critically extend social theory in a corporeal and gender aware light (Williams and Bendelow 1998).

Theoretically, an important gain from researching men concerns the emotional dimensions of social life and the status accorded to emotions. Contributors to embodied sociology make clear that emotions, like bodies, matter (Williams and Bendelow 1998) and this is a conclusion I would agree with after researching male bodies in the empirical world. Emotions are no less significant than the visceral or physiological, which are prioritized in the obesity discourse in ways that ignore the mutual imbrications of bodies and society. Indeed, as stated by Shilling (2005: 13) when underscoring the centrality of the multi-dimensional body to sociology, 'the embodied subject is possessed not only of a physical boundary and a metabolic network, but of feelings'. While Neckel (1996) relates socially produced feelings of inferiority to an 'emotional nexus' that is integral to the reproduction of social inequalities, Barbalet (2002: 1) states emotions are 'crucial' because 'all actions, and indeed reason itself, require facilitating emotions'. Hence, emotions are not simply good or bad, or a property of the atomized individual; they are multifaceted and social, arising out of symbolic interactions in fields of power. These interactions include self–body interactions that are not dependent on the presence of others (Shott 1979), though they may adversely affect well-being and internal physiological processes (Freund 2006, Shilling 2003). As observed, men identifying with weight problems may have felt weighed down by contrition and sometimes acted in ways that could be compared to holy folly, which invites disgust (Chapter 2). However, men's emotional bodies also constituted orderly gendered public performances. Rather than unreasonable displays, these enactments and associated affective states sometimes constituted a source of knowledge and even health and rationality. This is in a potentially injurious field where some bodies matter more than others because of how they look and the prejudicial meanings ascribed to and inferred from bodily appearance.

As might be expected in this realm of symbolic violence, men experienced, reported and enacted highly abrasive emotions. While self-disgust, shame, inferiority, fear, panic and anxiety were documented, more confrontational (and what could be typified as masculine) emotions included anger, annoyance, consternation, incredulity and a sense of injustice (Chapters 3 and 5). In Bourdieu's (2001) sense there was 'cognitive struggle' and 'antagonistic interpretations' that entailed the interplay of reason and emotion, mind and body, agency and structure, self and society. Ethical issues were a priority during this research – Chapter 1 talked about 'treading lightly on a potential minefield' – but emotions could not be avoided. Men's affective states or feelings emerged within a larger emotional economy where bodies are evaluated according to widely shared, and medically ratified, norms that facilitate stigma and discrimination (Rich and Evans 2005, Shilling 2003). As observed, men's negative but also insightful emotions emerged given their perceptions of imposed discipline, irrational rationalization and the routine belittlement of big people – which was also sometimes discursively amplified in men's shared narratives when conveying the message that they were more often sinned against rather than sinners. Given the weight of contrition, and associated 'shameful recognitions' (Skeggs 1997), these responses were understandable and I sought to empathize with big fellas in a critically informed way.

Men's emotional responses, similar to forms of repudiation and political ways of knowing fatness, sometimes captured their critically reflexive awareness of not-so-subtle symbolic violence. This was an awareness that societal degradation could undermine health, well-being and even contribute to weight-gain by making people turn to food for 'comfort' (Chapters 2 and 3). Here, and to quote Bourdieu (2001: 88) after discussing the paradox of doxa, or widespread acceptability of social injustice: 'masculine domination no longer imposes itself with the transparency of something taken for granted'. Bourdieu (2001: 88) attributes this awareness to 'the feminist movement'. Certainly, feminist writings on the body challenge these injustices, with cultural degradations of female fat read as a political backlash against women's growing autonomy in the public sphere (Wolf 1991). However, and without contradicting such claims, I would state that critical awareness of masculine domination among big fellas could be attributed to attacks on masculine status from androcentric institutions, mediated communications and everyday interactions. Analytically, I would suggest that the collective fight against female and feminizing fat seeks to maintain masculine status at a collective and macro-social level while, somewhat paradoxically, simultaneously threatening it, and promising to recoup it, at an individual and micro-interactional level. This paradox is easily understood when one recognizes that it is men embodying subordinated masculinities (Connell 1995) – men some academics call 'fat boys' (Gilman 2004) – who are both players and pawns in this political game. Similar to women and children who are constituted and constitute themselves as inferior bodies, it is men who are subordinated (or risk subordination and self-subordination) who most acutely 'feel the weight of the water' (Bourdieu and Wacquant 1992: 127) and risk being drowned by masculine domination.

By offering a theoretically informed study, I hope these grounded understandings help to challenge not only obesity warmongering but also the perpetuation of crude dichotomies in Western thinking. The latter issue is a key concern within embodied sociology, as explained by Williams and Bendelow (1998), and their important insights extend way beyond their theoretical foci. Empirically, crude dichotomies are clearly reproduced in everyday life (for example, men's use of the big/small dichotomy to justify their size and sense of masculinity), but at an analytical level, dichotomous thinking is problematic within and beyond sociology. As stated in Chapter 1, when reflecting on the university forum I organized and my engagement with the media, health professionals and the UK's Men's Health Forum, I have routinely encountered polarized dichotomies. These include the oversimplified idea of 'taking sides' where 'fat' is deemed good or bad and something to be attacked or defended. These oppositional dualities – which constrain productive discussion and developing more nuanced understandings – are part of an arbitrary, rather than natural, masculine worldview that is not tied to male bodies and is inseparable from gendered (and middle-class) power and privilege. Within this cosmology, female and feminizing fatness is positioned as the opposite of social and biological fitness and other 'distinctions that are reducible to the male/female opposition' (Bourdieu 2001: 30). However, in befuddling these dualities, this book has shown that masculinity, emotionality and corporeality are thoroughly entwined. This is in societies where rationalization and militarized medicine are often passionately endorsed by powerful social institutions, and their representatives, as a matter of faith while also fostering unfounded hope, transient warmth, virtue, irrationality, antagonism, belligerence, and emotional pain (Chapters 2, 3 and 4). Hence, this book not only critiques the institutional and emotionally charged 'bio-attack' on fat, as directed at practically everybody, but also crude and unreasonable dichotomies that help to sustain communicated violence and oppression (Chapter 1).

All of this is inseparable from politics. By bringing in men, this book hopefully furthers the politicization of sexed/gendered bodies. This is with a view to challenging iniquitous body norms, social structural antecedents and gendered/ institutional knowledges that sustain and even increase stigma, sizism, sexism and health inequalities. Researching men complements strands of feminist and fat activist thinking where fat has primarily been considered a woman's issue rather than a public health issue. In the remainder of this section I will underscore this book's political import, with an emphasis on gender, though, clearly, other considerations are important such as class and the political economic expediency of blaming people of lower social status for 'their' health problems (Scambler 2001). Before doing this, however, I will first briefly anticipate possible reservations about researching men.

Although historically truncated, the usual view is that fat and weight-loss issues are feminist or women's issues (Orbach 1978). Researching men could thus be read as an attempt to displace feminist work that seeks to challenge the degradation and regulation of female bodies. However, that is not my intention and it should be clear from the above that I have not offered 'a rhetoric of "competing victims" [which tries] to refute feminism by reciting men's disadvanatges' (Connell 1995: 248). My view, concordant with many men contacted during this study, is that the imperative to slim down generally hits females hardest (women, girls and perhaps children more generally). This is not contradicted by some men's slimming club attendance. Annandale and Hunt (2000: 21) could have been discussing this when writing: '[t]he relatively more fluid movement of men and women between what were once either male or female dominated social spheres is important, but it does not necessarily "make all things equal"'. For females throughout the gendered life course, slenderness is often a compulsory aspect of normative embodiment in a way that it is not for many men (Bordo 1993). The title of Seid's (1989) book, *Never Too Thin*, is unlikely to have much resonance among men even when attending a slimming club or exercising in a gym with the intention of developing a body that might be lean but is technically overweight or obese. Efforts to reduce the body and achieve a so-called 'healthy' weight remain heavily gendered, rendering it generally more difficult for females to accommodate levels of body mass that are acceptable and perhaps admirable for men. This is the 'double standard' (Germov and Williams 1996: 636) mentioned in Chapter 2. I certainly recognize the intensified commodification of men's bodies in consumer culture (Grogan 1999), and associated male body dissatisfaction (Chapter 3). However, the general consensus among social scientists is that fat – or what is contingently seen as fat in everyday life – is largely made into a problem for females, and I accept this view. Why, then, research men? Is this a distraction from the political task of challenging the degradation of female bodies and gender inequality?

In underscoring the political value of this book, I will make three points. First, because gender includes masculinities, 'bringing in' men affords the opportunity to critically engage medically ratified degradation that is occurring on a massive scale under the fiction of a 'gender equitable' approach, i.e. where everyone's health is presented as the central and seemingly incontestable rationale for communicated violence. If taken at face value, the war on obesity apparently negates feminist concerns that it is female fat that is despised. When proponents of public health emphasize men's health and 'adiposity' (or overweight and obesity) this seems caring and democratic – at least, it does if it is devoid of biting irony. The idea of a public health crisis merges with the idea that men are essentially in crisis and must be helped, or 'encouraged' to help themselves, regardless of what men might actually think about this. This apparently benevolent (paternalistic, potentially patronizing) action cannot be divorced from history, society, culture and gendered power. As feminist historians of science make clear, masculine or patriarchal medicine has played a central role in regulating female bodies from the nineteenth century onwards (Jacobus *et al.* 1990). This continues into the twenty-first century through the rationalized and instituted fight against medicalized fat. Because biomedicine is inseparable from the larger society and culture, it should be clear from this research that even when fat is defined as a problem for men the same misogynistic message is conveyed. Namely, feminized fat, and fat bodies positioned as passively feminine regardless of their actual sex, must be cut in line with militarized medicine that justifies aggressive intervention. And, because there are different gendered thresholds for what is considered 'fat' in everyday life (Monaghan 2007), power over female bodies is amplified. The beauty myth (Wolf 1991) is compounded by the obesity myth (Campos 2004), while also rationalizing and sustaining other prejudices such as racism, class disdain and ageism (Herndon 2005, Smith 1990).

Second, and following Wann (1998), if fat is equated with women and their presumed vanity then the seriousness of anti-fat prejudice will largely be trivialized. This trivialization is partly explicable in terms of ongoing gender inequality and associated sexist stereotypes; that is, where women are deemed overly emotional and naturally sensitive, with feminist and fat activists' complaints about social injustice dismissed as 'institutional victimhood' (*cf.* Ellen 2006). In line with the hegemony of masculinity, the pains of devalued bodies do not matter and are rationalized away as really being in the targets' best interests (Fumento 1997). Of course, given the intensity of obesity warmongering, and the explicit focus on men in public health, it is impossible to trivialize fat and fat hatred as a private and 'frivolous' woman's issue. Given the explicit focus on men's biomedical health in wartime, I would maintain public health officials have unwittingly made it difficult to ignore not only the seriousness but also the absurdity of anti-fat prejudice. By researching men and the war on obesity, this study has thrown into relief the irrationalities of this exercise in 'public health'. This project classifies the normal and even admirable as pathological, while fuelling fatphobia, sizism and oppression. It is unfortunate that this is an 'acceptable prejudice' (Smith 1990) (if it was unacceptable then we would not see the sort of campaigns mentioned in Chapter 5), but this research has hopefully gone some way in challenging this trivialization. The irrationality of the seemingly rational war on obesity cannot be ignored when most men are urged to lose weight for the sake of their health and ridiculed by caring, and publicly funded, institutions for not 'complying' with biomedical norms that label them overweight or obese.

Third, it should be clear that this study critiques a larger system of institutionalized meanings and practices within a gender order that provides different resources for doing gender and resisting, or attenuating the differential impact of, fat hatred. Again, this is an aspect of gender inequality in a world where things are not as they seem. Many men contacted during this study may have 'had it bad' but in some senses they were relatively privileged compared to others in the social structure. I would not trivialize men's experiences of fat oppression (especially common for 'really' big men), but justifiable resistance was a recurrent theme alongside forms of repudiation and expressed distance. This meant the cage of rationality was not always all encompassing, with men's ability to withstand or 'escape' imposed discipline reflecting and reproducing gendered power and inequality. Yet, despite the privileges of their gender and the meanings invested in their biological sex, it was not always easy for these men to express distance or resist the culture of slenderness. Many big fellas demonstrated skill at this, but their circumscribed resistance and limited size acceptance was a gendered practical accomplishment, or emergent property of the larger social body wherein fat is discredited as female/feminizing filth. These weighty constructions might be embodied and consequential for men, women and children in late modernity, but, as observed, they are also socially contingent and contestable. They are not fixed, 'natural' and inevitable even for male slimmers who sought to fulfil the embodied obligations of their habitus. Hence, they are clearly open to revision, at an interpersonal and institutional level, in ways that do not spoil or do violence to people's embodied identities and dimensions of health.

In sum, bringing in men and interpreting their views through a repudiating lens is intended to support feminists and fat activists when politicizing the sexed/ gendered body and fatness. This also connects with the political concern for social justice within masculinities literature (Connell 1995, Messner 1997), without endorsing the idea that overweight/obesity/fatness really is a massive health problem that should be tackled in order to ameliorate 'the costs of masculinity' (Messner 1997: 5). Bringing in men, I would maintain, throws into stark relief the irrationalities of the rationalized anti-fat campaign, the gendered distribution of socially constructed/embodied harms and the potential for meaningful resistances in everyday life. Hence, this study offers a political as well as empirical and theoretical contribution. It provides an alternative and hopefully well-rounded response to authoritative claimsmakers who exercise sizism and mandate fatphobia in the belief that they are simply promoting public health. It would be promising if, on the basis of this research and the burgeoning literature it complements, discussion could proceed with greater humility and without a dogged commitment to forms of violence that are anything but subtle.

Some policy recommendations: A different multi-levelled approach

In keeping with the religious theme, consider the following statement about policy discussions. This is from a medical doctor in *The British Journal of General Practice*:

> It seems that the effect of being drawn into policy discussions about obesity is to turn normally sensible clinicians and scientists into ranting prophets of doom and evangelical preachers of virtuous living.
>
> (Fitzpatrick 2004: 557)

While I want to promote productive dialogue, and I have no intention of name-calling, Fitzpatrick (2004) makes an important point when highlighting the difficulties in getting sensible policy recommendations heard and credited. To use Edgley and Brissett's (1999: 153) words, existing policy recommendations reflect the worries of 'Meddling Cassandras, named after the daughter of Priam in Greek mythology who was always going around prophesying some disaster or another'. Policy discourses largely reiterate the weight-centred approach to health where slimming is framed as obligatory, achievable and beneficial rather than optional, largely ineffective and risky. Existing recommendations range from taxation of people who are sedentary to the compulsory measuring and testing of schoolchildren's bodies and fitness levels (Gard and Wright 2005: 187). In some Australian schools, larger children are even made to run extra 'fat laps' during physical education (Rich and Evans 2006), while US government agencies expect their staff to diet and wear pedometers (Robison 2005a). Despite various proposals, the message is the same: fatness equals badness, sickness and immorality, and personal responsibility must be taken to bring about 'healthy' and objectively measurable change lest a calamity engulfs us all.

Of course, not all of this is 'blatantly' oppressive. Liberal academic commentators cite various mitigating factors, thus ostensibly removing direct blame from individuals (for example, social inequalities affecting people's access to affordable, nutritious food) (Harrington and Friel 2006). Nonetheless, this is fundamentally a medicalized discourse that pathologizes 'weight' arbitrarily judged excessive. It is a retrospective excuse-account that implies future contrition as a road to personal and collective salvation. Hence the logical if not 'final solution' is weight-loss, though, as observed in nations such as Ireland, this might be partially humanized through calls on government to tackle food poverty and what are called 'the wider determinants of obesity' (Harrington and Friel 2006).

This does not mean proponents of the obesity discourse have been particularly effective in the policy arena. Gard and Wright (2005) speculate on the general reluctance of governments, when they were writing, to heed obesity scientists' recommendations. They suggest perhaps not everybody outside of obesity science is convinced that this is a pressing public health problem. Possible reasons for government inertia include the suggestion that people recognize the tenuous relationship between weight and health; people in the West enjoy relatively good health, which appears to be improving; designating Western populations as 'sick' seems somewhat far-fetched; and everyday life is full of competing priorities and concerns (Gard and Wright 2005: 187). In short, they surmise that there is already much healthy scepticism and resistance out there. Based on this research, that is a fair assessment. However, in the short time since Gard and Wright

(2005) were writing, neo-liberal governments appear to be more proactive. Although, as explained by Campos (2006), the US government has generally taken an anti-regulatory stance, anti-obesity interventions have been introduced at a state level. These include 'BMI screenings' of schoolchildren and the requirement that schools inform parents of the health consequences of weight (Campos 2006: 22).

With the perpetuation of obesity epidemic psychology, governments and related organizations appear to be increasingly prepared to accept and authoritatively endorse the fight against obesity. This complicity is currently evidenced in the UK, which some commentators have described as a 'panic nation' (Feldman and Marks 2006) following recent government responses to matters ranging from Sudan 1 food dye to avian flu. In relation to obesity, institutional complicity is not simply about panic or infection but political and economic intention. It is expedient and, following Scambler's (2004) critical realist writing on stigma, is politically honed given the convenience of blaming individuals (overwhelmingly the new poor) for their own ills. In short, the obesity discourse serves government interests, comprising a neo-liberal agenda and depoliticizing healthism. The attack on fat can be used strategically to eclipse a policy focus on larger socio-economic realities affecting health, while paying lip service to social considerations in order to reiterate highly moralized ideas about personal and public responsibility. Retrospectively, individuals or groups of individuals as social categories might be excused; however, prospectively, they are ultimately expected to lose weight (Chapter 2). Hence, in England, one witnesses government-supported campaigns like Everyday Sport that aim to 'kick start the fight against obesity' by extolling people to stop being 'lazy' and a financial drain on public services (Chapter 5).

My policy recommendations aim to be more conducive to health, broadly defined, than those from organizations, obesity scientists and others wedded to militarized medicine. These recommendations are intended to work at various levels, incorporating the broader macro-social structure, organizational practices and micro-level interactions. My recommendations differ from the usual suggestions because they do not oblige individuals to slim down and measure 'success' using something as crude as the weighing scales, tape measure or BMI. Finally, what follows remains partial. For example, given the earlier reference to medical harms in the absence of informed consent, the legal dimensions could be more fully explored with the aim of affording people greater protection. Fortunately, others are discussing these issues (for example, Solovay 2000) and it is with a nod in their direction that I offer my contribution.

The first recommendation is that health promoters and organizations should not reproduce the obesity discourse as if it was based on uncontested and certain science. The primary research field does not support such a position. This means organizations should avoid making claims that pathologize the majority of the adult population (for example, two-thirds of men in England are overweight or obese and this is a major public health problem). Although largely respectful of science, the public often know a 'daft idea' when they hear it (Gregory and Miller 2001: 61) and those engaged in such definitional practices risk undermining their own credibility. Gard and Wright (2005) make a related point. After warning about unintended consequences, they state that prominent obesity scientists do themselves no favours when claiming the entire population of the USA, UK and Australia will be overweight or obese within the next 40 years. Of course, given the profits in fat fighting, such predictions could be fabricated if we witness yet another reduction in the threshold of what constitutes overweight among groups who are least able to resist this (Moynihan 2006a, b). Governments should resist such moves, which are often initiated by those who in some way profit from the war on obesity.

The second, related, recommendation concerns the unethical perpetuation of sizist imagery by publicly funded organizations – especially organizations that ostensibly care for public health. Similar to the tendency of racism (Porter 1993), sizism may be 'exercised unrealized' by health professionals and organizations but it draws from and reproduces a social environment that degrades and ineffectively seeks to 'cure' fatness. This should be deemed unacceptable and viewed in the same light as the projection of sexist, racist, ableist and homophobic attitudes. In the UK the publicly funded NHS repeatedly enacts sizism. As noted during this research, anti-obesity posters in north-east England featured a cartoon image of a man's large stomach and taut shirt that was intended to encourage people to lose weight and presumably become healthier by becoming slimmer. In the same year the UK's Men's Health Forum used similar imagery when promoting its Department of Health sponsored conference on 'male weight problems' (Chapter 1). Such imagery normalizes and ratifies fatphobia, with these ostensibly accept-able messages also finding expression in everyday interactions. I refer the reader back to Mike's 13-year-old son who expressed suicidal thoughts after being humiliated in class by a teacher who said his stomach was bursting out of his shirt (Chapter 3). This cruel act from a particular teacher is one thing, but, more broadly, is it acceptable for caring institutions to very publicly and graphically reproduce anti-fat sentiments, thereby contributing towards and solidifying the view that fatness is a deservedly ridiculed bodily state? Aphramor (2006) makes similar arguments with reference to imagery used by the British Dietetic Association and the UK's Royal College of Physicians.

The third recommendation has direct relevance for clinicians working with people whom they label obese. This is not simply about recognizing what clinical terms like 'obesity' mean to their patients. Nor is it about not infantilizing men who, despite stereotypes, may actually care about their health and perhaps seek dietetic advice because of health problems commonly, if misleadingly, assumed to be caused by fatness. This recommendation follows my point about the need for productive discussion among those working in this field. There is a substantial body of scientific evidence that could inform – and, as with the Health at Every Size paradigm, already is informing – clinical practice in a compassion-ate and sensitive manner. I would add that while patients may wish to lose weight and ask for medical assistance to achieve that goal, this acquiescent display of social fitness should not be confused with metabolic fitness (conflating the normative with the visceral). Also, it should be remembered that intentionally losing a significant amount of weight and keeping it off is unlikely for most people who try this. And, it is not without its risks. Hence, if patients request help to lose weight then they should be fully informed of the evidence base, while clinicians themselves should heed the Hippocratic Oath and above all else do no harm.

The fourth recommendation moves from clinical practice and connects with the massive literature on health inequalities (for example, Acheson 1998, Freund 2006, Marmot 2004, Williams 2003b). This is about macro-social and economic policy and the social gradient in health. Following Fitzpatrick's (2001) critique of Britain's New Labour government's efforts to tackle social inequality and exclusion, I am not referring to interventions that are targeted at individuals and communities in order to regulate personal behaviour. For example, I am not endorsing home visiting by health professionals to 'reinforce preventive health measures' (Fitzpatrick 2001: 95). Rather, this is about material factors such as income and different groups' unequal access to resources. It also relates to what Marmot (2004) calls the status syndrome; namely, people's experiences and autonomy in the workplace, their degree of control over their life circumstances, the presence or absence of meaningful social relationships and the ability to participate in society without shame. As made clear by medical sociologists and epidemiologists who are sociologically imaginative, these social and economic realities have the biggest impact upon health. This is not to detract from the value of clinical practice and a focus on individual metabolic profiles, as with Health at Every Size, assuming this fits with an individual's priorities and definition of a life worth living. However, it is to stress that larger social factors are more consequential for morbidity and mortality than supposedly free-floating 'lifestyle choices' like physical activity, diet and alcohol consumption. They are also more important than body mass, which can never be divorced from social organization and experiences in divided societies that abhor and denigrate fatness. Being a second-class citizen, or being made to feel like a second-class citizen, is not conducive to health, however defined. More broadly then, if policy makers wish significantly to improve public health under the rubric of ethically responsible science, the weight of evidence underscores the importance of tackling growing social inequalities (Acheson 1998) rather than tackling obesity. I would urge policy makers not to be blinded by fat. Otherwise they may fail to recognize or prioritize threats to health, such as social and economic marginalization, which extend way beyond individual control and which may actually be amplified by size discrimination.

Final words: Resisting and ending the war on obesity?

During the early stages of this research I undertook five months ethnography at a 'Health and Youth Project'. This project was mentioned at the end of Chapter 5 when talking with one of my respondents, Edward, who sounded like a fat activist. The project was aimed at a group of teenage schoolboys in an economically deprived area in north-east England. Various people and organizations supported this, including: health workers from the local council and NHS Primary Care Trust, a college sports lecturer and fitness centre staff. In order to attract resources, the project was aligned with the war on obesity during its backstage organization. Even so, most boys who subsequently participated in the scheme were thin. Some staff expressed concern that the boys were malnourished rather than overfed.

With the exception of two larger boys, the boys' weight could not really justify an anti-obesity initiative. That had little bearing on the viability of the project. As with the war on obesity, the project was an exercise in social fitness and disciplining bodies. It was about regulating unruly boys who risked school exclusion. Certainly, health was the overt message conveyed during this weekly pedagogic experience. And I have no doubt that the good people involved in organizing and delivering this project believed the boys would benefit from their education in many ways. However, in practice, the idea of health was a convenient rationale for attempting to control disorderly bodies that offended middle-class sensibilities. The irony is that this sugar-coated exercise set the stage for a cruel parody among the boys themselves: the discourse that served as the initial rationale for the project was directed at the two larger boys, who were labelled fat and gluttonous by their classmates. In short, these slimmer boys teased others for their weight and although staff members condemned this they nonetheless still supplied ammunition; i.e. 'health promotion' material that made 'weight' thematic. No doubt, such bullying may be read as a gross distortion of the messages conveyed by health professionals, promoters and representatives of the obesity industry. It could also be taken, through misrecognition, as evidence that the war on obesity should be intensified lest other children suffer. However, it would be unfortunate if readers left this book thinking that. Rather, what I observed at this 'Health and Youth Project' was a blunt and crude enactment of forms of violence that are routinely communicated by powerful institutions.

The question remains as to whether people working in key social organizations, especially those that are publicly funded and ostensibly in the business of caring, intend to continue lending authority to the war on obesity and reinforcing societal prejudices and phobias? Big fellas may be more or less able to resist, or distance themselves from, the more pernicious aspects of this metaphorical war even when they are willing recruits. However, women and children, differently located in the social structure, are likely to have a harder time accomplishing this, just as they may be less able to embrace activities that are fallaciously promoted for weight-loss (for example, the restricted ability of many mothers caring on a low income to regularly participate in exercise). Faced with this knowledge, it is my hope, but not necessarily my expectation, that more people and organizational representatives will become conscientious objectors and repudiate the attack on medicalized fat. While millions of people will still be willing recruits and stigma will not end, it would be a promising start if those in authority, and without such a vested interest, avoided targeting people and mandating fat hatred as acceptable and desirable.

This returns me to the constraints on critical, and ultimately productive, dialogue outlined in Chapter 1. Among other things, organizational representatives, who may otherwise align themselves with the war on obesity, will need to ask themselves which side is their bread buttered and whether they can afford to leave it without fear of going hungry. I know many organizations, including charities advocating men's health, have good economic reasons for joining the wartime effort. Objecting to and abandoning the war on obesity, then, is not simply a matter of changing a few people's minds that are somehow free-floating. It is about collectively challenging organizational interests and broader structures of power that render fat fighting politically and economically expedient and perhaps personally profitable. If conscientious objection and efforts to promote more peaceful relations are simply left to individuals then this will remain just as, if not more, difficult as trying to lose weight and keeping it off. And it may also have its own social risks, as indicated vis-à-vis the dietetic profession and accusations of insubordination and irresponsibility. Hence, there is the need for a collective and sociologically mindful response that is reflexive about constraints but open to productive possibilities. Such a response must work through the social hierarchy and connect in an informed and empathetic way with people in their contexts of everyday life.

At the same time, people who may or may not personally risk being discredited as overweight or worse can take steps, however fleeting and seemingly small, to resist institutional degradation. These moves are not confined to men or women; indeed, if men and women's experiences of sizism and fatphobia 'are more similar than different' then there is scope for 'articulating a universalist interest around health' (Carpenter 2000: 48). This, it should be added, is in a society where people, as relational bodies, care for others who are friends, lovers and kin – people who have perhaps encountered intolerance and insensitivity and feel inferior given the embodied meanings of their real or imagined fatness. Although these resistances are potentially awkward and might evoke antagonism in a field of power and domination, they *could* include: publicly treating sizism as the same as other socially unacceptable prejudices; challenging claims that fatness causes sickness or early death given that obesity science does not justify such certainty; asking people why they would recommend dieting given a 95 per cent chance of regaining the weight and evidence that weight-fluctuation may be more harmful than maintaining a higher stable weight; avoiding slimming clubs, or, if their promise of salvation is irresistible, not taking children along; refusing to be weighed by clinicians; asking clinicians who attribute health problems to one's weight (for example, hypertension, cardiac problems) how they would treat slim people diagnosed with these, then insisting on being treated the same; stressing the more pleasurable aspects of health, like eating a range of foods without being made to feel guilty, or enjoying physical activity as an end in itself, mentioning there are many 'big' or 'fat' people who are physically fit, active and healthy just as there are many 'slim' people who are not; pointing out that people denigrated as inappropriately fat, ugly and lazy may actually be considered sexually attractive, friendly and hardworking by those who know and love them; stressing that, according to the weight of scientific evidence, the risk of early death and illness in the population is overwhelmingly related to social inequalities rather than lifestyles and/or obesity; and repudiating publicly funded anti-obesity campaigns on the grounds that they are depoliticizing and stigmatizing. I do not want to be elitist because there is already much healthy scepticism among people in everyday life, including the man in the slimming club who ambivalently tries to fit in. I also do not want to eclipse the need for broader social structural and institutional change, which depends on political action and policy implementation. However, such resistance or expressed distance is possible knowing there is a burgeoning academic literature, fat activist movement and Health at Every Size paradigm that challenge the war on obesity and the violence it seeks to justify in the name of health.

Bibliography

Acheson, Sir D. (Chair) (1998) *Independent Inquiry into Inequalities in Health*. London: The Stationery Office.

Adler, P.A., Adler, P. and Fontana, A. (1987) Everyday Life Sociology. *Annual Review of Sociology* 13: 217–35.

Allen, K. (2004) Managing the Body: Health and the Experience of Children with Prader-Willi Syndrome. *The British Sociological Association Medical Sociology Group 36th Annual Conference*. University of York, UK, 16–18 September.

Angell, M. (2004) *The Truth About the Drug Companies: How They Deceive Us and What to Do About It*. New York: Random House.

Annandale, E. (2003) Gender and Health Status: Does Biology Matter? In S. Williams, L. Birke and G. Bendelow (eds) *Debating Biology: Sociological Reflections on Health, Medicine and Society*. London: Routledge.

Annandale, E. and Hunt, K. (eds) (2000) *Gender Inequalities in Health*. Buckingham: Open University Press.

Aphramor, L. (2005) Is a Weight-Centred Health Framework Salutogenic? Some Thoughts on Unhinging Certain Dietary Ideologies. *Social Theory & Health* 3 (4): 315–40.

—— (2006) *Report on Size Discrimination in Society and in Employment*. Unpublished Report Commissioned by the Welsh Development Agency SME Equality Project.

—— (2007) Has the Energy Balance Equation Had its Day? Remapping Fatness with Society in Mind. *Obesity and Extremes: What's the Problem?* Scottish Colloquium on Food and Feeding and BSA Food Study Group, University of Edinburgh, 26 January.

Aphramor, L. and Gingras, J. (2007) Sustaining Imbalance: Evidence of Neglect in the Pursuit of Nutritional Health. In S. Riley, M. Burns, H. Frith, S. Wiggins and P. Markula (eds) *Critical Bodies: Representations, Identities and Practices of Weight and Body Management*. Basingstoke. Palgrave Macmillan.

—— (2008) That Remains to Be Said: Disappeared Feminist Discourses on Fat in Dietetic Theory and Practice. In E. Rothblum and S. Solovay (eds) *The Fat Studies Reader*. Berkeley, CA: University of California Press.

Bacon, L. (2006) End the War on Obesity: Make Peace with Your Patients. *Medscape General Medicine* 8 (4): 40.

Barbalet, J. (2002) Introduction: Why Emotions are Crucial. In J. Barbalet (ed.) *Emotions and Sociology*. Oxford: Blackwell.

Bartky, S. (1990) *Femininity and Domination: Studies in the Phenomenology of Oppression*. New York: Routledge.

Bauman, Z. (1989) *Modernity and the Holocaust*. Cambridge: Polity.

—— (2005) Survival as a Social Construct. In M. Fraser and M. Greco (eds) *The Body: A Reader*. London: Routledge. (Orig. 1992)

BBC News Online (2006) *Army to Welcome 'Heavy' Soldiers*. 8 January. Online. Available HTTP: <http://news.bbc.co.uk/nolpda/ukfs_news/hi/newsid_4592000/4592230.stm> Accessed 12 January 2006.

BBC Online (2007) *Health, Obesity by Dr Rob Hicks*. Online. Available HTTP: <www.bbc.co.uk/health/mens/_health/issues_obesity.shtml> Accessed 28 March 2007.

Beck, U. (1992) *Risk Society: Towards a New Modernity*. London: Sage.

Bell, K. and McNaughton, D. (2007) Feminism and the Invisible Fat Man. *Body & Society* 13 (1): 107–31.

Berger, P. (1963) *Invitation to Sociology: A Humanistic Perspective*. Aylesbury: Penguin.

—— (1997) *Redeeming Laughter: The Comic Dimension of Human Experience*. New York: Walter de Gruyter.

Best J. (1995) *Images of Issues: Typifying Contemporary Social Problems*. New York: Aldine de Gruyter. (2nd edition.)

Blair, S. and Brodney, S. (1999) Effects of Physical Inactivity and Obesity on Morbidity and Mortality: Current Evidence and Research Issues. *Medicine and Science in Sports and Exercise* 31 (5) (Supplement): S646–S662.

Blaxter, M. (2004) Why do the Victims Blame Themselves? In M. Bury and J. Gabe (eds) *The Sociology of Health and Illness: A Reader*. London: Routledge.

Bloor, M. (1978) On the Analysis of Observational Data: A Discussion of the Worth and Uses of Inductive Techniques and Respondent Validation. *Sociology* 12: 542–52.

—— (1997) *Selected Writings in Medical Sociology Research*. Aldershot: Ashgate.

Bordo, S. (1993) *Unbearable Weight: Feminism, Western Culture and the Body*. Berkeley, CA: University of California Press.

Bourdieu, P. (1984) *Distinction: A Social Critique of the Judgement of Taste*. Cambridge, MA: Harvard University Press.

—— (2001) *Masculine Domination*. Cambridge: Polity Press.

Bourdieu, P. and Wacquant, L. (1992) *An Invitation to Reflexive Sociology*. Cambridge: Polity Press.

Brown, D. (2006) Pierre Bourdieu's 'Masculine Domination' Thesis and the Gendered Body in Sport and Physical Culture. *Sociology of Sport Journal* 23: 162–88.

Brown, L. (1989) Fat-Oppressive Attitudes and the Feminist Therapist: Directions for Change. In L. Brown and E. Rothblum (eds) *Fat Oppression and Psychotherapy: A Feminist Perspective*. New York: The Hawthorn Press.

Brown, L. and Rothblum, E. (eds) (1989) *Fat Oppression and Psychotherapy: A Feminist Perspective*. New York: The Hawthorn Press.

Brownell, K. (2005) Introduction: The Social, Scientific, and Human Context of Prejudice and Discrimination Based on Weight. In K. Brownell, R. Puhl, M. Schwartz and L. Rudd (eds) *Weight Bias: Nature, Consequences, and Remedies*. New York: The Guildford Press.

Brumberg, J. (1988) *Fasting Girls*. Cambridge, MA: Harvard University Press.

Bryman, A. (1999) The Disneyization of Society. *The Sociological Review* 47: 25–47.

BSA (British Sociological Association) (2002) *British Sociological Association – Statement of Ethical Practice*. Online. Available HTTP: <http://www.britsoc.co.uk> Accessed 22 May 2007.

Burnett, R. (1991) Accounts and Narratives. In B. Montgomery and S. Duck (eds) *Studying Interpersonal Interaction*. New York: The Guildford Press.

Burns, M. and Gavey, N. (2004) 'Healthy Weight' at What Cost? 'Bulimia' and a Discourse of Weight Control. *Journal of Health Psychology* 9 (4): 549–65.

Cahill, S. (1998) Toward a Sociology of the Person. *Sociological Theory* 16 (2): 131–48.

Campos, P. (2004) *The Obesity Myth: Why America's Obsession with Weight is Hazardous to Your Health*. New York: Gotham Books.

—— (2006) The Legalization of Fat: Law, Science and the Construction of a Moral Panic. *Legal Studies Research Paper Series*. Working Paper 06–16 March, University of Colorado Law School. Online. Available HTTP: <http://ssrn.com/abstract=902693> Accessed 28 April 2007.

Campos, P., Saguy, A., Ernsberger, P., Oliver, E. and Gaesser, G. (2006a) The Epidemiology of Overweight and Obesity: Public Health Crisis or Moral Panic? *International Journal of Epidemiology* 35: 55–60.

—— (2006b) Response: Lifestyle not Weight Should Be the Primary Target. *International Journal of Epidemiology* 35: 81–2.

Carmona, R. (2003) Reducing Racial and Cultural Disparities in Health Care: What Actions Now? *Keynote Speech for National Healthcare Congress Summit*, Washington DC, 11 March. Online. Available HTTP: <www.surgeongeneral.gov/news/speeches/managed care031103.htm> Accessed 15 February 2007.

Carpenter, M. (2000) Reinforcing the Pillars: Rethinking Gender, Social Divisions and Health. In E. Allendale and K. Hunt (eds) *Gender Inequalities in Health*. Buckingham: Open University Press.

Carryer, J. (2001) Embodied Largeness: A Significant Women's Health Issue. *Nursing Inquiry* 8 (2): 90 7.

Cash, T. and Roy, R. (1999) Pounds of Flesh: Weight, Gender, and Body Images. In J. Sobal and D. Maurer (eds) *Interpreting Weight: The Social Management of Fatness and Thinness*. New York: Aldine de Gruyter.

Cavanagh, K., Dobash, R.E., Dobash, R.P. and Lewis, R. (2001) 'Remedial Work': Men's Strategic Response to their Violence against Intimate Female Partners. *Sociology* 35 (3): 695–714.

Chamberlain, M. (2001) Oscar Zeta Acosta's Autobiography of a Brown Buffalo: A Fat Man's Recipe for Chicano Revolution. In J. Braziel and K. LeBesco (eds) (2001) *Bodies Out of Bounds: Fatness and Transgression*. California: University of California Press.

Chang, V. and Christakis, N. (2002) Medical Modelling of Obesity: A Transition from Action to Experience in a 20th Century American Textbook, *Sociology of Health & Illness* 24 (20): 151–77.

Chandola, T., Brunner, E. and Marmot, M. (2006) Chronic Stress at Work and the Metabolic Syndrome. *British Medical Journal* 332: 521–4.

Chapman, G. (1999) From 'Dieting' to 'Healthy Eating': An Exploration of Shifting Constructions of Eating for Weight Control. In J. Sobal and D. Maurer (eds) *Interpreting Weight: The Social Construction of Fatness and Thinness*. New York: Aldine de Gruyter.

Charmaz, K., and Mitchell, R. (2001) Grounded Theory in Ethnography. In P. Atkinson, A. Coffey, S. Delamont, J. Lofland, and L. Lofland (eds) *Handbook of Ethnography*. London: Sage.

Chernin, K. (1981) *The Obsession: Reflections on the Tyranny of Slenderness*. New York: Harper.

Cogan, J. (1999) Re-evaluating the Weight-Centered Approach Toward Health: The Need for a Paradigm Shift. In J. Sobal and D. Maurer (eds) *Interpreting Weight: The Social Management of Fatness and Thinness*. New York: Aldine de Gruyter.

Cohen, L., Perales, D. and Steadman, C. (2005) The O Word: Why the Focus on Obesity is Harmful to Community Health. *Californian Journal of Health Promotion* 3 (3): 154–61.

Connell, R. (1987) *Gender and Power*. Oxford: Polity Press.

—— (1995) *Masculinities*. Cambridge: Polity Press.

—— (2000) *The Men and the Boys*. Cambridge: Polity Press.

Connell, R. and Wood, J. (2005) Globalization and Business Masculinities. *Men and Masculinities* 7 (4): 347–64.

Conrad, P. (2004) The Shifting Engines of Medicalization. *The British Sociological Association Medical Sociology Group 36th Annual Conference*. University of York, 16 to 18 September.

Conrad, P. and Schneider, J. (1992) *Deviance and Medicalization: From Badness to Sickness*. Philadelphia, PA: Temple University Press.

Cooley, C. (1983) *Human Nature and Social Order*. London: Transaction. (Orig. 1902)

Cooper, C. (1997) Can a Fat Woman Call Herself Disabled? *Disability and Society* 12 (1): 31–41.

—— (1998) *Fat and Proud: The Politics of Size*. London: The Women's Press.

Crawford, R. (1980) Healthism and the Medicalization of Everyday Life. *International Journal of Health Services* 10 (3): 365–89.

Critser, G. (2003) *Fat Land: How Americans Became the Fattest People in the World*. London: Allen Lane.

Crossley, N. (2001) *The Social Body: Habit, Identity and Desire*. London: Sage.

—— (2004) Fat is a Sociological Issue: Obesity Rates in Late Modern, 'Body Conscious' Societies. *Social Theory & Health* 2 (3): 222–53.

Davison, C., Frankel, S. and Davey Smith, G. (1992) The Limits of Lifestyle: Reassessing 'Fatalism' in the Popular Culture of Illness Prevention. *Social Science & Medicine* 34 (6): 675–85.

Degher, D. and Hughes, G. (1999) The Adoption and Management of a 'Fat' Identity. In J. Sobal and D. Maurer (eds) *Interpreting Weight: The Social Management of Fatness and Thinness*. New York: Aldine de Gruyter.

Dhurandhar, N., Israel, B., Kolesar, J., Mayhew, G., Cook, M. and Atkinson, R. (2000) Increased Adiposity in Animals Due to a Human Virus. *International Journal of Obesity* 24: 989–96.

Discovery Health (2004) *Fat Man Slim*. Screened 9 May, UK Sky TV.

Duneier, M. (1992) *Slim's Table: Race, Respectability and Masculinity*. Chicago, IL: University of Chicago Press.

Edgley, C. (2006) The Fit and Healthy Body: Consumer Narratives and the Management of Postmodern Corporeity. In D. Waskul and P. Vannini (eds) *Body/Embodiment: Symbolic Interaction and the Sociology of the Body*. Aldershot: Ashgate.

Edgley, C. and Brissett, D. (1990) Health Nazis and the Cult of the Perfect Body: Some Polemical Observations. *Symbolic Interaction* 13 (2): 257–79.

—— (1999) *A Nation of Meddlers*. Boulder, CO: Westview Press.

Elias, N. (2000) *The Civilizing Process: Sociogenetic and Psychogenetic Investigations*. (Revised edition) Oxford: Blackwell Publishers. (Orig. 1939)

Ellen, A. (2006) Big People on Campus. *The New York Times* 26 November.

Emslie, C., Hunt, K. and Watt, G. (2001) Invisible Women? The Importance of Gender in Lay Beliefs about Heart Problems. *Sociology of Health & Illness* 23 (2): 203–33.

Ernsberger, P. and Haskew, P. (1987) Health Implications of Obesity: An Alternative View. *Journal of Obesity and Weight Regulation* 6 (67): 58–137.

Evans, J., Rich, E., Allwood, R. and Davies, B. (forthcoming) *Fat Fabrications*. London: Routledge.

Everyday Sport (2004) *Everyday Sport: Every Body Feels Better For It*. Online. Available HTTP: <www.everydaysport.com./> Accessed 26 August 2004.

Featherstone, M. (1991) The Body in Consumer Culture. In M. Featherstone, M. Hepworth and B. Turner (eds) *The Body: Social Process and Cultural Theory*. London: Sage.

Feldman, S. and Marks, V. (2006) *Panic Nation: Exposing the Myths We're Told about Food and Health*. London: John Blake.

Fikkan, J. and Rothblum, E. (2005) Weight Bias in Employment. In K. Brownell, R. Puhl, M. Schwartz and L. Rudd (eds) *Weight Bias: Nature, Consequences, and Remedies*. New York: The Guildford Press.

Fitzpatrick, M. (2001) *The Tyranny of Health: Doctors and the Regulation of Lifestyle*. London: Routledge.

—— (2004) The Obesity Time Bomb. *The British Journal of General Practice* 54 (504): 557.

Flegal, K., Graubard, B., Williamson, D. and Gail, M. (2005) Excess Deaths Associated with Underweight, Overweight, and Obesity. *Journal of the American Medical Association* 293 (15): 1861–7.

Flum, D., Salem, L., Elrod, A., Dellinger, E., Cheadle, A., Chan, L. (2005) Early Mortality among Medicare Beneficiaries Undergoing Bariatric Surgical Procedures. *Journal of the American Medical Association* 294 (15): 1903–8.

Food Standards Agency (2007) *Low Income Diet and Nutrition Survey*. Online. Available HTTP: <http://www.food.gov.uk/news/newsarchive/2007/jul/lowincome> Accessed 16 July 2007.

Foucault, M. (1978) Politics and the Study of Discourse. *Ideology and Consciousness* 3: 7–26.

Frank, A. (1991) For a Sociology of the Body: An Analytical Review. In M. Featherstone, M. Hepworth and B. Turner (eds) *The Body: Social Process and Cultural Theory*. London: Sage.

Freespirit, J. and Aldebaran, S. (1973) *Fat Liberation Manifesto*. Online. Available HTTP: <www.largesse.ne/Archives/FU/manifesto.html> Accessed 5 December 2006.

Freund, P. (2006) Socially Constructed Embodiment: Neurohormonal Connections as Resources for Theorizing about Health Inequalities. *Social Theory & Health* 4 (2): 85–108.

Friedman, J. (2003) A War on Obesity, Not the Obese. *Science* 299: 856–8.

Fumento, M. (1997) *The Fat of the Land: Our Health Problem Crisis and How Overweight Americans Can Help Themselves*. New York: Penguin.

Gaesser, G. (1998) The Obesity Problem [Correspondence]. *The New England Journal of Medicine* 338 (16): 1156–8.

—— (2002) *Big Fat Lies: The Truth About Your Weight and Your Health*. Carlsbad, CA: Gurze Books.

—— (2005) Fit and Fat, Still a Solid Concept Despite Recent Challenges. *Health at Every Size Journal* 19 (1): 54–61.

Gard, M. (2003) An Elephant in the Room and a Bridge Too Far, or Physical Education and the 'Obesity Epidemic'. In J. Evans, B. Davies and J. Wright (eds) *Body, Knowledge and Control: Studies in the Sociology of Physical Education and Health*. London: Routledge.

Gard, M. and Wright, J. (2005) *The Obesity Epidemic*. London: Routledge.

Garfinkel, H. (1967) *Studies in Ethnomethodology*. Englewood Cliffs, NJ: Prentice Hall.

Germov, J. and Williams, L. (eds) (1996) The Sexual Division of Dieting: Women's Voices. *The Sociological Review* 44 (4): 630–47.

—— (1999) Dieting Women: Self-Surveillance and the Body Panopticon. In J. Sobal and D. Maurer (eds) *Weighty Issues: Fatness and Thinness as Social Problems*. New York: Aldine de Gruyter.

—— (2004) *A Sociology of Food and Nutrition: The Social Appetite*. Oxford: Oxford University Press. (2nd edition)

Giddens, A. (1991) *Modernity and Self-Identity: Self and Society in the Late Modern Age*. Cambridge: Polity Press.

—— (1992) *The Transformation of Intimacy: Love, Sexuality and Eroticism in Modern Societies*. Cambridge: Polity Press.

—— (2006) Big Britain. *Guardian Unlimited*. 26 November. Online. Available HTTP: <www.commentisfree.guardian.co.uk/anthony_giddens/2006/11/post_661.> Accessed 28 November 2006.

Gill, R., Henwood, K. and McLean, C. (2005) Body Projects and the Regulation of Normative Masculinity. *Body & Society* 11 (1): 37–62.

Gilman, S. (2004) *Fat Boys: A Slim Book*. Lincoln, NE: University of Nebraska Press.

Gimlin, D. (2002) *Body Work: Beauty and Self Image in American Culture*. Berkeley, CA: University of California Press.

—— (2007a) Accounting for Cosmetic Surgery in the USA and Great Britain: A Cross-cultural Analysis of Women's Narratives. *Body & Society* 13 (1): 41–60.

—— (2007b) Constructions of Ageing and Narrative Resistance in a Commercial Slimming Group. *Ageing & Society* 27: 407–24.

Glaser, B. and Strauss, A. (1967) *The Discovery of Grounded Theory*. Chicago, IL: Aldine.

Goffman, E. (1961a) *Asylums: Essays on the Social Situation of Mental Patients and Other Inmates*. Middlesex: Penguin Books.

—— (1961b) *Encounters: Two Studies in the Sociology of Interaction*. Indianapolis, IN: Bobbs-Merrill.

—— (1963) *Behavior in Public Places: Notes on the Social Organization of Gatherings*. New York: Free Press.

—— (1967) *Interaction Ritual: Essays on Face-to-Face Behavior*. New York: Pantheon.

—— (1968) *Stigma: Notes on the Management of Spoiled Identity*. Middlesex: Penguin Books.

—— (1971) *Relations in Public: Microstudies of the Public Order*. New York: Basic Books.

Graham, H. (1995) Cigarette Smoking: A Light on Gender and Class Inequality in Britain. *Journal of Social Policy* 24: 509–27.

Gregory, J. and Miller, S. (2001) Caught in the Crossfire? The Public's Role in the Science Wars. In J. Labinger and H. Collins (eds) *The One Culture? A Conversation About Science*. Chicago, IL: University of Chicago Press.

Gregg, E., Cheng, Y., Cadwell, B., Imperatore, G., Williams, D., Flegal, K., Narayan, K. and Williamson, D. (2005) Secular Trends in Cardiovascular Disease Risk Factors According to Body Mass Index in US Adults. *Journal of the American Medical Association* 293 (15): 1868–74.

Gremillion, H. (2005) The Cultural Politics of Body Size. *The Annual Review of Anthropology* 34: 13–32.

Grogan, S. (1999) *Body Image: Understanding Body Dissatisfaction in Men, Women and Children*. London: Routledge.

Grogan, S. and Richards, H. (2002) Body Image: Focus Groups with Boys and Men. *Men and Masculinities* 4 (3): 219–32.

Gross, J. (2005) Phat. In D. Kulick and A. Meneley (eds) (2005) *Fat: The Anthropology of an Obsession.* New York: Penguin Books.

Guthman, J. and DuPuis, M. (2006) Embodying Neoliberalism: Economy, Culture, and the Politics of Fat. *Environment and Planning* 24 (3): 427–48

Harrington, J. and Friel, S. (2006) Obesity: The Wider Determinants. Paper presented at *Expanding the Obesity Debate.* University of Limerick, 9 January.

Haslam, D. (2005) Taking Sides: Can Being Fat Be Good For You? No. *MHF* 7: 8–9.

Hepworth, J. (1999) *The Social Construction of Anorexia Nervosa.* London: Sage.

Herndon, M. (2005) Collateral Damage from Friendly Fire? Race, Nation, Class and the 'War Against Obesity'. *Social Semiotics* 15 (2): 127–41.

Heyes, C. (2006) Foucault Goes to Weight Watchers. *Hypatia* 21 (2): 126–49.

Hine, C. (2000) *Virtual Ethnography.* London: Sage.

Hochschild, A. (1983) *The Managed Heart: Commercialization of Human Feelings.* Berkeley, CA: University of California Press.

Honeycutt, K. (1999) Fat World/Thin World: 'Fat Busters', 'Equivocators', 'Fat Boosters', and the Social Construction of Obesity. In J. Sobal and D. Maurer (eds) *Interpreting Weight: The Social Management of Fatness and Thinness.* New York: Aldine de Gruyter.

Huff, J. (2001) A 'Horror of Corpulence': Interrogating Bantingism and Mid-Nineteenth Century Fat-Phobia. In J. Braziel and K. LeBesco (eds) *Bodies Out of Bounds: Fatness and Transgression.* Berkeley, CA: University of California Press.

Hunter, C. (1984) Aligning Actions: Types and Social Distribution. *Symbolic Interaction* 7 (2): 155–74.

Illich, I. (1975) *Medical Nemesis: The Expropriation of Health.* London: Marion Boyars.

Imperato, J. (1998) Correspondence: The Obesity Problem. *New England Journal of Medicine* 338 (16): 1158.

Innanen, M. (1999) Secret Life in the Culture of Slenderness: A Man's Story. In A. Sparkes and M. Silvennoinen (eds) *Talking Bodies: Men's Narratives of the Body and Sport.* Jyväskylä, Finland: SOPHI.

Jacobus, M., Fox Keller, E. and Shuttleworth, S. (eds) (1990) *Body/Politics: Women and the Discourses of Science.* London: Routledge.

Joanisse, L. and Synnott, A. (1999) Fighting Back: Reactions and Resistance to the Stigma of Obesity. In J. Sobal and D. Maurer (eds) *Interpreting Weight: The Social Management of Fatness and Thinness.* New York: Aldine de Gruyter.

Jutel, J. (2005) Weighing Health: The Moral Burden of Obesity. *Social Semiotics* 15 (2): 113–25.

Kassirer, J. (2005) *On the Take: How Medicine's Complicity with Big Business Can Endanger Your Health.* Oxford: Oxford University Press.

Kassirer, J. and Angell, M. (1998) Losing Weight: An Ill fated New Year's Resolution. *The New England Journal of Medicine* 338 (1): 52–4.

Keith, S., Redden, D., Katzmarzyk, P., Boggiano, M., Hanlon, E., Benca, R., Ruden, D., Pietrobelli, A., Barger, J., Fontaine, K., Wang, C., Aronne, L., Wright, S., Baskin, M., Dhurandhar, N., Lijoi, M., Grilo, C., DeLuca, M., Westfall, A. and Allison, D. (2006) Review: Putative Contributors to the Secular Increase in Obesity: Exploring the Roads Less Travelled. *International Journal of Obesity* 1 10. Advance online publication, 27 June 2006.

Klein, R. (1996) *Eat Fat.* New York: Pantheon.

Klein, S. (1999) The War Against Obesity: Attacking a New Front. *American Journal of Clinical Nutrition* 69: 1061–3.

Knapp, T. (1983) A Methodological Critique of the 'Ideal Weight' Concept. *Journal of the American Medical Association* 250 (4): 506–10.

Kulick, D. and Meneley, A. (eds) (2005) *Fat: The Anthropology of an Obsession*. New York: Penguin Books.

Laville, S. (2004) The Question Mark Over McDonald's. *Guardian*, 13 October.

Lawler, S. (2005) Disgusted Subjects: The Making of Middle-Class Identities. *The Sociological Review* 53 (3): 429–66.

LeBesco, K. (2004) *Revolting Bodies? The Struggle to Redefine Fat Identity*. Boston, MA: University of Massachusetts Press.

Leder, D. (1990) *The Absent Body*. Chicago, IL: University of Chicago Press.

Lee, C., Blair, S. and Jackson, A. (1999) Cardiorespiratory Fitness, Body Composition, and All-Cause and Cardiovascular Disease Mortality in Men. *American Journal of Clinical Nutrition* 69: 373–80.

Lester, R. (1999) Let Go and Let God: Religion and the Politics of Surrender in Overeaters Anonymous. In J. Sobal and D. Maurer (eds) *Interpreting Weight: The Social Management of Fatness and Thinness*. New York: Aldine de Gruyter.

Longhurst, R. (2005a) 'Man-Breasts': Spaces of Sexual Difference, Fluidity and Abjection. In B. van Hoven and K. Hörschelmann (eds) *Spaces of Masculinities*. London: Routledge.

—— (2005b) Fat Bodies: Developing Geographical Research Agendas. *Progress in Human Geography* 29 (3): 247–59.

Lyman, S. and Scott, M. (1970) *A Sociology of the Absurd*. New York: Appleton-Century-Crofts, Inc.

Lyons, P. (1989) Fitness, Feminism and the Health of Fat Women. In L. Brown and E. Rothblum (eds) *Fat Oppression and Psychotherapy: A Feminist Perspective*. New York: The Hawthorn Press.

Mann, T., Tomiyama, J., Westling, E., Lew, A., Samuels, B. and Chatman, J. (2007) Medicare's Search for Effective Obesity Treatments: Diets are Not the Answer. *American Psychologist* 62 (3): 220–33.

Martin, D. (2002) From Appearance Tales to Oppression Tales: Frame Alignment and Organizational Identity. *Journal of Contemporary Ethnography* 31 (2): 158–206.

Marmot, M. (2004) *The Status Syndrome: How Your Social Standing Directly Affects Your Health*. London: Bloomsbury.

Matza, D. (1969) *Becoming Deviant*. New Jersey: Prentice-Hall.

Mayer, K. (2004) An Unjust War: The Case Against the Government's War on Obesity. *Georgetown Law Journal* 92 (5): 999–1031.

McDowell, L. (1997) *Capital Culture: Gender at Work*. Oxford: Blackwell.

Mead, G. (1934) *Mind, Self, and Society*. Chicago, IL: University of Chicago Press.

MHF (Men's Health Forum) (2005) *Hazardous Waist? Tackling the Epidemic of 'Excess' Weight in Men. National Men's Health Week 2005 Policy Report*. London: Men's Health Forum.

Mennell, S. (1991) On the Civilizing of Appetite. In M. Featherstone, M. Hepworth and B. Turner (eds) *The Body: Social Process and Cultural Theory*. London: Sage.

Messner, M. (1997) *Politics of Masculinity: Men in Movements*. London: Sage.

Miller, W. (1999) Fitness and Fatness in Relation to Health: Implications for a Paradigm Shift. *Journal of Social Issues* 55 (2): 207–19.

Mills, C. Wright (1940) Situated Actions and Vocabularies of Motive. *American Sociological Review* 5 (5): 904–13.

—— (1970) *The Sociological Imagination*. New York: Penguin Books. (Orig. 1959)

Mitchell, A. (2005) Pissed Off. In D. Kulick and A. Meneley (eds) *Fat: The Anthropology of an Obsession*. New York: Penguin Books.

Monaghan, L. (1999) Challenging Medicine? Bodybuilding, Drugs and Risk. *Sociology of Health & Illness* 21 (6): 707–34.

—— (2001) *Bodybuilding, Drugs and Risk*. London: Routledge.

—— (2002) Hard Men, Shop Boys and Others: Embodying Competence in a Masculinist Occupation. *The Sociological Review* 50 (3): 334–55.

—— (2005a) Discussion Piece: A Critical Take on the Obesity Debate. *Social Theory & Health* 3 (4): 302–14.

—— (2005b) Big Handsome Men, Bears and Others: Virtual Constructions of 'Fat Male Embodiment'. *Body & Society* 11 (2): 81–111.

—— (2006) Corporeal Indeterminacy: The Value of Embodied, Interpretive Sociology. In D. Waskul and P. Vannini (eds) *Body/Embodiment: Symbolic Interaction and the Sociology of the Body*. Aldershot: Ashgate.

—— (2007) Body Mass Index, Masculinities and Moral Worth: Men's Critical Understandings of 'Appropriate' Weight-for-Height. *The Sociology of Health & Illness*. 29 (4): 584–609.

Morgan, D. (1993) You Too Can Have a Body Like Mine: Reflections on the Male Body and Masculinities. In S. Scott and D. Morgan (eds) *Body Matters: Essays on the Sociology of the Body*. London: The Falmer Press.

Moynihan, R. (2006a) Expanding Definitions of Obesity May Harm Children. *British Medical Journal* 332: 1412.

—— (2006b) Obesity Task Force Linked to WHO takes 'Millions' from Drug Firms. *British Medical Journal* 332: 1412.

Muhr, T. (1997) *Atlas.ti*. Berlin: Scolari and Scientific Software Development.

Murray, L. (2005) *The State of the F-Word: Three Letters that Still Shock*. Online. Available HTTP: <http://www.maadwomen.com/lynnemurray/essays/fword.html> Accessed 25 January 2006.

Murray, S. (2005) Doing Politics or Selling Out? Living the Fat Body. *Women's Studies* 34: 265–77.

NAO (National Audit Office) (2001) *Tackling Obesity in England*. London: The Stationery Office.

Neckel, A. (1996) Inferiority: From Collective Status to Deficient Individuality. *The Sociological Review* 44 (1): 17–34.

Oliver, E. (2006) *Fat Politics: The Real Story Behind America's Obesity Epidemic*. Oxford: Oxford University Press.

Oliver, M. (2004) Defining Impairment and Disability: Issues at Stake. In M. Bury and J. Gabe (eds) *The Sociology of Health and Illness: A Reader*. (Orig. 1996)

Orbach, S. (1978) *Fat is a Feminist Issue: The Anti-Diet Guide for Women*. New York: Berkeley.

—— (2006) Commentary: There is a Public Health Crisis – it's not Fat on the Body but Fat in the Mind and the Fat of Profits. *International Journal of Epidemiology* 35: 67–9.

Orbuch, T. (1997) People's Accounts Count: The Sociology of Accounts. *Annual Review of Sociology* 23: 455–78.

Packer, J. (1989) The Role of Stigmatization in Fat People's Avoidance of Exercise. In L. Brown and E. Rothblum (eds) *Fat Oppression and Psychotherapy: A Feminist Perspective*. New York: The Hawthorn Press.

Petersen, A. and Lupton, D. (1996) *The New Public Health: Health and Self in the Age of Risk.* London: Sage.

Porter, S. (1993) Critical Realist Ethnography: The Case of Racism and Professionalism in a Medical Setting. *Sociology* 27 (4): 591–609.

Probyn, E. (2000) *Carnal Appetites: FoodSexIdentities.* London: Routledge.

Rich, E. and Evans, J. (2005) 'Fat Ethics': The Obesity Discourse and Body Politics. *Social Theory & Health* 3 (4): 341–58.

—— (2006) Fat Ethics: Exploring the Negative Implications of the 'Anti-Obesity' Discourse. Paper presented at *Expanding the Obesity Debate.* University of Limerick, 9 January.

Rich, E., Harjunen, H., and Evans, J. (2006) 'Normal Gone Bad': Health Discourses, Schools and the Female Body. In V. Kalitzkus and P. Twohig (eds) *Bordering Biomedicine: Probing the Boundaries.* New York: Rodopi.

Ritenbaugh, C. (1982) Obesity as a Culture Bound Syndrome. *Culture, Medicine and Psychiatry* 6: 347–61.

Ritzer, G. (2004) *The McDonaldization of Society: Revised New Century Edition.* London: Sage.

Robertson, S. (2006) 'I've Been Like a Coiled Spring this Last Week': Embodied Masculinity and Health. *Sociology of Health & Illness* 28 (4): 433–56.

Robison, J. (1999) Weight, Health, and Culture: Shifting the Paradigm for Alternative Health Care. *Alternative Health Practitioner* 5 (1): 45–69.

—— (2005a) Editorial: Health at Every Size: Antidote for the 'Obesity Epidemic'. *Health at Every Size Journal* 19 (1): 3–10.

—— (2005b) Health at Every Size: Toward a New Paradigm of Weight and Health. *Medscape General Medicine* 7 (3): 13.

Rose, N. (2004) Emergent Forms of Life. Paper presented at *Making Sense of Transformations and Transitions*, School of Geography, Politics and Sociology, Newcastle University. 14 May.

Ruppel Shell, E. (2003) *Fat Wars: The Inside Story of the Obesity Industry.* London: Atlantic Books.

Saguy, A. and Riley, K. (2005) Weighing Both Sides: Morality, Mortality and Framing Contests over Obesity. *Journal of Health Politics, Policy and Law* 30 (5): 869–921.

Saporta, I. and Halpern, J. (2002). Being Different Can Hurt: Effects of Deviation from Physical Norms on Lawyers' Salaries. *Industrial Relations* 41(3): 442–66.

Savill, R. (2006) Gym Bans 21-stone Man for Being 'Unfit'. *Telegraph* 29 June.

Scambler, G. (2001) Critical Realism, Sociology and Health Inequalities: Social Class as a Generative Mechanism and its Media of Enactment. *Journal of Critical Realism* 4 (1): 35–42.

—— (2002) *Health and Social Change: A Critical Theory.* Buckingham: Open University Press.

—— (2004) Re-framing Stigma: Felt and Enacted Stigma and Challenges to the Sociology of Chronic and Disabling Conditions. *Social Theory & Health* 2 (1): 29–46.

Scambler, G. and Hopkins, A. (1986) Being Epileptic: Coming to Terms with Stigma. *Sociology of Health & Illness* 8 (1): 26–43.

Schauss, A. (2006) *Obesity: Why are Men Getting Pregnant?* Laguna Beach, CA: Basic Health Publications.

Schutz, A. (1962) *Collected Papers I: The Problem of Social Reality.* The Hague: Martinus Nijhoff.

—— (1964) *Collected Papers II: Studies in Social Theory.* The Hague: Martinus Nijhoff.

—— (1970) *On Phenomenology and Social Relations*. Chicago, IL: University of Chicago Press.

Schwartz, H. (1986) *Never Satisfied: A Cultural History of Diets, Fantasies and Fat*. New York: The Free Press.

Scott, M. and Lyman, S. (1968) Accounts. *American Sociological Review* 33 (1): 46–62.

Seid, R. (1989) *Never Too Thin: Why Women Are at War with their Bodies*. New York: Prentice Hall.

Shakespeare, T. (1999) Joking a Part. *Body & Society* 5 (4): 47–52.

—— (2006) *Disability Rights and Wrongs*. London: Routledge.

Shilling, C. (2003) *The Body and Social Theory*. London: Sage. (2nd edition)

—— (2005) *The Body in Culture, Technology and Society*. London: Sage.

Shott, S. (1979) Emotion and Social Life: A Symbolic Interactionist Analysis. *The American Journal of Sociology* 84 (6): 1317–34.

Shriver, T. and Waskul, D. (2006) Managing the Uncertainties of Gulf War Illness: The Challenge of Living with Chronic Illness. *Symbolic Interaction* 29 (4): 465–86.

Silverman, D. (2001) *Interpreting Qualitative Data: Methods for Analysing Talk, Text and Interaction*. London: Sage.

Simpson, M. (2005) Sexualising the City. Paper presented at the University of Newcastle upon Tyne. 3 March.

Skeggs, B. (1997) *Formations of Class and Gender*. London: Sage.

Smart, B. (ed.) (1999) *Resisting McDonaldization*. London: Sage.

Smith, S. (1990) Sizism: One of the Last 'Safe' Prejudices. *The California Now Activist*. Online. Available HTTP: <www.naafa.org/press_room/sizism.html> Accessed 6 December 2006.

Sobal, J. (1995) The Medicalization and Demedicalization of Obesity. In D. Maurer and J. Sobal (eds) *Eating Agendas: Food and Nutrition as Social Problems*. New York: Aldine de Gruyter.

Sobal, J. and Maurer, D. (eds) (1999a) *Weighty Issues: Fatness and Thinness as Social Problems*. New York: Aldine de Gruyter.

—— (eds) (1999b) *Interpreting Weight: The Social Management of Fatness and Thinness*. New York: Aldine de Gruyter.

Sobal, J., Rauschenbach, B. and Fongillo, E. (2003) Marital Status and Body Weight Changes: A US Longitudinal Analysis. *Social Science & Medicine* 56 (7): 1543–55.

Solovay, S. (2000) *Tipping the Scales of Justice: Fighting Weight-Based Discrimination*. New York: Prometheus Books.

Sontag, S. (1978) *Illness as Metaphor*. New York: Penguin Books.

de Souza, P. and Ciclitira, K. (2005) Men and Dieting: A Qualitative Analysis. *Journal of Health Psychology* 10 (6): 793–804.

Spurlock, M. (2004) Director's Statement. *Supersize Me: A Film of Epic Proportions*. Online. Available HTTP: <http://www.supersizeme.com/home.aspx?page=about director> Accessed 21 September 2004.

Stanley, L. (2005) A Child of its Time: Hybridic Perspectives on Othering in Sociology. *Sociological Research Online* 10 (3). Online. Available HTTP: <www.socres online.org.uk/10/3/stanley.html> Accessed 10 January 2006.

Stearns, P. (1997) *Fat History: Bodies and Beauty in the Modern West*. New York: New York University Press.

Stinson, K. (2001) *Women and Dieting Culture: Inside a Commercial Weight Loss Group*. New Brunswick, NJ: Rutgers University Press.

Stokes, R. and Hewitt, J. (1976) Aligning Actions. *American Sociological Review.* 41 (5): 838–49.

Strong, P. (1990) Epidemic Psychology: A Model. *Sociology of Health & Illness* 12 (3): 249–59.

Sykes, G. and Matza, D. (1957) Techniques of Neutralization: A Theory of Delinquency. *American Sociological Review* 22 (6): 664–70.

Taylor, L. (1979) Vocabularies, Rhetoric and Grammar. In D. Downes and P. Rock (eds) *Deviant Interpretations: Problems in Criminological Theory.* New York, NY: Barnes & Noble.

Tenzer, S. (1989) Fat Acceptance Therapy (F.A.T.): A Non-Dieting Group Approach to Physical Wellness, Insights and Self-Acceptance. In L. Brown and E. Rothblum (eds) *Fat Oppression and Psychotherapy: A Feminist Perspective.* New York: The Hawthorn Press.

Textor, A. (1999) Organization, Specialization, and Desires in the Big Men's Movement: Preliminary Research in the Study of Subculture-Formation. *Journal of Gay, Lesbian, and Bisexual Identity* 4 (3): 217–39.

The Report of the National Taskforce on Obesity (2005) *Obesity – The Policy Challenges.* Online. Available HTTP: <www.healthpromotion.ie> Accessed 12 September 2005.

Thomas, C. (2001) The Body and Society: Some Reflections on the Concepts of 'Disability' and 'Impairment'. In N. Watson and S. Cunningham-Burley (eds) *Reframing the Body.* Basingstoke: Palgrave.

Throsby, K. (2007) 'Dieting Like a Normal Person': Obesity, Risk and Responsibility in Accounts of Weight-Loss Surgery. *Obesity and Extremes: What's the Problem?* Scottish Colloquium on Food and Feeding and BSA Food Study Group, University of Edinburgh, 26 January.

Turner, B. (1991) The Discourse of Diet. In M. Featherstone, M. Hepworth, and B. Turner (eds) *The Body: Social Process and Cultural Theory.* London: Sage.

—— (1992) *Regulating Bodies: Essays in Medical Sociology.* London: Routledge.

—— (1995) *Medical Power and Social Knowledge.* London: Sage. (2nd edition)

—— (1996) *The Body and Society.* London: Sage. (2nd edition)

Turner, V. (1969) *The Ritual Process: Structure and Anti-Structure.* Chicago, IL: Aldine.

UK Parliament (2004) *House of Commons Health Committee: Obesity.* Third Report of Session 2003–4, volume 1. Ordered by The House of Commons, 10 May 2004. Online. Available HTTP: <www.publications.parliament.uk/pa/cm200304/cmselect/cmhealth/23/2302.htm> Accessed 8 September 2004.

Vannini, P. and Waskul, D. (2006) Body Ekstasis: Socio-Semiotic Reflections on Surpassing the Dualism of Body-Image. In D. Waskul and P. Vannini (eds) *Body/Embodiment: Symbolic Interaction and the Sociology of the Body.* Aldershot: Ashgate.

Wadden, R. and Didie, E. (2003) What's in a Name? Patients' Preferred Terms for Describing Obesity. *Obesity Research* 11 (9): 1140–46.

Wann, M. (1998) *FAT!SO? Because You Don't Have to Apologize For Your Size!* Berkeley, CA: Ten Speed Press.

Waskul, D. and Vannini, P. (eds) (2006) *Body/Embodiment: Symbolic Interaction and the Sociology of the Body.* Aldershot: Ashgate.

Watson, J. (2000) *Male Bodies: Health, Culture and Identity.* Buckingham: Open University Press.

Weber, M. (1930) *The Protestant Ethic and the Spirit of Capitalism.* London: Unwin Hyman. (Orig. 1905)

Weight Watchers (2003) Success Story: Richard Walters. In *Weight Watchers Magazine* October/November: 74–9.

Weinstein, D. and Weinstein, A. (1999) McDonaldization Enframed. In B. Smart (ed.) *Resisting McDonaldization*. London: Sage.

Weinstein, R. (1980) Vocabularies of Motive for Illicit Drug Use: An Application of the Accounts Framework. *The Sociological Quarterly* 21: 577–93.

West, C. and Zimmerman, H. (2002) Doing Gender. In S. Fenstermaker and C. West (eds) *Doing Gender, Doing Difference: Inequality, Power, and Institutional Change*. New York: Routledge.

White, M. (2006) Where Do You Want to Sit Today? Computer Programmers' Static Bodies and Disability. *Information, Communication & Society* 9 (3): 396–416.

WHO (World Health Organization) (1998) *Obesity: Preventing and Managing the Global Epidemic*. Geneva: World Health Organization.

Williams, L. and Germov, J. (2004) The Thin Ideal: Women, Food, and Dieting. In Germov, J. and Williams, L. (eds) *A Sociology of Food and Nutrition: The Social Appetite*. Oxford: Oxford University Press. (2nd edition)

Williams, S. (1999) Is Anybody There? Critical Realism, Chronic Illness and the Disability Debate. *Sociology of Health & Illness* 21 (6): 797–819.

—— (2003a) *Medicine and the Body*. London: Sage.

—— (2003b) Beyond Meaning, Discourse and the Empirical World: Critical Realist Reflections on Health. *Social Theory & Health* 1: 42–71.

Williams, S. and Bendelow, G. (1998) *The Lived Body: Sociological Themes, Embodied Issues*. London: Routledge.

Williams, S., Birke, L. and Bendelow, G. (eds) (2003) *Debating Biology: Sociological Reflections on Health, Medicine and Society*. London: Routledge.

Wolf, N. (1991) *The Beauty Myth: How Images of Beauty are Used Against Women*. London: Vintage.

Young, E. (1997) *World Hunger*. London: Routledge.

Zimmerman, M. (2006) Guys and Guts. *USA WEEKEND.com*. 4 June. Online. Available HTTP: <usaweekend.com/06_issues/060604/060604menshealth.html> Accessed 6 June 2006.

Zola, E. (1972) Medicine as an Institution of Social Control. *Sociological Review* 20 (4): 487–504.

—— (1973) Pathways to the Doctor – From Person to Patient. *Social Science & Medicine* 7: 677–89.

Index

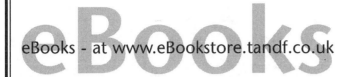

eBooks - at www.eBookstore.tandf.co.uk

A library at your fingertips!

eBooks are electronic versions of print books. You can store them onto your PC/laptop or browse them online.

They have advantages for anyone needing rapid access to a wide variety of published, copyright information.

eBooks can help your research by enabling you to bookmark chapters, annotate and use instant searches to find specific words or phrases. Several eBook files would fit on even a small laptop or PDA.

NEW: Save money by eSubscribing: cheap, online acess to any eBook for as long as you need it.

Annual subscription packages

We now offer special low cost bulk subscriptions to packages of eBooks in certain subject areas. These are available to libraries or to individuals.

For more information please contact webmaster.ebooks@tandf.co.uk

We're continually developing the eBook concept, so keep up to date by visiting the website.

www.eBookstore.tandf.co.uk